AF148550

Neurogenic Bowel Dysfunction

Neurogenic Bowel Dysfunction

Editor

Klaus Krogh

MDPI • Basel • Beijing • Wuhan • Barcelona • Belgrade • Manchester • Tokyo • Cluj • Tianjin

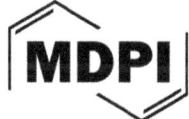

Editor
Klaus Krogh
Department of Hepatology
and Gastroenterology, Aarhus
University Hospital
Denmark

Editorial Office
MDPI
St. Alban-Anlage 66
4052 Basel, Switzerland

This is a reprint of articles from the Special Issue published online in the open access journal *Journal of Clinical Medicine* (ISSN 2077-0383) (available at: https://www.mdpi.com/journal/jcm/special_issues/Bowel_Dysfunction).

For citation purposes, cite each article independently as indicated on the article page online and as indicated below:

LastName, A.A.; LastName, B.B.; LastName, C.C. Article Title. *Journal Name* **Year**, *Volume Number*, Page Range.

ISBN 978-3-0365-4797-8 (Hbk)
ISBN 978-3-0365-4798-5 (PDF)

© 2022 by the authors. Articles in this book are Open Access and distributed under the Creative Commons Attribution (CC BY) license, which allows users to download, copy and build upon published articles, as long as the author and publisher are properly credited, which ensures maximum dissemination and a wider impact of our publications.

The book as a whole is distributed by MDPI under the terms and conditions of the Creative Commons license CC BY-NC-ND.

Contents

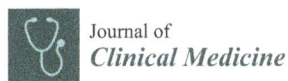

Journal of
Clinical Medicine

MDPI

Article

Neurogenic Bowel in Acute Rehabilitation Following Spinal Cord Injury: Impact of Laxatives and Opioids

Andrew M. Round [1,2,3,†], Min Cheol Joo [4,†], Carolyn M. Barakso [1], Nader Fallah [2,5], Vanessa K. Noonan [1,5] and Andrei V. Krassioukov [1,6,7,*]

1   International Collaboration on Repair Discoveries (ICORD), Department of Medicine, University of British Columbia, Vancouver, BC V5Z 1M9, Canada; drewround@gmail.com (A.M.R.); cbarakso@alumni.ubc.ca (C.M.B.); vnoonan@praxisinstitute.org (V.K.N.)
2   Department of Medicine, University of British Columbia, Vancouver, BC V5Z 1M9, Canada; nfallah@praxisinstitute.org
3   Department of Physical Medicine and Rehabilitation, University of Ottawa, Ottawa, ON K1H 8M2, Canada
4   Department of Rehabilitation Medicine and Institute of Wonkwang Medical Science, Wonkwang University School of Medicine, Iksan 570-749, Korea; jmc77@daum.net
5   Praxis Spinal Cord Institute, Vancouver, BC V5Z 1M9, Canada
6   Division of Physical Medicine and Rehabilitation, Department of Medicine, University of British Columbia, Vancouver, BC V5Z 2G9, Canada
7   GF Strong Rehabilitation Centre, Vancouver Coastal Health, Vancouver, BC V5Z 2G9, Canada
*   Correspondence: krassioukov@icord.org; Tel.: +1-604-675-8819
†   Co-first authors.

Citation: Round, A.M.; Joo, M.C.; Barakso, C.M.; Fallah, N.; Noonan, V.K.; Krassioukov, A.V. Neurogenic Bowel in Acute Rehabilitation Following Spinal Cord Injury: Impact of Laxatives and Opioids. *J. Clin. Med.* 2021, 10, 1673. https://doi.org/10.3390/jcm10081673

Academic Editors: Mark A. Korsten and Gian Paolo Caviglia

Received: 26 February 2021
Accepted: 10 April 2021
Published: 14 April 2021

Publisher's Note: MDPI stays neutral with regard to jurisdictional claims in published maps and institutional affiliations.

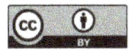

Copyright: © 2021 by the authors. Licensee MDPI, Basel, Switzerland. This article is an open access article distributed under the terms and conditions of the Creative Commons Attribution (CC BY) license (https://creativecommons.org/licenses/by/4.0/).

Abstract: Objective: To explore the association between bowel dysfunction and use of laxatives and opioids in an acute rehabilitation setting following spinal cord injury (SCI). Methods: Data was collected regarding individuals with acute traumatic/non-traumatic SCI over a two-year period (2012–2013) during both the week of admission and discharge of their inpatient stay. Results: An increase in frequency of bowel movement (BM) ($p = 0.003$) and a decrease in frequency of fecal incontinence (FI) per week ($p < 0.001$) between admission and discharge was found across all participants. There was a reduction in the number of individuals using laxatives ($p = 0.004$) as well as the number of unique laxatives taken ($p < 0.001$) between admission and discharge in our cohort. The number of individuals using opioids and the average dose of opioids in morphine milligram equivalents (MME) from admission to discharge were significantly reduced ($p = 0.001$ and $p = 0.02$, respectively). There was a positive correlation between the number of laxatives and frequency of FI at discharge ($r = 0.194$, $p = 0.014$), suggesting that an increase in laxative use results in an increased frequency of FI. Finally, there was a significant negative correlation between average dose of opioids (MME) and frequency of BM at discharge, confirming the constipating effect of opioids ($r = -0.20$, $p = 0.009$).

Keywords: bowel dysfunction; acute rehabilitation; spinal cord injury; laxatives; opioids; SCI bowel management

1. Introduction

Spinal cord injury (SCI) is a devastating event, which affects multiple facets of an individual's life with far-reaching implications and dangerous complications. Although paralysis is the most obvious and visible outcome of SCI, individuals have reported neurogenic bowel dysfunction (NBD) as being one of the greatest contributors to disability [1–5]. NBD occurs in up to 80% of individuals with SCI and has significant negative impacts on quality of life [6,7]. Bowel management is a key concern in this population as it frequently interferes with independence, causes embarrassment and social isolation, and alters relationships [8,9].

Bowel dysfunction following SCI is closely correlated with the level and severity of SCI, involving impaired abdominal and pelvic floor muscle control, impaired rectal sensation, and delayed colonic transit time (CTT) [10]. Two main patterns of bowel dysfunction in individuals with SCI who have recovered from spinal shock have been described in detail, known as upper motor neuron (UMN) and lower motor neuron (LMN) bowel syndromes [4] (Figure 1). UMN bowel syndrome, otherwise known as hyperreflexic bowel, is attributed to supraconal injury and has the predominant feature of constipation. Clinically, these individuals suffer from significant constipation and fecal retention with a reliance on rectal irritation to encourage stool propulsion via intact enteric/sacral reflexes. LMN bowel syndrome, otherwise known as areflexic bowel, is attributed to injury at the conus or cauda equina level and has the predominant features of fecal incontinence (FI) and decreased frequency of bowel movement (BM) due to constipation. Constipation is most often defined as fewer than two to three bowel movements per week [3,11]. These issues are explained by atonic external anal sphincter (EAS) and pelvic floor musculature secondary to disrupted alpha motor neurons in the sacral spinal segments.

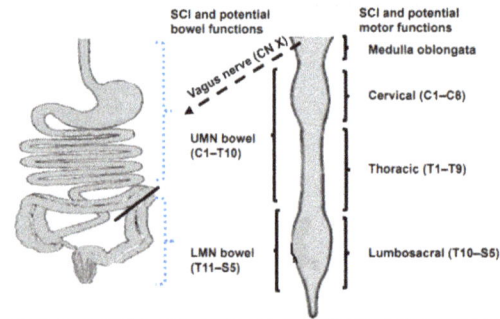

Figure 1. Schematic diagram of the gastrointestinal tract innervation and potential functional bowel and motor outcomes.

Innervation of GI tract: Parasympathetic innervation to the portion of the GI tract extending from the esophagus to the splenic flexure of the colon (solid line), which modulates peristalsis, is provided by the vagus nerve (CN X). Parasympathetic innervation to the descending colon and rectum is provided by the pelvic splanchnic nerves, which exit from the spinal cord at segments S2–S4. Sympathetic innervation to the upper GI tract is provided by the sympathetic preganglionic neurons (SPN) localized within the upper thoracic spinal cord segments (T1–T5); the small and large intestine are controlled by SPNs localized within the T6–L2 spinal segments. Somatic innervation and voluntary control of the external anal sphincter and pelvic floor musculature is originating from S2–S4 spinal cord segments.

Bowel functional outcomes and level of SCI: A SCI that damages segments above the sacral segments (above T10) produces a hyperreflexive or UMN bowel, in which defecation cannot be initiated by voluntary relaxation of the external anal sphincter, although there can be reflex-mediated colonic peristalsis. In contrast, a SCI that includes destruction of the lumbar/sacral spinal cord segments produces an areflexic or LMN bowel, in which there is no reflex-mediated colonic peristalsis. The anal sphincter of an LMN bowel is typically atonic and prone to leakage of stool.

Motor functional outcomes and SCI: Functional abilities of individuals with cervical and thoracic SCI ranges significantly. Meaningful functional categories include: independence in activities of daily living, wheelchair independence, bed mobility, voluntary weight shifting, and independent transfers. However, most of these individuals do not have abdominal, pelvic muscle or anal sphincter control. Finally, although individuals with lower thoracic/lumbar and sacral SCI (below T11 spinal segment) have full control of their upper extremities, core/abdominal musculature and may be able to stand or ambulate with assistive devices, individuals with complete spinal cord lesion do not have control to their pelvic floor muscles or anal sphincter.

Abbreviations: C—cervical; T—thoracic; L—Lumbar; S—sacral; GI—gastrointestinal; SCI—spinal cord injury; SPNs—sympathetic preganglionic neurons; UMN—upper motor neuron; LMN—lower motor neuron.

Strict and detailed bowel management protocols delineated by UMN and LMN injuries have become recognized as essential in management of NBD in individuals with SCI [12]. The main goal of such regimens is to achieve a regular and efficient bowel evacuation within a reasonable and regular time frame [4,13]. The components of a successful bowel protocol commonly include regulation of diet (fiber intake), abdominal massage, digital rectal stimulation, manual evacuation, oral laxatives, transanal irrigation, rectal suppository, and other pharmacological agents (stool softeners, colonic stimulants, contact irritants, bulk formers) [14–16]. The management of NBD is further hindered by the presence of secondary complications such as chronic pain, requiring pharmacologic treatment. Chronic neuropathic pain, which affects approximately one-third of people with SCI, is often managed using analgesic-narcotics (opioids); unfortunately, constipation is a common side effect [17,18]. Other commonly prescribed medications that can contribute to constipation in individuals with SCI are anticholinergics [3].

Lynch et al. [19] suggested that in uninjured individuals, the average frequency of BM per week is estimated at 9.3, while the average for individuals with chronic SCI was estimated at 6.6. Despite the growing body of literature that focuses on various issues related to NBD following SCI [20,21], there is a paucity of data on the progression of bowel function (frequency of BM and FI) during an acute period of rehabilitation, and upon discharge to the community. It is also unknown how the use of laxatives and opioids (number of laxatives and average dose of opioids) during the acute period of rehabilitation impacts bowel management.

The objective in this study was to examine the impact of inpatient rehabilitation and the use of various medications on bowel dysfunctions of individuals with acute traumatic/non-traumatic SCI. Two questions guided our investigation: (1) How does the frequency of BM and the frequency of FI change during the acute period of rehabilitation and how does it pertain to injury-related characteristics of individuals with SCI? (2) What are the impacts of laxatives and opioids on overall bowel dysfunction during the acute period of rehabilitation of individuals with SCI?

2. Methods

The protocol for this study was reviewed and approved by the University of British Columbia Clinical Research Ethics Board, conforming to the Declaration of Helsinki.

2.1. Setting and Participants

We conducted a retrospective chart review using electronic medical records from a single, tertiary rehabilitation centre (GF Strong Rehabilitation Centre (GFSRC) in Vancouver, Canada) during a two-year period (January 2012 to December 2013) to identify a cohort of 161 patients. Only individuals with acute traumatic/non-traumatic SCI admitted for inpatient rehabilitation were included into the study. Upon admission to the rehabilitation centre, an order form with the bowel management protocol was completed for each individual. The frequency of BM, which included date and time of bowel routine was documented by nursing staff; frequency of FI was documented according to the patient report. The protocol specific to our centre included the following crucial components: diet recommendations, medications (e.g., osmotic laxatives, stimulant laxatives, suppositories and enemas) and specific bowel manipulations to assist with bowel movements (e.g., digital evacuation, digital stimulation). The decision to use diet, medication and/or various manipulations was based on the treating physician's knowledge of UMN/LMN bowel syndrome in combination with frequency of BM and FI as documented in the patient's chart.

2.2. Measures

The following demographic and injury-related characteristics were collected: age, sex, duration of SCI, mechanism of injury (traumatic vs. non-traumatic), neurological level of injury, and severity of SCI according to the International Standards for Neurological Classification of SCI (ISNCSCI) [22]. Clinical data regarding medications (including laxatives and opioids) and bowel function/management (bowel movement (BM), fecal incontinence (FI), digital stimulation (DS), digital evacuation (DE)) were measured daily during the first week of admission and the last week prior to discharge from inpatient rehabilitation. These measures were compared from admission to discharge in the whole cohort as well as in subdivision of three neurological and two functional bowel groups. The neurological level of injury groups was defined with consideration to potential motor functionality: cervical (C1-C8), thoracic (T1–T9), and lumbosacral (T10–S5). Functional bowel groups were selected based on upper motor neuron and lower motor neuron bowel syndrome: UMN (T10 and above) and LMN (T11 and below).

Following review of the participants' medication regimen, data on laxative and opioid use was analyzed. The dose of all opioids was converted to morphine milligram equivalents (MME) for purposes of analysis, using an established opioid analgesic conversion table [23]. None of the individuals in this study used methadone. Finally, the frequency of BM and FI were measured by calculating the mean values during the week of admission and week of discharge.

2.3. Statistical Analysis

Bivariate analysis of age, sex, medication use, injury severity and level was done to determine the relationship of these variables with BM status. Spearman or Pearson correlation test was used to assess association of continuous variables with outcomes and an independent t-test or Mann-Whitney U test were used to compare two groups. After the bivariate analyses, a repeated measures analysis of variance (ANOVA) was used to investigate the effect of each medication on outcome by adjusting for other demographics and clinical variables.

A p-value of <0.05 was considered statistically significant. All statistical analyses were performed using SPSS (version 23).

3. Results

3.1. Characteristics of Cohort of SCI Individuals

A total of 161 individuals with acute traumatic/non-traumatic SCI were included in the study. The majority of individuals in our cohort were male (112 (69.6%) and sustained traumatic cervical SCI (45.9%; Table 1). Individuals were admitted to inpatient rehabilitation on average within 52.83 ± 56.8 days of onset of SCI. The average period of inpatient rehabilitation was 79.1 ± 39.7 days.

3.2. Bowel Function Variables

3.2.1. Changes in Bowel Function from Admission to Discharge in Whole Cohort

When all participants were analyzed as a group, there was an increase in frequency of BM per week between admission and discharge ($p = 0.003$; Figure 2A; Table 2). There were decreases in both the number of individuals experiencing FI (78 vs. 34) as well as frequency of FI ($p < 0.001$; Table 2) between admission and discharge, respectively. There was a decrease in the number of individuals using DS between admission and discharge (71 vs. 48). Finally, there was a decrease in the number of individuals using DE between admission and discharge (70 vs. 32).

Table 1. Demographic characteristics of participants.

Characteristics	Mean ± s.d. or N (%)
Total number of participants	161 (100.0%)
Age (Years)	48.1 ± 19.1
Sex (Male/Female)	112 (69.6%)/49 (30.4%)
Time since injury (Days)	52.8 ± 56.8
Mechanism of injury (% Traumatic)	103 (64.0%)
Neurological level of injury on admission	
Cervical	74 (45.9%)
AIS A + B	25 (15.5%)
AIS C + D	49 (30.4%)
Thoracic	39 (24.2%)
AIS A + B	21 (13.0%)
AIS C + D	18 (11.2%)
Lumbosacral	48 (29.8%)
AIS A + B	18 (11.2%)
AIS C + D	30 (18.6%)
Neurological level of injury at discharge	
Cervical	69 (42.8%)
AIS A + B	20 (12.4%)
AIS C + D	49 (30.4%)
Thoracic	34 (21.1%)
AIS A + B	13 (8.1%)
AIS C + D	21 (13.0%)
Lumbosacral	58 (36.1%)
AIS A + B	12 (7.5%)
AIS C + D	45 (28.0%)
AIS E	1 (0.6%)
Functional bowel levels on admission	
UMN	119 (73.9%)
LMN	42 (26.1%)
Functional bowel levels at discharge	
UMN	111 (68.9%)
LMN	50 (31.1%)

Abbreviations: s.d—standard deviation; N—number of participants; AIS—ASIA Impairment Scale.

Table 2. Change in bowel dysfunctions from admission to discharge in individuals with SCI during acute rehabilitation.

Frequency	Whole Cohort	Neurological Level of Injury Groups			Functional Bowel Groups	
		Cervical	Thoracic	Lumbosacral	UMN	LMN
			Admission vs. Discharge, *p*-Value			
BM (Mean ± s.d)	3.38 ± 1.85 vs. 3.84 ± 1.15, $p = 0.003$	3.39 ± 1.84 vs. 3.83 ± 1.16, $p = 0.113$	3.59 ± 2.10 vs. 4.06 ± 1.59, $p = 0.174$	3.24 ± 1.73 vs. 3.74 ± 1.07, $p = 0.025$	3.43 ± 1.88 vs. 3.87 ± 1.18, $p = 0.029$	3.26 ± 1.73 vs. 3.78 ± 1.11, $p = 0.039$
FI (Mean ± s.d)	1.57 ± 2.43 vs. 0.49 ± 1.26, $p < 0.001$	1.72 ± 2.59 vs. 0.71 ± 1.59, $p = 0.001$	1.62 ± 2.85 vs. 0.5 ± 1.26, $p = 0.015$	1.34 ± 1.93 vs. 0.22 ± 0.62, $p < 0.001$	1.69 ± 2.56 vs. 0.61 ± 1.45, $p < 0.001$	1.21 ± 1.92 vs. 0.22 ± 0.62, $p < 0.001$

Abbreviations: BM—bowel movement; FI—fecal incontinence; UMN—upper motor neuron; LMN—lower motor neuron; s.d.—standard deviation.

3.2.2. Changes in Bowel Function from Admission to Discharge Depending on Level/Completeness of SCI

There was no difference in frequency of BM between the three neurological level of injury groups at admission or discharge ($p = 0.46$ and $p = 0.15$, respectively). There was no difference in frequency of BM within the cervical or thoracic neurological level of injury groups between admission and discharge. However, there was a significant increase in frequency of BM within the lumbosacral neurological level of injury group between admission and discharge ($p = 0.025$; Table 2).

A

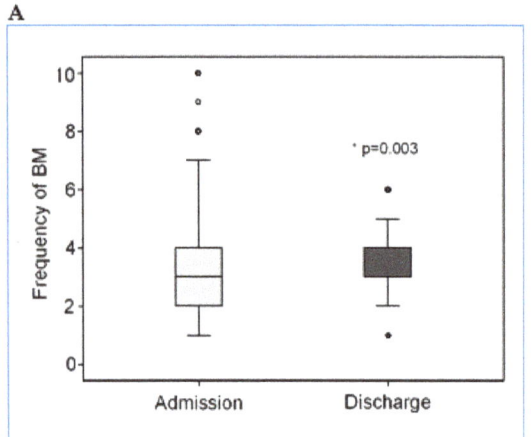

B

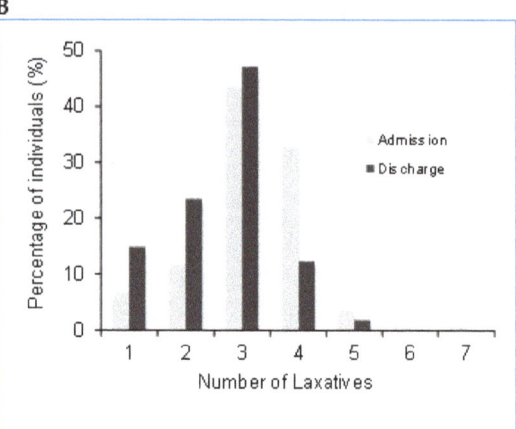

C

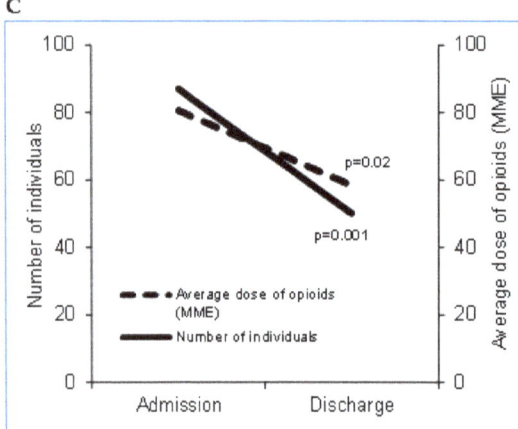

D

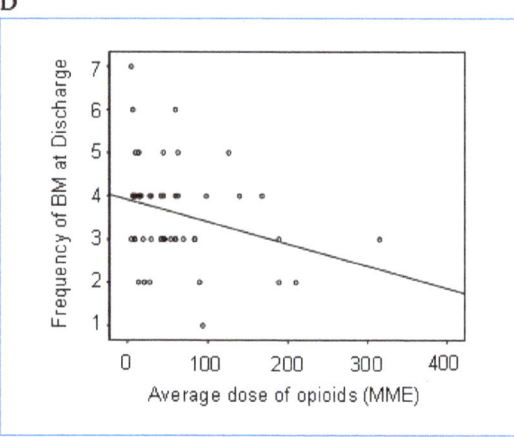

Figure 2. Changes in bowel function and medication use from admission to discharge in our whole cohort of individuals with SCI at an acute rehabilitation setting. (**A**) Frequency of BM at admission and discharge. (**B**) Total number of laxatives taken at admission and discharge. (**C**) Number of individuals taking opioids and average dose of opioids (MME) at admission and discharge. (**D**) Correlation between frequency of BM and average dose of opioids (MME) at discharge. Abbreviations: SCI—spinal cord injury; BM—bowel movement; MME—morphine milligram equivalents. * *p*-values < 0.01 are considered statistically significant.

There was no difference in frequency of FI between the three neurological level of injury groups at admission or discharge ($p = 0.33$ and $p = 0.096$, respectively). However, there was a significant decrease in frequency of FI between admission and discharge within the cervical ($p = 0.001$; Table 2), thoracic ($p = 0.015$; Table 2) and lumbosacral neurological level of injury groups ($p < 0.001$; Table 2).

There was no difference in the number of individuals using DS between the three neurological level of injury groups at admission ($p = 0.19$); however, there was a significant difference at discharge (cervical: 29, thoracic: 9, lumbosacral: 10; $p = 0.009$). There was no difference in the number of individuals using DE between the three neurological level of injury groups at admission or discharge ($p = 0.22$ and $p = 0.175$, respectively).

There was no difference between frequency of BM in motor complete vs. incomplete injury groups at admission and discharge ($p = 0.88$ and $p = 0.06$, respectively). There was no difference between frequency of FI in motor complete vs. incomplete injury groups at admission and discharge (p = 0.36 and p = 0.21, respectively).

3.2.3. Changes in Bowel Function from Admission to Discharge Depending on UMN vs. LMN Bowel Syndrome

There was no difference in frequency of BM between the two functional bowel groups at admission or discharge (p = 0.63 and p = 0.63, respectively). However, there was a significant increase in frequency of BM between admission and discharge within the UMN functional bowel group (p = 0.029; Table 2) and LMN functional bowel group (p = 0.039; Table 2).

There was no difference in frequency of FI between the two functional bowel groups at admission (p = 0.27); however, there was a significant decrease at discharge between the UMN and LMN functional bowel groups (0.61 ± 1.45 vs. 0.22 ± 0.62, p = 0.017). There was a significant decrease in frequency of FI between admission and discharge within the UMN functional bowel group (p < 0.001; Table 2) and LMN functional bowel group (p < 0.001; Table 2).

There was no difference in the number of individuals using DS between the two functional bowel groups at admission (p = 0.075); however, there was a significant difference at discharge (p = 0.002). Of those who were using DS at discharge, 85.4% were individuals in the UMN functional bowel group vs. 14.6% who were in the LMN functional bowel group. There was no difference in the number of individuals using DE between the two functional bowel groups at admission or discharge (p = 0.063 and p = 0.068); however, there does show a trend toward significance.

3.3. Medication Use—Laxatives

3.3.1. Laxatives in Whole Cohort, Three Neurological Level of Injury Groups, and Two Functional Bowel Groups

A variety of laxatives were used between admission and discharge among the participants such as stimulant (86.3% vs. 64.6%), polyethylene glycol (42.9% vs. 31.1%) and bisacodyl suppository (32.9% vs. 29.8%). The majority of individuals in our study used laxatives during their rehabilitation at admission and discharge (150 (93%) vs. 137 (85%)). Various laxatives were commonly combined with average use of 2.19 ± 1.00 vs. 1.63 ± 0.95 at admission and discharge respectively (Figure 2B). There was a reduction in the number of individuals using laxatives (p = 0.004) as well as the number of unique laxatives taken (p < 0.0001) between admission and discharge respectively when the cohort was analyzed as a whole.

There was no difference in the numbers of individuals using laxatives between the three neurological level of injury groups at admission and discharge (p = 0.82 and p = 0.097). However, there was a significant decrease in the number of laxatives used between admission and discharge within the thoracic (p = 0.001; Table 3) and lumbosacral neurological level of injury groups (p < 0.001; Table 3).

There was no difference in the number of individuals using laxatives between the two functional bowel groups at admission. However, there was a significant difference in the number of UMN and LMN functional bowel group (82 vs. 55) laxative users at discharge (p = 0.016).

There was a significant decrease in the number of laxatives taken between admission and discharge within the UMN (p = 0.017; Table 3) and LMN functional bowel groups (p < 0.001; Table 3).

3.3.2. Frequency of BM with Laxatives in Whole Cohort and Two Functional Bowel Groups

Regarding the whole cohort, the frequency of BM was negatively correlated with the number of laxatives used both at admission (r = −0.28, p < 0.001) and discharge (r = −0.16, p = 0.035).

Regarding the functional bowel groups, the frequency of BM was negatively correlated with the number of laxatives used at admission for the UMN (r = −0.218, p = 0.022) and LMN functional bowel groups (r = −0.384, p = 0.006). This correlation was not present at discharge in either UMN or LMN functional bowel groups.

Table 3. Change in laxative and opioids use from admission to discharge in individuals with SCI during acute rehabilitation.

Medication	Whole Cohort	Neurological Level of Injury Groups			Functional Bowel Groups	
		Cervical	Thoracic	Lumbosacral	UMN	LMN
		Admission vs. Discharge, *p*-Value				
Laxatives (Mean ± s.d)	2.19 ± 1.00 vs. 1.63 ± 0.95, p < 0.001	2.00 ± 0.92 vs. 1.83 ± 0.89, p = 0.159	2.35 ± 1.04 vs. 1.68 ± 0.98, p = 0.001	2.33 ± 1.03 vs. 1.36 ± 0.95, p < 0.001	2.09 ± 0.98 vs. 1.81 ± 0.90, p = 0.017	2.32 ± 1.01 vs. 1.39 ± 0.96, p < 0.001
Opioids (Average MME ± s.d)	80.58 ± 96.65 vs. 58.38 ± 63.65, p = 0.02	58.30 ± 56.61 vs. 43.74 ± 46.58, p = 0.83	109.37 ± 143.12 vs. 61.58 ± 56.44, p = 0.29	82.94 ± 84.57 vs. 67.28 ± 77.35, p = 0.49	99.10 ± 110.41 vs. 70.97 ± 72.61, p = 0.13	87.50 ± 73.64 vs. 60.90 ± 57.88, p = 0.034

Abbreviations: UMN—upper motor neuron; LMN—lower motor neuron; s.d.—standard deviation; MME—morphine milligram equivalents.

3.3.3. Frequency of FI with Laxatives in Whole Cohort

Regarding the whole cohort, there was no correlation between the number of laxatives and frequency of FI at admission; however, there was a positive correlation at discharge (r = 0.194, p = 0.014).

3.4. Medication Use—Opioids

3.4.1. Opioids in Whole Cohort, Three Neurological Level of Injury Groups, and Two Functional Bowel Groups

A total of 87/161 (54.0%) and 50/161 (31.1%) from the whole cohort were taking opioid medications at admission and discharge respectively (Figure 2C). The average dose of opioids (MME) taken at admission and discharge was 80.58 ± 96.65 and 58.38 ± 63.65 respectively (Figure 2C; Table 3). The number of individuals using opioids and the average dose of opioids (MME) from admission to discharge were significantly reduced (p = 0.001 and p = 0.02, respectively).

There was a significant decrease in the number of individuals taking opioids from admission to discharge within the cervical neurological of injury group only (33 vs. 16, p = 0.016); however, there was no difference between admission and discharge within the thoracic (33 vs. 16, p = 0.20) and lumbosacral neurological level of injury groups (31 vs. 22, p = 0.32).

There was no difference in the average dose of opioids (MME) from admission to discharge within the cervical (p = 0.83; Table 3), thoracic (p = 0.29; Table 3), and lumbosacral levels of injury (p = 0.49; Table 3)

There was a significant decrease in the number of individuals taking opioids from admission to discharge within the UMN functional bowel group (61 vs. 31, p = 0.001); however, there was no difference for the LMN functional bowel group (26 vs. 19, p = 0.42).

There was no difference in the average dose of opioids (MME) taken from admission to discharge within the UMN functional bowel group; however, there was a significant decrease from admission to discharge within the LMN functional bowel group (87.50 mg vs. 60.90 mg, p = 0.034).

3.4.2. Opioids and Frequency of Bowel Movement in the Whole Cohort and Two Functional Bowel Groups

Regarding the whole cohort, there was no correlation between average dose of opioids (MME) and frequency of BM at admission. However, there was a significant negative correlation between average dose of opioids (MME) and frequency of BM at discharge, confirming the constipating effect of opioids (r = −0.20, p = 0.009; Figure 2D).

In the UMN functional bowel group, there was a significant positive correlation between the frequency of BM and the average dose of opioids (MME) at admission (r = 0.350, p = 0.006). However, this correlation was not present in the LMN bowel group. The correlation was trending negatively in both the UMN and LMN functional bowel groups at discharge; however, it was not significant.

3.4.3. Opioids and Frequency of Fecal Incontinence in the Whole Cohort and Two Functional Bowel Groups

Regarding the whole cohort, there was no correlation between average dose of opioids (MME) and frequency of FI at admission or discharge.

Regarding the functional bowel groups, there was no correlation between average dose of opioids (MME) and frequency of FI at admission or discharge for the UMN or LMN functional bowel groups.

4. Discussion

It is well recognized that SCI can impede the autonomic circuits responsible for normal GI function and result in the typical neurogenic bowel dysfunctions including decreased colonic motility, delayed gastric emptying, difficult defecation and FI [4,14]. To our knowledge, this is the first study to provide insight into the changes in bowel dysfunctions of individuals with acute traumatic/non-traumatic SCI during the rehabilitation period. Studies assessing bowel dysfunctions following SCI are typically conducted with chronically (>1 year) injured individuals [24]. Investigators have previously agreed that following SCI, a period of at least one year was required for bowel functions to stabilize [25,26]. Therefore, our data documents a crucial period of bowel dysfunction and subsequent bowel routine implementation during early rehabilitation and the challenge faced by these individuals and their caregivers.

Our data demonstrated that although there was an increase in frequency of BM and decrease in frequency of FI per week between admission and discharge in our cohort of individuals (Figure 2A), we were not able to detect the impact of the level and severity of SCI on these measures. Previously, Liu and colleagues [6] used the NBD score to demonstrate that the level and completeness, as well as duration of injury (>10 years), could predict the severity of NBD in individuals with chronic SCI [6]. However, other studies show conflicting data with respect to NBD [22]. A study by Pavese et al. [27] showed that the level of injury and AIS were not main predictors of severe NBD. The same investigators found that the total motor score reflected by the degree of neurological injury after SCI, was the main predictor for the severity of bowel dysfunctions following SCI, suggesting that completeness of cord injury would be a potential risk factor for severe bowel dysfunctions following SCI [27].

As evidenced by Lynch et al. [28], up to 56% of individuals with chronic SCI are affected by FI and it is crucial to recognize its negative impact on their quality of life. Our data corroborated Lynch et al. [28] in demonstrating that 48% of individuals experienced FI prior to inpatient rehabilitation, though only 21% were still experiencing FI upon discharge. Additionally, the frequency of FI in our study was significantly higher than in the study by Yim et al. [29], where investigators reported on a group of individuals with chronic SCI (injuries more than 2 years). However, our analysis of the cohort as a whole did show the frequency of FI drop dramatically from admission to discharge (1.57 ± 2.43 vs. 0.49 ± 1.26, p < 0.001). It is most likely that the high frequency of FI in our study was related to the early stages of rehabilitation following acute traumatic/non-traumatic SCI, as individuals are adjusting to their bowel needs and ongoing recovery of neurological functions [30]. Finally, we hypothesize that the high frequency of FI in our cohort may have been related to antibiotic-associated diarrhea that is common in SCI patients during the acute rehabilitation period [31].

As was expected, we found that there was a positive correlation between the number of laxatives and frequency of FI at discharge (r = 0.194, p = 0.014). This suggests that laxative use correlates with an increased frequency of FI, which was interestingly only obvious at discharge. The initiation of laxatives during acute rehabilitation after SCI is a crucial component for development of effective bowel management protocol [4]. However, clinicians need to be aware of the potential negative impact of laxatives, especially if multiple laxatives are combined with other modalities for bowel management. As evident from the study by Coggrave et al. [32], frequency of FI was significantly higher in an intervention group that used a combination of laxative and various interventions to ensure effective BM.

Similar to able-bodied individuals [33,34], opioid medications would be expected to increase CTT in individuals with SCI in a dose dependent manner and are known to result in various side effects including constipation [35]. Numerous studies examining the use of opioids following SCI have suggested chronic opioid use as less desirable [36] due to its effects on cognition [37], chronic pain [38], and tendency of habit formation. The bowel related side effects of opioids are likely related to enteric, opioid specific receptors (gamma, kappa, mu) that reduce gastrointestinal mobility through neuronal inhibition [39]. In addition to common constitutional side effects such as nausea and drowsiness observed in able-bodied individuals, opioid use in individuals with SCI can be associated with respiratory depression and further delay of gastric emptying already affected by the injury [40]. While laxatives are considered safe and are commonly included as part of bowel management protocol following SCI, their use is not innocuous. Many laxatives can result in undesirable side effects such as nausea, loose stools, abdominal cramps, excess gas, dehydration, and electrolyte imbalance [41]. Furthermore, in individuals with SCI, stimulant laxatives can be associated with unplanned bowel evacuation and an increase in the duration of time it takes to complete an evacuation [41]. As evidenced from our study, the medical team made a significant effort to decrease the number of individuals treated with opioids (54.0% at admission vs. 31.1% at discharge; Figure 2C) as well as their average dose of opioid (MME) from admission to the time of discharge. Despite the relatively large doses of opioids at admission among our cohort (average 80.58 ± 96.65 MME) we were not able to detect the impact on frequency of BM at admission. It is reasonable to expect that the risk of developing opioid induced constipation does increase over time. As demonstrated by FitzHenry et al. [42] in able-bodied individuals, the risk of opioid induced constipation is higher after six months of continuous opioid use. The majority of individuals in our cohort were admitted to acute rehabilitation within two months of injury, and therefore had only a short period of opioid exposure. However, at the time of discharge, where the majority of individuals had been using opioids for >6 months, the constipating effect of opioids was evident. This was shown by the significant negative correlation between average dose of opioids (MME) and frequency of BM at the time of discharge ($r = -0.20$, $p = 0.009$; Figure 2D). We postulate that additional exposures of acute illness (as in our cohort) and use of other medications could potentially increase rates of opioid-induced constipation.

We would like to acknowledge several limitations in this study. We attempted to analyze clinically relevant injuries with respect to medication use and bowel function, but due to sample size it was challenging to have sufficient power. Unfortunately, the issue of small sample size accompanies most SCI research, as this area of study pertains to relatively rare conditions of which large data are not always available. This was compounded by the incomplete data we encountered at times given the study's retrospective nature. Finally, lumbosacral injuries were particularly underrepresented in our patient sample, which limited us in intergroups comparison. However, the low number of patients with lumbosacral level of injury reflects the epidemiology of SCI, where only 11–22% of individuals present with lumbosacral injuries [43–45].

The authors would also like to acknowledge that the selected LMN functional bowel group in this study (T11 and below) may potentially include a combination of mixed and LMN injury. While the group of individuals with T10 and above had true UMN bowel dysfunction.

J. Clin. Med. **2021**, *10*, 1673

The authors also recognize the fact that multiple factors could influence bowel function including activity level, fluid intake, and diet. We did not collect information regarding food and oral liquid intake in our study, factors known to contribute to constipation. However, it has to be noted that all individuals in this study were on a hospital-based diet and inpatient bladder management protocol in which patients were given at least 2000 cc of fluid per day. With respect to activity level, all individuals during inpatient rehabilitation for acute traumatic/non-traumatic SCI have very similarly structured rehabilitation activities depending on their level of injury. Furthermore, their physical activity outside of structured therapy within the inpatient SCI rehabilitation setting is relatively low as a substantial amount of time is spent in sedentary leisure time activities [46].

Acknowledging the great distress that bowel dysfunction contributes to the quality of life of those with spinal cord injury, it is unfortunate we could not collect data on the satisfaction of medication use, bowel dysfunction, and implemented bowel retraining.

5. Conclusions

In conclusion, we examined bowel function evolution during the sensitive time of acute rehabilitation. NBD presents significant challenges for individuals with SCI and medical professionals in the community. Clinicians should be aware of the negative impact of laxatives, especially if multiple laxatives are being combined with other modalities for bowel management. Opioid use should be minimized where possible; however, many individuals still require opioid analgesics for pain management. As this study was restricted to the acute traumatic/non-traumatic SCI patients, further research studying laxative use, opioid use, and bowel dysfunction in individuals with chronic SCI is needed.

Author Contributions: Conceptualization, A.M.R., M.C.J. and A.V.K.; methodology, A.M.R., M.C.J., C.M.B., N.F., V.K.N. and A.V.K.; formal analysis, A.M.R., M.C.J., C.M.B., N.F., V.K.N. and A.V.K.; resources, A.V.K.; data curation, A.M.R., M.C.J., C.M.B. and A.V.K.; writing—original draft preparation, A.M.R., M.C.J., C.M.B. and A.V.K.; writing—review and editing, A.M.R., M.C.J., C.M.B., N.F., V.K.N. and A.V.K.; supervision, A.V.K.; project administration, A.V.K. All authors have read and agreed to the published version of the manuscript.

Funding: The study was supported by an educational grant from Coloplast, Denmark.

Institutional Review Board Statement: The study was conducted according to the guidelines of the Declaration of Helsinki, and approved by the Clinical Research Ethics Board of the University of British Columbia (H14-02724, approved on 20 October 2014).

Informed Consent Statement: Patient consent was waived due to the retrospective nature of this minimal risk study. The data used in the study is part of routine assessment upon each patient and part of medical records. Permission to obtain the data and use for publication was given by Health Records, GF Strong Rehabilitation Centre.

Data Availability Statement: The data presented in this study are available on request from the corresponding author. The data are not publicly available due to their containing information that could compromise the privacy of research participants.

Acknowledgments: We would like to acknowledge the following organizations for their contribution in making this research possible: Praxis Spinal Cord Institute, ICORD, and administrative support staff at the Health Records at GF Strong Rehabilitation Centre. M.C.J. was supported by fellowship from Wonkwang University. A.V.K. holds an Endowed Chair in Spinal Cord Rehabilitation Research, Department of Medicine, UBC.

Conflicts of Interest: The authors declare no conflict of interest. V.K.N. and N.F. are employees of the Praxis Spinal Cord Institute. The funders had no role in the design of the study; in the collection, analyses, or interpretation of data; in the writing of the manuscript, or in the decision to publish the results.

References

1. Glickman, S.; Kamm, M. Bowel dysfunction in spinal-cord-injury patients. *Lancet* **1996**, *347*, 1651–1653. [CrossRef]
2. Krogh, K.; Nielsen, J.; Djurhuus, J.C.; Mosdal, C.; Sabroe, S.; Laurberg, S. Colorectal function in patients with spinal cord lesions. *Dis. Colon Rectum* **1997**, *40*, 1233–1239. [CrossRef] [PubMed]
3. De Looze, D.; Van Laere, M.; De Muynck, M.; Beke, R.; Elewaut, A. Constipation and other chronic gastrointestinal problems in spinal cord injury patients. *Spinal Cord* **1998**, *36*, 63–66. [CrossRef] [PubMed]
4. Stiens, S.A.; Bergman, S.B.; Goetz, L.L. Neurogenic bowel dysfunction after spinal cord injury: Clinical evaluation and rehabilitative management. *Arch. Phys. Med. Rehabil.* **1997**, *78* (Suppl. 3), S86–S102. [CrossRef]
5. Faaborg, P.M.; Christensen, P.; Finnerup, N.; Laurberg, S.; Krogh, K. The pattern of colorectal dysfunction changes with time since spinal cord injury. *Spinal Cord* **2007**, *46*, 234–238. [CrossRef]
6. Liu, C.W.; Huang, C.C.; Chen, C.H.; Yang, Y.H.; Chen, T.W.; Huang, M.H. Prediction of severe neurogenic bowel dysfunction in persons with spinal cord injury. *Spinal Cord* **2010**, *48*, 554–559. [CrossRef]
7. Inskip, J.A.; Lucci, V.-E.M.; McGrath, M.S.; Willms, R.; Claydon, V.E. A community perspective on bowel management and quality of life after spinal cord injury: The influence of autonomic dysreflexia. *J. Neurotrauma* **2018**, *35*, 1091–1105. [CrossRef]
8. Anderson, K.D. Targeting Recovery: Priorities of the spinal cord-injured population. *J. Neurotrauma* **2004**, *21*, 1371–1383. [CrossRef]
9. Braaf, S.; Lennox, A.; Nunn, A.; Gabbe, B. Social activity and relationship changes experienced by people with bowel and bladder dysfunction following spinal cord injury. *Spinal Cord* **2017**, *55*, 679–686. [CrossRef]
10. Vallès, M.; Mearin, F. Pathophysiology of bowel dysfunction in patients with motor incomplete spinal cord injury: Comparison with patients with motor complete spinal cord injury. *Dis. Colon Rectum* **2009**, *52*, 1589–1597. [CrossRef]
11. Tramonte, S.M.; Brand, M.B.; Mulrow, C.D.; Amato, M.G.; O'Keefe, M.E.; Ramirez, G. The treatment of chronic constipa-tion in adults. A systematic review. *J. Gen. Intern. Med.* **1997**, *12*, 15–24. [CrossRef]
12. Consortium for Spinal Cord Medicine. Clinical practice guidelines: Neurogenic bowel management in adults with spinal cord injury. *J. Spinal Cord Med.* **1998**, *21*, 248–293. [CrossRef]
13. Correa, G.I.; Rotter, K.P. Clinical evaluation and management of neurogenic bowel after spinal cord injury. *Spinal Cord* **2000**, *38*, 301–308. [CrossRef]
14. Sezer, N.; Akkuş, S.; Uğurlu, F.G. Chronic complications of spinal cord injury. *World J. Orthop.* **2015**, *6*, 24–33. [CrossRef]
15. Krassioukov, A.; the SCIRE Research Team; Eng, J.J.; Claxton, G.; Sakakibara, B.M.; Shum, S. Neurogenic bowel management after spinal cord injury: A systematic review of the evidence. *Spinal Cord* **2010**, *48*, 718–733. [CrossRef] [PubMed]
16. Hughes, M. Bowel Management in spinal cord injury patients. *Clin. Colon Rectal Surg.* **2014**, *27*, 113–115. [CrossRef]
17. Woller, S.A.; Hook, M.A. Opioid administration following spinal cord injury: Implications for pain and locomotor recovery. *Exp. Neurol.* **2013**, *247*, 328–341. [CrossRef] [PubMed]
18. Pappagallo, M. Incidence, prevalence, and management of opioid bowel dysfunction. *Am. J. Surg.* **2001**, *182*, S11–S18. [CrossRef]
19. Lynch, A.C.; Wong, C.; Anthony, A.; Dobbs, B.R.; Frizelle, F.A. Bowel dysfunction following spinal cord injury: A descrip-tion of bowel function in a spinal cord-injured population and comparison with age and gender matched controls. *Spinal Cord* **2000**, *38*, 717–723. [CrossRef] [PubMed]
20. Holmes, G.M.; Hubscher, C.H.; Krassioukov, A.; Jakeman, L.B.; Kleitman, N. Recommendations for evaluation of bladder and bowel function in pre-clinical spinal cord injury research. *J. Spinal Cord Med.* **2020**, *43*, 165–176. [CrossRef] [PubMed]
21. Wheeler, T.L.; de Groat, W.; Eisner, K.; Emmanuel, A.; French, J.; Grill, W.; Kennelly, M.J.; Krassioukov, A.; Gallo Santacruz, B.; Biering-Sørensen, F.; et al. Translating promising strategies for bowel and bladder management in spinal cord injury. *Exp. Neurol.* **2018**, *306*, 169–176. [CrossRef] [PubMed]
22. Kirshblum, S.C.; Burns, S.P.; Biering-Sorensen, F.; Donovan, W.; Graves, D.E.; Jha, A.; Johansen, M.; Jones, L.; Krassioukov, A.; Mulcahey, M.J.; et al. International standards for neurological classification of spinal cord injury (revised 2011). *J. Spinal Cord Med.* **2011**, *34*, 535–546. [CrossRef] [PubMed]
23. Kahan, M.; Mailis-Gagnon, A.; Wilson, L.; Srivastava, A. Canadian guideline for safe and effective use of opioids for chronic noncancer pain: Clinical summary for family physicians. Part 1: General population. *Can. Fam. Physician* **2011**, *57*, 1257–1266.
24. Kirshblum, S.C.; Gulati, M.; O'Connor, K.C.; Voorman, S.J. Bowel care practices in chronic spinal cord injury patients. *Arch. Phys. Med. Rehabil.* **1998**, *79*, 20–23. [CrossRef]
25. Furlan, J.C.; Urbach, D.R.; Fehlings, M.G. Optimal treatment for severe neurogenic bowel dysfunction after chronic spinal cord injury: A decision analysis. *BJS* **2007**, *94*, 1139–1150. [CrossRef]
26. Han, T.R.; Kim, J.H.; Kwon, B.S. Chronic gastrointestinal problems and bowel dysfunction in patients with spinal cord injury. *Spinal Cord* **1998**, *36*, 485–490. [CrossRef]
27. Pavese, C.; Bachmann, L.M.; Schubert, M.; Curt, A.; Mehnert, U.; Schneider, M.P.; Scivoletto, G.; Agrò, E.F.; Maier, D.; Abel, R.; et al. Bowel outcome prediction after traumatic spinal cord injury: Longitudinal cohort study. *Neurorehabilit. Neural. Repair* **2019**, *33*, 902–910. [CrossRef]
28. Lynch, A.C.; Antony, A.; Dobbs, B.R.; Frizelle, F.A. Bowel dysfunction following spinal cord injury. *Spinal Cord* **2001**, *39*, 193–203. [CrossRef] [PubMed]
29. Yim, S.Y.; Yoon, S.H.; Lee, I.Y.; Rah, E.W.; Moon, H.W. A comparison of bowel care patterns in patients with spinal cord injury: Upper motor neuron bowel vs lower motor neuron bowel. *Spinal Cord* **2001**, *39*, 204–207. [CrossRef]

30. Steeves, J.D.; Kramer, J.K.; Fawcett, J.W.; Cragg, J.; Lammertse, D.P.; Blight, A.R.; Marino, R.J.; Ditunno, J.F.; Coleman, W.P.; Geisler, F.H.; et al. Extent of spontaneous motor recovery after traumatic cervical sensorimotor complete spinal cord injury. *Spinal Cord* **2011**, *49*, 257–265. [CrossRef] [PubMed]

31. Wong, S.; Santullo, P.; O'Driscoll, J.; Jamous, A.; Hirani, S.P.; Saif, M. Use of antibiotic and prevalence of antibiotic-associated diarrhoea in-patients with spinal cord injuries: A UK national spinal injury centre experience. *Spinal Cord* **2017**, *55*, 583–587. [CrossRef]

32. Coggrave, M.J.; Norton, C. The need for manual evacuation and oral laxatives in the management of neurogenic bowel dysfunction after spinal cord injury: A randomized controlled trial of a stepwise protocol. *Spinal Cord* **2009**, *48*, 504–510. [CrossRef]

33. Gyawali, B.; Hayashi, N.; Tsukuura, H.; Honda, K.; Shimokata, T.; Ando, Y. Opioid-induced constipation. *Scand. J. Gastroenterol.* **2015**, *50*, 1331–1338. [CrossRef] [PubMed]

34. Sridharan, K.; Sivaramakrishnan, G. Drugs for treating opioid-induced constipation: A mixed treatment comparison network meta-analysis of randomized controlled clinical trials. *J. Pain Symptom Manag.* **2018**, *55*, 468–479.e1. [CrossRef]

35. Barrera-Chacon, J.M.; Mendez-Suarez, J.L.; Jáuregui-Abrisqueta, M.L.; Palazon, R.; Barbara-Bataller, E.; García-Obrero, I. Oxycodone improves pain control and quality of life in anticonvulsant-pretreated spinal cord-injured patients with neuro-pathic pain. *Spinal Cord* **2011**, *49*, 36–42. [CrossRef]

36. Cardenas, D.D.; Jensen, M.P. Treatments for chronic pain in persons with spinal cord injury: A survey study. *J. Spinal Cord Med.* **2006**, *29*, 109–117. [CrossRef] [PubMed]

37. Norrbrink, C.; Lundeberg, T. Tramadol in neuropathic pain after spinal cord injury: A randomized, double-blind, place-bo-controlled trial. *Clin. J. Pain* **2009**, *25*, 177–184. [CrossRef] [PubMed]

38. Stampas, A.; Pedroza, C.; Bush, J.N.; Ferguson, A.R.; Kramer, J.L.K.; Hook, M. The first 24 h: Opioid administration in people with spinal cord injury and neurologic recovery. *Spinal Cord* **2020**, *58*, 1080–1089. [CrossRef] [PubMed]

39. Camilleri, M. Opioid-induced constipation: Challenges and therapeutic opportunities. *Am. J. Gastroenterol.* **2011**, *106*, 835–842. [CrossRef] [PubMed]

40. Bryce, T.N. Opioids should not be prescribed for chronic pain after spinal cord injury. *Spinal Cord Ser. Cases* **2018**, *4*, 66. [CrossRef] [PubMed]

41. Haas, U.; Geng, V.; Evers, G.C.M.; Knecht, H. Bowel management in patients with spinal cord injury—A multicentre study of the German speaking society of paraplegia (DMGP). *Spinal Cord* **2005**, *43*, 724–730. [CrossRef] [PubMed]

42. FitzHenry, F.; Eden, S.K.; Denton, J.; Cao, H.; Cao, A.; Reeves, R.; Chen, G.; Gobbel, G.; Wells, N.; Matheny, M.E. Prevalence and risk factors for opioid-induced constipation in an older national veteran cohort. *Pain Res. Manag.* **2020**, *2020*, 5165682. [CrossRef] [PubMed]

43. Yang, R.; Guo, L.; Wang, P.; Huang, L.; Tang, Y.; Wang, W.; Chen, K.; Ye, J.; Lu, C.; Wu, Y.; et al. Epidemiology of apinal cord injuries and risk factors for complete injuries in Guangdong, China: A retrospective study. *PLoS ONE* **2014**, *9*, e84733. [CrossRef]

44. Ning, G.-Z.; Mu, Z.-P.; Shangguan, L.; Tang, Y.; Li, C.-Q.; Zhang, Z.-F.; Zhou, Y. Epidemiological features of traumatic spinal cord injury in Chongqing, China. *J. Spinal Cord Med.* **2015**, *39*, 455–460. [CrossRef]

45. Fehlings, M.G.; Singh, A.; Tetreault, L.; Kalsi-Ryan, S.; Nouri, A. Global prevalence and incidence of traumatic spinal cord injury. *Clin. Epidemiology* **2014**, *6*, 309–331. [CrossRef]

46. Zbogar, D.; Eng, J.J.; Miller, W.C.; Krassioukov, A.V.; Verrier, M.C. Physical activity outside of structured therapy during inpatient spinal cord injury rehabilitation. *J. Neuroeng. Rehabil.* **2016**, *13*, 1–11. [CrossRef] [PubMed]

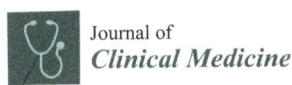

Journal of
Clinical Medicine

MDPI

Article

Postprandial Hypotension and Spinal Cord Injury

Rikke Middelhede Hansen [1],*, Klaus Krogh [2], Joan Sundby [1], Andrei Krassioukov [3] and Ellen Merete Hagen [4,5]

[1]   Spinal Cord Injury Centre of Western Denmark, Department of Neurology, Regional Hospital,
      DK-8800 Viborg, Denmark; joan.sundby@midt.rm.dk
[2]   Department of Hepatology and Gastroenterology, Aarhus University Hospital, DK-8200 Aarhus, Denmark;
      klaukrog@rm.dk
[3]   University of British Columbia and GF Strong Rehabilitation Centre, Department of Medicine, International
      Collaboration on Repair Discovery, Vancouver, BC V5Z 1MP, Canada; krassioukov@icord.org
[4]   National Hospital for Neurology and Neurosurgery, Queens Square, UCLH, London WC 1N 3BG, UK;
      ellenmerete.hagen@nhs.net
[5]   Institute of Neurology, University College London, London WC 1N 3BG, UK
*   Correspondence: rikke.m.hansen@viborg.rm.dk; Tel.: +45-78-44-61-50

Abstract: Postprandial hypotension (PPH) is defined as a fall of $\geq$20 mmHg in systolic blood pressure (SBP) or a SBP of <90 mmHg after having been >100 mmHg before the meal within two hours after a meal. The prevalence of PPH among persons with spinal cord injury (SCI) is unknown. Ambulatory blood pressure measurement was performed in 158 persons with SCI, 109 men, median age was 59.1 years (min.:13.2; max.: 86.2). In total, 78 persons (49.4%) had PPH after 114 out of 449 meals (25.4%). The median change in SBP during PPH was −28 mmHg (min.: −87; max.: −15 mmHg) and 96% of the PPH episodes were asymptomatic. The occurrence of PPH was correlated to older age (p = 0.001), level of injury (p = 0.023), and complete SCI (p = 0.000), but not, gender or time since injury. Further studies are needed to elucidate if PPH contributes to the increased cardiovascular mortality in the SCI population.

Keywords: spinal cord injury; postprandial hypotension; food ingestion; ambulatory blood pressure measurement; cohort study

Citation: Hansen, R.M.; Krogh, K.; Sundby, J.; Krassioukov, A.; Hagen, E.M. Postprandial Hypotension and Spinal Cord Injury. *J. Clin. Med.* **2021**, *10*, 1417. https://doi.org/10.3390/jcm10071417

Academic Editor: Bruno Annibale

Received: 26 February 2021
Accepted: 27 March 2021
Published: 1 April 2021

Publisher's Note: MDPI stays neutral with regard to jurisdictional claims in published maps and institutional affiliations.

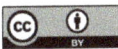

Copyright: © 2021 by the authors. Licensee MDPI, Basel, Switzerland. This article is an open access article distributed under the terms and conditions of the Creative Commons Attribution (CC BY) license (https://creativecommons.org/licenses/by/4.0/).

1. Introduction

In most individuals, the intake of a meal increases blood flow to the gut with no or very minor effects on systemic blood pressure. Abnormally low systolic blood pressure (SBP) following a meal is termed postprandial hypotension (PPH). Usually PPH is defined as a fall of $\geq$20 mmHg in SBP or a SBP of <90 mmHg after having been >100 mmHg before the meal within two hours after ingesting a meal [1–3]. The prevalence of PPH increases with age and may occur as a side-effect to various medications [4–6]. In addition, PPH is associated with increased risk of falls, syncope, coronary events, stroke, asymptomatic lacunar infarction, asymptomatic cerebrovascular damage, and death [7]. The above mentioned are associated with a risk of vascular cognitive impairment and dementia [8].

Spinal cord injury (SCI) has profound effects on autonomic function, including disruption of baroreflex and cardiovascular regulation [9–11]. Loss of supraspinal control may cause increased blood pressure (BP) variability, orthostatic hypotension (OH), exercise-induced hypotension, post-exercise induced hypotension, autonomic dysreflexia, and reduced quality of life [12–21]. Ambulatory blood pressure measurement (ABPM) has been used in several studies of fluctuations in the BP in various groups of patients, including persons with SCI [22–24]. Case reports have indicated that PPH occurs in persons with SCI, but the prevalence is unknown and potential associations with level and type of SCI remain uncertain [25–29].

In the western world, the incidence of non-traumatic SCI and the age at time of injury have increased significantly [30–32]. Fortunately, the expected longevity of persons with

SCI has also increased dramatically over the last five decades. Today, cardiovascular disease, urinary tract infection, and septicemia are the leading causes of increased mortality in persons surviving acute SCI [33]. It is plausible that BP instability and PPH may contribute to the increased cardiovascular mortality and increased risk of dementia seen in the SCI population [34].

Spinal cord injury severely affects gastrointestinal function, causing delayed gastric emptying and colonic transit time [35–39]. Splanchnic blood flow is under autonomic control, but it remains unknown how SCI affects postprandial blood flow to the intestines.

The primary aim of the present study was to describe the prevalence of PPH in a large group of persons with SCI by means of ABPM. The secondary aim was to determine whether PPH is associated with age, gender, time since SCI, or the level and completeness of lesions.

2. Materials and Methods

2.1. Subjects

The present study is a cohort study based on ABPM performed among persons with SCI admitted to The Spinal Cord Injury Centre of Western Denmark. The center covers the western half of Denmark with an underlying population of 3.1 million inhabitants and receives persons with both non-traumatic and traumatic SCI in all age groups for specialized rehabilitation after the acute phase. ABPM is part of the systematic routine assessment of hospitalized persons with a new SCI. It is also used as part of outpatient follow-up when persons with SCI report symptoms of autonomic dysfunction. Subjects included in the present paper were investigated from January 2017 to May 2017 or from October 2019 until restrictions due to the COVID-19 pandemic were instituted in March 2020. From medical records, data were obtained regarding date of birth, gender, date of injury and ABPM, type of injury (traumatic/non-traumatic), neurological level of injury, and ASIA Impairment Scale (AIS) grade according to International Standards of Neurological Classification of Spinal Cord Injuries [40]. Information of gastrointestinal morbidity and surgery was obtained from the medical records or the International Spinal Cord Injury Bowel Function Basic Data Set (version 2.0) when available [41]. Data on diabetes and other neurological diseases (i.e., Parkinson's disease, multiple system atrophy, and stroke) as well as number of medications used on the day of the ABPM were obtained for each patient.

Use of data for publication was granted from the Hospital Management, Regional Hospital Central Jutland. The project was reported to The Scientific Ethical Committees of Region Central Jutland (case number 1-10-72-181-20) and The Legal Office of the Central Denmark Region (reference number 706735, case number 1-16-02-590-20).

2.2. Ambulatory Blood Pressure Measurements

The ABPM was recorded using Meditech Card(X)plore device and Cardiovision 1.1.8.22 software (Meditech Ltd., Budapest, Hungary). The sampling frequency was four times per hour during the daytime (07:00–22:00) and two times per hour during the night. Figure 1 shows an example of an ABPM with three episodes of PPH in a 69-year old male with a C 1, AIS B SCI four months and eight days post injury. The person was one of seven persons having three or four episodes of PPH during the ABPM.

Each person with SCI was instructed to fill in a diary of activities, including time of meals and symptoms of hypo- and hypertension i.e., dizziness, headache, feeling weak, sweating, and blurred vision. Patients unable to fill in the diary were assisted by the staff. At the centre, three main meals are served at 08:00 (breakfast), 12:00 (lunch), and 17:30 (dinner). These time points were used as time of assumed meal intake, unless comments from the diary confirmed meals at another time. If eating was noted in the diary, this was considered the correct time of a meal. The following activities were noted in the diary as well: physical activity e.g., physical exercise, physiotherapy and occupational therapy, transfer (transfers with and without lift), eating at other times than the main meals, and nutrition through percutaneous endoscopic gastrostomy-tube (PEG-tube). Information of clean intermittent catheterization, bowel management, dressing/personal care, reposition in bed, smoking, administration of medication, drinking at other times than at meals, fluid through PEG-tube, procedures related to tracheostomy, continuous positive airway pressure (CPAP)/Bilevel Positive Airway Pressure (BiPAP), and resting were obtained as well, but not used in the present study.

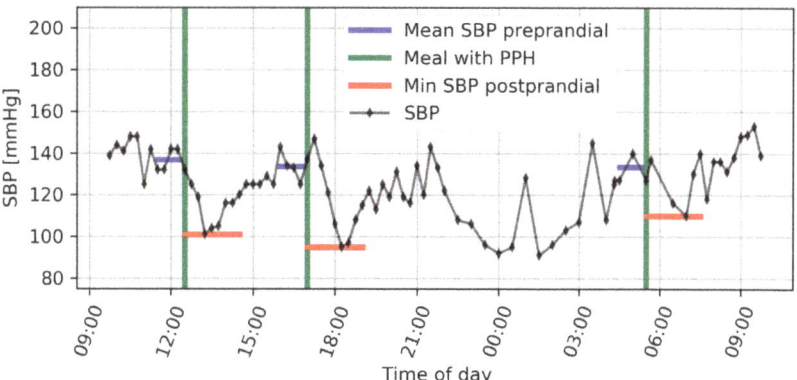

Figure 1. ABPM showing systolic blood pressure (SBP) in a 69-year old male with C1, AIS B SCI four months and eight days post injury. He had three episodes of PPH after lunch, dinner, and early breakfast.

2.3. Statistical Analysis

The applied definition of PPH was a decrease in SBP ≥20 mmHg or SBP <90 mmHg if SBP before the meal was ≥100 mm Hg within two hours after ingesting a meal [1–3]. The mean value of SBP measurements one hour before a meal and with at least two measurements was used as the reference SBP. Logged SBP data, including diary notes of activities, were transferred to Excel, and coded into the defined activities. Data from Excel were augmented with a calculated SBP drop indicator for each time-stamped SBP measurement using a Python script and in addition enriched with demographic and medication data prior to importing the data in STATA via Stat Transfer 14. STATA version 16 was used for preprocessing the data and statistical analysis. Various Python scripts were used on csv exported data to generate figures and extract counting statistics for physical activity and transfer events before and after meals. Logistic regression was performed using PPH as the dependent variable. Independent variables were gender, age at ABPM, number of meals, number of medications on the day of ABPM, time since injury, complete/incomplete SCI, gastrointestinal morbidity and surgery, other neurological diseases, diabetes and level of injury defined as: (1) high tetraplegia with neurological level of injury from C1–C3, (2) low tetraplegia C4–C8, (3) high paraplegia (T1–T6), and (4) low paraplegia (T7 and below).

3. Results

Valid recordings of pre- and postprandial SBP were available for a total of 449 meals in 158 subjects. Data regarding demography, comorbidity, and use of medications are shown in Table 1. The median observational time of the ABPMs was 24 h. The median SBP was 120 mmHg before breakfast, 125 mmHg before lunch, 125 mmHg before dinner, and 118 mmHg during the night.

Table 1. Demographics, comorbidity, and medications when ABPM was performed.

N= 158	Number (*n*)	Frequency (%)
Male/Female	109/49	69%/31%
Tetraplegia		
High/low tetraplegia [1]	49/45	31%/28%
AIS A	14	9%
AIS B	8	5%
AIS C	13	8%
AIS D	59	37%
Paraplegia		
High/low paraplegia [1]	26/38	16%/24%
AIS A	15	9%
AIS B	3	2%
AIS C	12	8%
AIS D	34	22%
Non-traumatic SCI	85	54 %
Diabetes	16	10%
Other neurological diseases	20	13%
Number of medications	Median: 10	(min: 0; max: 22)
Time since injury	Median: 0.24 years	(min: 0.02; max: 56.7)
Age	Median: 59.1 years	(min: 13.2; max: 86.2)
Duration of ABPM	Median: 24.0 h	(min: 10.5; max: 49.4)

[1] High Tetraplegia C1–C3, low tetraplegia C4–C8, high paraplegia T1–T6, low paraplegia T7 and below. ABPM: Ambulatory blood pressure measurement. SCI: Spinal Cord Injury. AIS: ASIA Impairment Scale.

A total of 114 (25.3%) episodes of decrease in SBP within two hours after a meal meet the criteria of PPH in 78 (49.4%) subjects. In only seven (4.4%) subjects, the decrease in SBP was associated with symptoms of hypotension. The median time from ingestion of the meal until PPH was registered was 60 min (min 15, max 120 min). The median change in SBP during PPH was −28 mmHg (min: −87; max: −15 mmHg). Twenty of 114 (17%) episodes interpreted as PPH occurred simultaneously with transfers noted in the diary, while 26 (23%) occurred simultaneously with physical activity e.g., physical exercise, physiotherapy, and occupational therapy. Logistic regression analysis revealed that PPH was associated with age when ABPM was performed, higher levels of injury, and complete SCI (Table 2).

Table 2. Logistic regression analysis.

Independent Variable	Odds Ratio	Standard Error	*p*-Value	95% Confidence Interval
Age when ABPM performed	1.039	0.012	0.001 *	1.015–1.063
Gender	0.950	0.434	0.906	0.404–2.231
Time since spinal cord injury	1.068	0.466	0.132	0.980–1.163
Level of injury [1]	1.512	0.120	0.023 *	1.060–2.160
Complete/incomplete SCI	9.482	5.941	0.000 *	2.776–32.380

Statistical method: Logistic regression with PPH as the dependent variable. Number of medications on the day of the ABPM, gastrointestinal morbidity and surgery, other neurological diseases and diabetes were used as independent variable as well but did not show statistically significant association with PPH. [1] Level of injury was divided into four groups: high tetraplegia C1–C3, low tetraplegia C4–C8, high paraplegia T1–T6, low paraplegia T7 and below. * p-values < 0.01 are considered statistically significant.

4. Discussion

The main finding from the present study is that PPH is common among persons with SCI. In our setting, the prevalence of PPH was 49% and the risk increased with increasing age, higher levels of SCI, and completeness of the lesion. Surprisingly, concomitant medication, other neurological diseases or diabetes did not increase the risk. To the best of our knowledge, the present study is the first to provide data on PPH in a large group of persons with SCI.

Our results are in contrast to some earlier publications. Catz et al. found that PPH can occur in thoracic paraplegia, but not in tetraplegia [29]. Baliga et al. did not find PPH in neither para- nor tetraplegic patients [28]. The present study is by far the largest but also differs from previous by having a high proportion of incomplete and non-traumatic lesions and especially by including significantly older patients. The previous studies were performed under standardized conditions with liquid test-meals and supine position during study and with a post prandial observational time of 45 min. In contrast, our data were collected during the patient's daily routine and most recordings lasted 24 h. In support of our findings, two case reports on persons with SCI and age 62 and 66 years also found PPH [26,27]. It is therefore likely that age is an important factor for developing PPH in persons with SCI.

The cardiovascular response to a meal is mediated through the sympathetic gastrovascular reflex, whereby gastric distension elicits a vasoconstrictive response. In addition, the plasma levels of glucose, insulin, and norepinephrine rises. In supine young able-bodied subjects, ingestion of a meal leads to minor, if any change, in SBP. The increased splanchnic blood flow in the superior mesenteric artery is counterbalanced by increased heartrate, cardiac output, and systemic peripheral resistance. In supine elderly subjects, ingestion of a meal leads to the same changes, but the SBP decreases if the subject is sitting.

The pathophysiology of PPH is not fully understood but it represents an imbalance between increased splanchnic blood flow and the needed adjustment from the cardiovascular system. Impaired peripheral vasoconstrictor response, lack of increase in heartrate by activation of the sympathetic nervous system i.e., reduced baroreflex function and diminished function of the gastrovascular reflex are factors known to contribute. The temperature of the meal is important, as fluid with a temperature of 50 °C affects the SBP more than a fluid meal of 5 °C [42]. PPH is more frequent after breakfast than lunch and dinner due to circadian changes in BP [43]. Furthermore, a high content of mono-saccharides, primarily glucose, and a high number of calories transported to the duodenum also increases risk of PPH [44].

In other groups of patients, PPH is often asymptomatic [3]. Despite the lack of symptoms, PPH is associated with an increased risk of falls, syncope, coronary events, stroke, asymptomatic lacunar infarction, asymptomatic cerebrovascular damage, and death [4,7,45]. In our study, PPH was observed in 49% of patients, but only 4% had symptoms. Worldwide, people with SCI are living longer and the risk of cardiovascular diseases is high [46]. Furthermore, persons with SCI are at an increased risk of developing non-Alzheimer's dementia [34]. Thus, PPH may be clinically important, even if asymptomatic. PPH is defined as occurring within two hours after a meal [1]. Our study shows that a drop in SBP can occur from 15–120 min after ingesting a meal. We have not examined if a decrease in SBP could last more than 120 min after a meal. Studies have found the most pronounced fall in SBP after 60 min [47,48]. These studies show that the lowering of BP post meal continues, to a lesser extent, after two hours in persons with autonomic failure and essential hypertension. Persons with SCI have delayed gastric emptying [35]. This could raise the question if the observation time post meal should be longer than two hours. However, the findings from the present study need to be confirmed and clinically relevant interventions developed before changes in daily practice of persons with SCI and PPH are recommended. Thus, the definition of PPH must be validated for the SCI-population. This includes definitions for a standard test-meal, test position, sampling intervals, length of observational time after ingesting a meal, time of day for the test, and which medication should be paused. Possibly, this could be performed as an addition to the International Standards to Document Remaining Autonomic Function after Spinal Cord Injury [49]. Long-term observational studies are needed to elucidate if PPH is associated with increased morbidity and mortality in persons with SCI. Further investigations are needed to explore the mechanisms that trigger PPH, specifically in the SCI population.

There are several limitations to the present study. We performed ABPM for approximately 24 h. Among patients in hospital, we assumed that they actually ate their meals at

J. Clin. Med. **2021**, *10*, 1417

the time it was served. In addition, we do not know the exact composition of each meal and the amount of liquid ingested. At our institution, meals are served at specific time points and patients were encouraged to write in the diary, if they deviated from this daily routine. Since we defined PPH as a decrease in SBP occurring within 2 h after a meal and most episodes occurred within this time frame, we find that the exact timing of the meal is of lesser importance. However, the fall in SBP in the postprandial observational time could arise from other activities known to trigger hypotensive episodes i.e., transfers and physical activity. In our study, such activity could potentially explain up to 50% of episodes interpreted as PPH. In spite of this, our data indicate that PPH is very common in persons with SCI. Another limitation is the medication taken by the subjects during the study period. Thus, some cases of PPH may be explained by medication taken, rather that SCI per se. Taken as a whole, the use of medication was not associated with PPH, but we did not go into details with each type of drug or combination of medications.

In conclusion, we found that PPH is common among persons with SCI. We also found that PPH is associated with higher levels of SCI, complete lesions, and age of the patient.

Author Contributions: Conceptualization, R.M.H., E.M.H., and K.K.; methodology, R.M.H., E.M.H., K.K., and A.K.; formal analysis J.S. and R.M.H., investigation R.M.H.; writing—original draft preparation, R.M.H. and K.K.; writing—review and editing, K.K., E.M.H., A.K., and J.S.; funding acquisition, K.K. All authors have read and agreed to the published version of the manuscript.

Funding: The study was supported by an educational grant from Coloplast, Denmark.

Institutional Review Board Statement: The study was conducted according to the guidelines of the Declaration of Helsinki. Use of data for publication was granted from the Hospital Management, Regional Hospital Central Jutland. The project was reported to The Scientific Ethical Committees of Region Central Jutland (case number 1-10-72-181-20) and The Legal Office of the Central Denmark Region (reference number 706735, case number 1-16-02-590-20).

Informed Consent Statement: Patient consent was waived due to Danish legislation since the study is a quality control study to which written informed consent is not needed. The data used in the study is part of routine assessment upon each patient and part of medical records. Permission to obtain the data and use for publication was given by the Hospital Management, Regional Hospital Central Jutland.

Data Availability Statement: The data presented in this study are available on request from the corresponding author. The data are not publicly available due to language.

Acknowledgments: The authors would like to thank Kim Hansen for his technical assistance.

Conflicts of Interest: The authors declare no conflict of interest. The funders had no role in the design of the study; in the collection, analyses, or interpretation of data; in the writing of the manuscript, or in the decision to publish the results.

References

1. Jansen, R.W.; Lipsitz, L.A. Postprandial hypotension: Epidemiology, pathophysiology, and clinical management. *Ann. Intern. Med.* **1995**, *122*, 286–295. [CrossRef] [PubMed]
2. Pavelic, A.; Krbot Skoric, M.; Crnosija, L.; Habek, M. Postprandial hypotension in neurological disorders: Systematic review and meta-analysis. *Clin. Auton. Res.* **2017**, *27*, 263–271. [CrossRef]
3. Trahair, L.G.; Horowitz, M.; Jones, K.L. Postprandial hypotension: A systematic review. *J. Am. Med. Dir. Assoc.* **2014**, *15*, 394–409. [CrossRef]
4. Luciano, G.L.; Brennan, M.J.; Rothberg, M.B. Postprandial hypotension. *Am. J. Med.* **2010**, *123*, e281–e286. [CrossRef]
5. Aronow, W.S.; Ahn, C. Postprandial hypotension in 499 elderly persons in a long-term health care facility. *J. Am. Geriatr. Soc.* **1994**, *42*, 930–932. [CrossRef]
6. Cohen, I.; Rogers, P.; Burke, V.; Beilin, L.J. Predictors of medication use, compliance and symptoms of hypotension in a community-based sample of elderly men and women. *J. Clin. Pharm. Ther.* **1998**, *23*, 423–432. [CrossRef] [PubMed]
7. Aronow, W.S.; Ahn, C. Association of postprandial hypotension with incidence of falls, syncope, coronary events, stroke, and total mortality at 29-month follow-up in 499 older nursing home residents. *J. Am. Geriatr. Soc.* **1997**, *45*, 1051–1053. [CrossRef] [PubMed]

8. Gorelick, P.B.; Scuteri, A.; Black, S.E.; Decarli, C.; Greenberg, S.M.; Iadecola, C.; Launer, L.J.; Laurent, S.; Lopez, O.L.; Nyenhuis, D.; et al. Vascular contributions to cognitive impairment and dementia: A statement for healthcare professionals from the american heart association/american stroke association. *Stroke* **2011**, *42*, 2672–2713. [CrossRef]
9. Biering-Sorensen, F.; Biering-Sorensen, T.; Liu, N.; Malmqvist, L.; Wecht, J.M.; Krassioukov, A. Alterations in cardiac autonomic control in spinal cord injury. *Auton. Neurosci.* **2018**, *209*, 4–18. [CrossRef]
10. Phillips, A.A.; Krassioukov, A.V.; Ainslie, P.N.; Warburton, D.E. Baroreflex function after spinal cord injury. *J. Neurotrauma* **2012**, *29*, 2431–2445. [CrossRef] [PubMed]
11. Teasell, R.W.; Arnold, J.M.; Krassioukov, A.; Delaney, G.A. Cardiovascular consequences of loss of supraspinal control of the sympathetic nervous system after spinal cord injury. *Arch. Phys. Med. Rehabil.* **2000**, *81*, 506–516. [CrossRef]
12. Frisbie, J.H. Unstable baseline blood pressure in chronic tetraplegia. *Spinal Cord* **2007**, *45*, 92–95. [CrossRef]
13. Claydon, V.E.; Steeves, J.D.; Krassioukov, A. Orthostatic hypotension following spinal cord injury: Understanding clinical pathophysiology. *Spinal Cord* **2006**, *44*, 341–351. [CrossRef] [PubMed]
14. Claydon, V.E.; Krassioukov, A.V. Orthostatic hypotension and autonomic pathways after spinal cord injury. *J. Neurotrauma* **2006**, *23*, 1713–1725. [CrossRef]
15. King, M.L.; Lichtman, S.W.; Pellicone, J.T.; Close, R.J.; Lisanti, P. Exertional hypotension in spinal cord injury. *Chest* **1994**, *106*, 1166–1171. [CrossRef] [PubMed]
16. Machač, S.; Radvanský, J.; Kolář, P.; Kříž, J. Cardiovascular response to peak voluntary exercise in males with cervical spinal cord injury. *J. Spinal Cord Med.* **2016**, *39*, 412–420. [CrossRef]
17. Claydon, V.E.; Hol, A.T.; Eng, J.J.; Krassioukov, A.V. Cardiovascular responses and postexercise hypotension after arm cycling exercise in subjects with spinal cord injury. *Arch. Phys. Med. Rehabil.* **2006**, *87*, 1106–1114. [CrossRef] [PubMed]
18. Karlsson, A.K. Autonomic dysreflexia. *Spinal Cord* **1999**, *37*, 383–391. [CrossRef]
19. Eldahan, K.C.; Rabchevsky, A.G. Autonomic dysreflexia after spinal cord injury: Systemic pathophysiology and methods of management. *Auton. Neurosci.* **2018**, *209*, 59–70. [CrossRef]
20. Carlozzi, N.E.; Fyffe, D.; Morin, K.G.; Byrne, R.; Tulsky, D.S.; Victorson, D.; Lai, J.S.; Wecht, J.M. Impact of blood pressure dysregulation on health-related quality of life in persons with spinal cord injury: Development of a conceptual model. *Arch. Phys. Med. Rehabil.* **2013**, *94*, 1721–1730. [CrossRef] [PubMed]
21. Adriaansen, J.J.; Ruijs, L.E.; van Koppenhagen, C.F.; van Asbeck, F.W.; Snoek, G.J.; van Kuppevelt, D.; Visser-Meily, J.M.; Post, M.W. Secondary health conditions and quality of life in persons living with spinal cord injury for at least ten years. *J. Rehabil. Med.* **2016**, *48*, 853–860. [CrossRef]
22. Hubli, M.; Gee, C.M.; Krassioukov, A.V. Refined assessment of blood pressure instability after spinal cord injury. *Am. J. Hypertens.* **2015**, *28*, 173–181. [CrossRef]
23. Hubli, M.; Krassioukov, A.V. Ambulatory blood pressure monitoring in spinal cord injury: Clinical practicability. *J. Neurotrauma* **2014**, *31*, 789–797. [CrossRef]
24. Kohara, K.; Uemura, K.; Takata, Y.; Okura, T.; Kitami, Y.; Hiwada, K. Postprandial hypotension: Evaluation by ambulatory blood pressure monitoring. *Am. J. Hypertens.* **1998**, *11*, 1358–1363. [CrossRef]
25. Catz, A.; Mendelson, L.; Solzi, P. Symptomatic postprandial hypotension in high paraplegia. Case report. *Paraplegia* **1992**, *30*, 582–586. [CrossRef]
26. Farrehi, C.; Pazzi, C.; Stillman, M. A case of postprandial hypotension in an individual with cervical spinal cord injury: Treatment with acarbose. *Spinal Cord Ser. Cases* **2019**, *5*, 75. [CrossRef]
27. Ishikawa, J.; Watanabe, S.; Harada, K. Awakening Blood Pressure Rise in a Patient with Spinal Cord Injury. *Am. J. Case Rep.* **2016**, *17*, 177–181. [CrossRef] [PubMed]
28. Baliga, R.R.; Catz, A.B.; Watson, L.D.; Short, D.J.; Frankel, H.L.; Mathias, C.J. Cardiovascular and hormonal responses to food ingestion in humans with spinal cord transection. *Clin. Auton. Res.* **1997**, *7*, 137–141. [CrossRef]
29. Catz, A.; Bluvshtein, V.; Pinhas, I.; Akselrod, S.; Gelernter, I.; Nissel, T.; Vered, Y.; Bornstein, N.M.; Korczyn, A.D. Hemodynamic effects of liquid food ingestion in mid-thoracic paraplegia: Is supine postprandial hypotension related to thoracic spinal cord damage? *Spinal Cord* **2007**, *45*, 96–103. [CrossRef] [PubMed]
30. New, P.W.; Cripps, R.A.; Bonne Lee, B. Global maps of non-traumatic spinal cord injury epidemiology: Towards a living data repository. *Spinal Cord* **2014**, *52*, 97–109. [CrossRef] [PubMed]
31. New, P.W.; Sundararajan, V. Incidence of non-traumatic spinal cord injury in Victoria, Australia: A population-based study and literature review. *Spinal Cord* **2008**, *46*, 406–411. [CrossRef]
32. Halvorsen, A.; Pettersen, A.L.; Nilsen, S.M.; Halle, K.K.; Schaanning, E.E.; Rekand, T. Non-traumatic spinal cord injury in Norway 2012–2016: Analysis from a national registry and comparison with traumatic spinal cord injury. *Spinal Cord* **2019**, *57*, 324–330. [CrossRef]
33. Buzzell, A.; Chamberlain, J.D.; Gmünder, H.P.; Hug, K.; Jordan, X.; Schubert, M.; Brinkhof, M.W.G. Survival after non-traumatic spinal cord injury: Evidence from a population-based rehabilitation cohort in Switzerland. *Spinal Cord* **2019**, *57*, 267–275. [CrossRef]
34. Huang, S.W.; Wang, W.T.; Chou, L.C.; Liou, T.H.; Lin, H.W. Risk of Dementia in Patients with Spinal Cord Injury: A Nationwide Population-Based Cohort Study. *J. Neurotrauma* **2017**, *34*, 615–622. [CrossRef]
35. Holmes, G.M.; Blanke, E.N. Gastrointestinal dysfunction after spinal cord injury. *Exp. Neurol.* **2019**, *320*, 113009. [CrossRef]

36. Krogh, K.; Nielsen, J.; Djurhuus, J.C.; Mosdal, C.; Sabroe, S.; Laurberg, S. Colorectal function in patients with spinal cord lesions. *Dis. Colon Rectum* **1997**, *40*, 1233–1239. [CrossRef]
37. Faaborg, P.M.; Christensen, P.; Finnerup, N.; Laurberg, S.; Krogh, K. The pattern of colorectal dysfunction changes with time since spinal cord injury. *Spinal Cord* **2008**, *46*, 234–238. [CrossRef]
38. Fynne, L.; Worsøe, J.; Gregersen, T.; Schlageter, V.; Laurberg, S.; Krogh, K. Gastric and small intestinal dysfunction in spinal cord injury patients. *Acta Neurol. Scand.* **2012**, *125*, 123–128. [CrossRef]
39. Kao, C.H.; Ho, Y.J.; Changlai, S.P.; Ding, H.J. Gastric emptying in spinal cord injury patients. *Dig. Dis. Sci.* **1999**, *44*, 1512–1515. [CrossRef]
40. The 2019 revision of the International Standards for Neurological Classification of Spinal Cord Injury (ISNCSCI)—What's new? *Spinal Cord* **2019**, *57*, 815–817. [CrossRef]
41. Krogh, K.; Emmanuel, A.; Perrouin-Verbe, B.; Korsten, M.A.; Mulcahy, M.J.; Biering-Sorensen, F. International spinal cord injury bowel function basic data set (Version 2.0). *Spinal Cord* **2017**, *55*, 692–698. [CrossRef] [PubMed]
42. Kuipers, H.M.; Jansen, R.W.; Peeters, T.L.; Hoefnagels, W.H. The influence of food temperature on postprandial blood pressure reduction and its relation to substance-P in healthy elderly subjects. *J. Am. Geriatr. Soc.* **1991**, *39*, 181–184. [CrossRef] [PubMed]
43. Puisieux, F.; Bulckaen, H.; Fauchais, A.L.; Drumez, S.; Salomez-Granier, F.; Dewailly, P. Ambulatory blood pressure monitoring and postprandial hypotension in elderly persons with falls or syncopes. *J. Gerontol. A Biol. Sci. Med. Sci.* **2000**, *55*, M535–M540. [CrossRef] [PubMed]
44. Sidery, M.B.; Macdonald, I.A. The effect of meal size on the cardiovascular responses to food ingestion. *Br. J. Nutr.* **1994**, *71*, 835–848. [CrossRef] [PubMed]
45. Jang, A. Postprandial Hypotension as a Risk Factor for the Development of New Cardiovascular Disease: A Prospective Cohort Study with 36 Month Follow-Up in Community-Dwelling Elderly People. *J. Clin. Med.* **2020**, *9*, 345. [CrossRef]
46. Groah, S.L.; Weitzenkamp, D.; Sett, P.; Soni, B.; Savic, G. The relationship between neurological level of injury and symptomatic cardiovascular disease risk in the aging spinal injured. *Spinal Cord* **2001**, *39*, 310–317. [CrossRef]
47. Mathias, C.J.; da Costa, D.F.; Fosbraey, P.; Bannister, R.; Wood, S.M.; Bloom, S.R.; Christensen, N.J. Cardiovascular, biochemical and hormonal changes during food-induced hypotension in chronic autonomic failure. *J. Neurol. Sci.* **1989**, *94*, 255–269. [CrossRef]
48. Kohara, K.; Jiang, Y.; Igase, M.; Takata, Y.; Fukuoka, T.; Okura, T.; Kitami, Y.; Hiwada, K. Postprandial hypotension is associated with asymptomatic cerebrovascular damage in essential hypertensive patients. *Hypertension* **1999**, *33*, 565–568. [CrossRef]
49. Krassioukov, A.; Biering-Sorensen, C.F.; Donovan, W.; Kennelly, M.; Kirshblum, S.; Krogh, K.; Alexander, M.S.; Vogel, L.; And Wecht, J. International Standards to document remaining Autonomic Function after Spinal Cord Injury (ISAFSCI), First Edition 2012. *Top. Spinal Cord Inj. Rehabil.* **2012**, *18*, 282–296. [CrossRef]

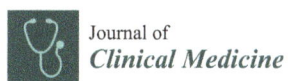

Journal of
Clinical Medicine

MDPI

Review

Assessment of Gastrointestinal Autonomic Dysfunction: Present and Future Perspectives

Ditte S. Kornum [1,2,*], Astrid J. Terkelsen [3], Davide Bertoli [4], Mette W. Klinge [1], Katrine L. Høyer [1,2], Huda H. A. Kufaishi [5], Per Borghammer [6], Asbjørn M. Drewes [4,7], Christina Brock [4,7] and Klaus Krogh [1,2]

[1] Department of Hepatology and Gastroenterology, Aarhus University Hospital, DK8200 Aarhus, Denmark; meteader@rm.dk (M.W.K.); kathoeye@rm.dk (K.L.H.); klaukrog@rm.dk (K.K.)
[2] Steno Diabetes Centre Aarhus, Aarhus University Hospital, DK8200 Aarhus, Denmark
[3] Department of Neurology, Aarhus University Hospital, DK8200 Aarhus, Denmark; astrterk@rm.dk
[4] Mech-Sense, Department of Gastroenterology and Hepatology, Aalborg University Hospital, DK9100 Aalborg, Denmark; d.bertoli@rn.dk (D.B.); amd@rn.dk (A.M.D.); christina.brock@rn.dk (C.B.)
[5] Steno Diabetes Centre Copenhagen, Gentofte Hospital, DK2820 Gentofte, Denmark; huda.kufaishi@regionh.dk
[6] Department of Nuclear Medicine and PET-Centre, Aarhus University Hospital, DK8200 Aarhus, Denmark; perborgh@rm.dk
[7] Steno Diabetes Centre North Jutland, Aalborg University Hospital, DK9100 Aalborg, Denmark
* Correspondence: Dittiver@rm.dk

Citation: Kornum, D.S.; Terkelsen, A.J.; Bertoli, D.; Klinge, M.W.; Høyer, K.L.; Kufaishi, H.H.A.; Borghammer, P.; Drewes, A.M.; Brock, C.; Krogh, K. Assessment of Gastrointestinal Autonomic Dysfunction: Present and Future Perspectives. *J. Clin. Med.* **2021**, *10*, 1392. https://doi.org/10.3390/jcm10071392

Academic Editor: Bruno Annibale

Received: 27 February 2021
Accepted: 27 March 2021
Published: 31 March 2021

Publisher's Note: MDPI stays neutral with regard to jurisdictional claims in published maps and institutional affiliations.

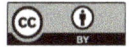

Copyright: © 2021 by the authors. Licensee MDPI, Basel, Switzerland. This article is an open access article distributed under the terms and conditions of the Creative Commons Attribution (CC BY) license (https://creativecommons.org/licenses/by/4.0/).

Abstract: The autonomic nervous system delicately regulates the function of several target organs, including the gastrointestinal tract. Thus, nerve lesions or other nerve pathologies may cause autonomic dysfunction (AD). Some of the most common causes of AD are diabetes mellitus and α-synucleinopathies such as Parkinson's disease. Widespread dysmotility throughout the gastrointestinal tract is a common finding in AD, but no commercially available method exists for direct verification of enteric dysfunction. Thus, assessing segmental enteric physiological function is recommended to aid diagnostics and guide treatment. Several established assessment methods exist, but disadvantages such as lack of standardization, exposure to radiation, advanced data interpretation, or high cost, limit their utility. Emerging methods, including high-resolution colonic manometry, 3D-transit, advanced imaging methods, analysis of gut biopsies, and microbiota, may all assist in the evaluation of gastroenteropathy related to AD. This review provides an overview of established and emerging assessment methods of physiological function within the gut and assessment methods of autonomic neuropathy outside the gut, especially in regards to clinical performance, strengths, and limitations for each method.

Keywords: autonomic dysfunction; gastrointestinal; motility; investigations; manometry; breath test; imaging; Parkinson's disease; diabetes mellitus

1. Introduction

Autonomic disorders may involve the parasympathetic, sympathetic, and enteric nervous systems with extensive, multisystemic consequences [1]. Among several other organ manifestations, pan-enteric gastrointestinal (GI) dysmotility is frequently seen [2]. Not only do the motility disturbances contribute to GI symptoms, they may also affect the absorption of medication used to treat the underlying disease [3,4].

Methods for assessment of GI motility are generally applicable across autonomic dysfunction (AD) etiologies despite different underlying pathophysiology. Verification of the extent of GI involvement is important to support diagnosis and guide effective treatment, especially because gastrointestinal symptoms and objective measures correlate poorly [5–8]. However, commercially available assessment methods have different inherent limitations, and better techniques are needed for evaluating GI dysfunction. Thus, the main focus of this review is to describe established and emerging methods for assessment of enteric dysfunction in patients with AD.

2. Clinical Presentation

2.1. Autonomic Neuropathy in Neurological Disorders

The autonomic nervous system involves sympathetic and parasympathetic neural structures in the central and peripheral nervous systems that innervate all internal organs [1]. Moreover, and often under-recognized, is the enteric nervous system that is also part of the autonomic nervous system [9]. Centrally, the autonomic nervous system is regulated by areas localized at the forebrain pontomescencephalic and bulbopontine level, and in the spinal cord. The peripheral autonomic nervous system acts via the postganglionic parasympathetic and sympathetic nervous systems, which interact with the enteric nervous system in a complex and delicately coordinated network [10,11]. Thus, central and peripheral nerve lesions and pathology may induce AD [1]. Pure AD can manifest acutely or sub-acutely such as seen in autoimmune autonomic ganglionopathy or treatment-induced neuropathy of diabetes mellitus (DM). The latter can be caused by a too fast downregulation of blood glucose in a dysregulated DM patient [12]. On the other hand, the presentation can be slowly progressing as seen in α-synucleinopathies or neuropathy of various etiologies. α-synucleinopathies are neurodegenerative diseases characterized by abnormal accumulation of aggregates of α-synuclein protein in nerve fibers or glial cells. The main types of α-synucleinopathies are Parkinson's disease (PD), dementia with Lewy bodies, multiple-system atrophy, and pure autonomic failure [13]. Large and small fiber sensory and autonomic neuropathy is seen in metabolic disorders (DM, hypothyroidism, uremia), cobalamin deficiency, infections, immune-mediated conditions (gammopathies, vasculitis, and coeliac disease), neurotoxic exposure (alcoholism, and pharmacological treatment), and in hereditary conditions (hereditary sensory and autonomic neuropathy, Fabry's disease, and hereditary transthyretin-mediated amyloidosis) [14]. Autonomic dysfunction is also seen in patients with postural orthostatic tachycardia syndrome (POTS) defined by an abnormal increase in heart rate of at least 30 beats/min within 10 min of standing or during a tilt table test. The rise in heart rate is seen in the absence of orthostatic hypotension and symptoms of orthostatic intolerance must be present for at least 6 months [15]. POTS has been associated with small fiber neuropathy, Ehlers–Danlos syndrome and mast cell activation syndrome [16,17].

2.2. Clinical Presentation of Autonomic Neuropathy in General

The symptoms of autonomic neuropathy are numerous and the condition is multisystemic due to the extensive parasympathetic and sympathetic innervation of multiple organs and structures such as the cardiovascular, gastrointestinal, thermoregulatory, respiratory, urogenital, pupillomotor, and sudomotor systems [2]. Thus, diagnosis, treatment, and follow-up may involve multiple specialties. Parasympathetic dysfunction may cause the sicca syndrome with dry eyes and mouth, light intolerance due to dilated non-responding pupils, urine retention, erectile dysfunction, resting tachycardia, and reduced GI motility. Sympathetic dysfunction is characterized by miotic pupils, orthostatic intolerance with dizziness or syncope, exercise intolerance, anhidrosis, and heat intolerance [18]. GI dysfunction may cause gastroparesis and enteropathy with constipation, diarrhea, and fecal incontinence, and may affect absorption of oral medication, see below.

Recognizing AD is important because of the increased morbidity and mortality associated with reduced heart rate variability, arrhythmias, increased blood pressure variability, and neurogenic orthostatic hypotension [19,20]. Acute development of AD can be the first sign of an underlying paraneoplastic condition. Furthermore, early recognition is important to ensure early initiation of conservative or pharmacological treatments targeting orthostatic or postprandial hypotension, supine hypertension, erectile dysfunction, and gastroenteropathy as these conditions may have a negative impact on the quality of life if left untreated. Finally, autonomic testing can monitor the course of dysautonomia and the response to treatment.

2.3. Clinical Presentation of Gastrointestinal Autonomic Neuropathy

Studies of GI function in patients with AD have mainly included patients with DM or PD. However, pan-enteric autonomic neuropathy is also seen in the less commonly described etiologies, and principles for clinical evaluation and treatment will be largely similar across etiologies. All segments of the GI tract may be affected, contributing to a highly variable inter-individual clinical presentation and intra-individual symptom fluctuation with time, the latter especially seen in patients with DM [21]. Common GI symptoms, such as dysphagia, nausea, vomiting, bloating, early satiety, abdominal pain, constipation, diarrhea, weight loss, and fecal incontinence may be present, combined or solitary, and they may substantially affect the quality of life [22–24]. In patients with DM, symptoms of gastroparesis are present in up to 18%, diarrhea in 20%, and constipation in up to 60%. Furthermore, fecal incontinence is frequently reported [25,26]. The prevalence of symptoms of gastroparesis and constipation in PD reaches 50%. Furthermore, 72% have anorectal dysfunction expressed as straining for defecation, but also incomplete emptying, with symptoms becoming more severe during disease progression [27,28]. Constipation is reported in 50% of patients with pure autonomic failure and in up to 82% of patients with multiple system atrophy [3]. Orthostatic symptoms in POTS often coexist with severe GI symptoms, with nausea, abdominal pain and constipation reported in more than 70% [29,30]. Prominent multi-segmental GI symptoms are also commonly seen in the hypermobile Ehlers–Danlos syndrome and in the mast cell activation syndrome, which is relevant as a differential diagnosis [16,17]. However, prevalence measures vary across studies in all the above-mentioned disorders. While several AD etiologies are associated with GI symptoms, studies on motility across multiple GI segments are primarily performed in PD and DM. Thus, motility disturbances in PD and DM will gain most attention in this review, but dysmotility findings in other diseases will be mentioned when available.

Pan-enteric dysmotility has been documented, and the abnormalities in each segment of the GI tract are presented in Figure 1. Aperistalsis and uncoordinated contractions are common in the esophagus [7,31]. Gastric dysmotility presents as delayed or accelerated gastric emptying time and reduced postprandial accommodation [21,30]. Dysmotility, prolonged transit time, and a higher prevalence of small intestinal bacterial overgrowth (SIBO) are seen within the small intestine [32,33]. Delayed colonic transit time is frequently seen in PD and primarily caused by a combination of slow transit constipation and anorectal outlet obstruction [27]. Anorectal dysfunction in PD is primarily due to dystonia and pathological contractions of the external sphincter during defecation [27]. Both colonic hypo- and hypermotility have been shown in DM and a dysfunctional internal sphincter combined with rectal hyposensitivity contributes to fecal incontinence [34–36].

Widespread dysmotility and varying transit times, especially prolonged gastric emptying time, can make the absorption of oral medication unpredictable and reduce the effectiveness of some drugs [3,4]. Additionally, abnormal postprandial fluctuations in blood glucose, related to a mismatch between insulin administration and food availability in the small intestine, may be harmful to patients with DM [21]. Postprandial hypotension, mainly related to autonomic neuropathy, is also more frequent in patients with DM than in healthy controls [37].

No commercially available in vivo diagnostic test of enteric neuropathy exists. Furthermore, GI symptoms are generally not predictive of the objective motility dysfunction, with objective dysmotility occurring more frequently than subjective symptoms. This necessitates objective assessment to verify the extent of GI dysmotility to support the diagnosis of enteric neuropathy and guide treatment [5–8]. However, even though a verification of GI dysmotility in a patient with AD significantly increases the likelihood of enteric neuropathy, some patients may have enteric neuropathy despite normal motility measurements.

The underlying pathophysiology of AD varies across patient groups, but assessment methods of the pan-enteric dysfunction are overall identical. Thus, established and emerging methods for assessment of gut function in autonomic disorders and the most relevant general assessment methods of autonomic neuropathy will be reviewed below. The assessment-guided treatment approach will be described at the end of this review.

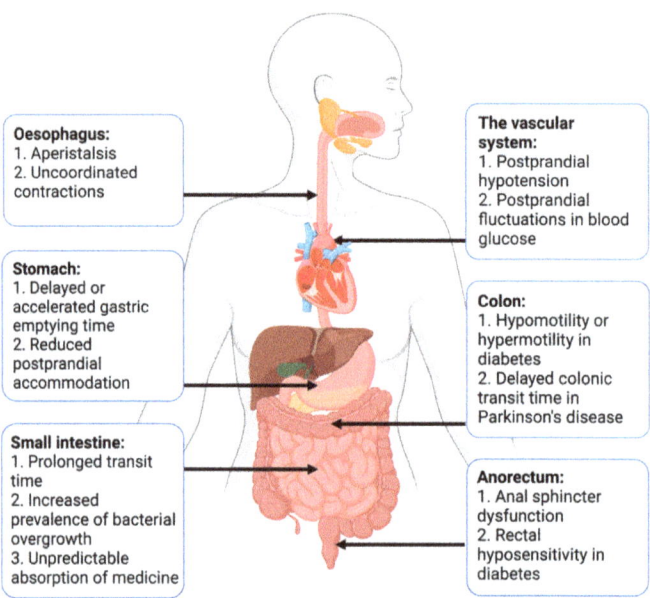

Oesophagus:
1. Aperistalsis
2. Uncoordinated contractions

Stomach:
1. Delayed or accelerated gastric emptying time
2. Reduced postprandial accommodation

Small intestine:
1. Prolonged transit time
2. Increased prevalence of bacterial overgrowth
3. Unpredictable absorption of medicine

The vascular system:
1. Postprandial hypotension
2. Postprandial fluctuations in blood glucose

Colon:
1. Hypomotility or hypermotility in diabetes
2. Delayed colonic transit time in Parkinson's disease

Anorectum:
1. Anal sphincter dysfunction
2. Rectal hyposensitivity in diabetes

Figure 1. Motility disturbances related to autonomic dysfunction in each gastrointestinal segment.

3. Established Methods for Assessment of Gastroenteropathy

3.1. Exclusion of Differential Diagnoses

When enteric neuropathy is suspected in a patient with an autonomic disorder, the primary approach is to exclude other plausible causes of the gastrointestinal symptoms, such as gastrointestinal cancer, inflammatory bowel disease, exocrine pancreas insufficiency, bile acid malabsorption, coeliac disease, and porphyria. Furthermore, it is important to substitute medication if side effects are suspected to be the cause of GI symptoms.

3.2. Assessment of Symptoms

In spite of several scoring systems being used in the literature, no questionnaire has been validated specifically for assessment of AD-related gastroenteropathy, except for the GI sub-score within the Composite Autonomic Symptom Score (COMPASS-31) questionnaire, see Section 5 [38].

The Gastroparesis Cardinal Symptom Index is a sub-score in the larger questionnaire PAGI-SYM (patient assessment of upper gastrointestinal disorders-symptom severity index) [39]. It is a symptom severity scale assessing gastroparesis and consists of nine items grouped into three subscales including nausea/vomiting, postprandial fullness/early satiety, and bloating. The severity of each symptom is rated on a Likert scale ranging from 0 (no symptoms) to 5 (very severe symptoms), and the recall period is two weeks. The Gastroparesis Cardinal Symptom Index is reliable, valid, and responsive to change [40,41]. However, gastroparesis can be asymptomatic and previous studies suggest that delayed gastric emptying cannot be predicted by the severity of symptoms alone [42,43].

The Gastrointestinal Symptom Rating Scale is a well-validated, responsive, and reliable instrument for assessing GI symptoms. It has been used in several clinical trials mainly for dyspepsia and gastroesophageal reflux disease, but also in patients with DM [44–46]. It consists of 15 items covering five symptom clusters: reflux, abdominal pain, indigestion, diarrhea, and constipation. A 7-point Likert-type response scale is used to grade the severity of symptoms, ranging from 1 (no symptoms) to 7 (very troublesome symptoms), and the recall period is the past week [44].

Specific constipation scoring systems have also been used in autonomic disorders. The Cleveland Constipation Score consists of eight items, and a total score above 15 represents constipation. Symptoms are graduated from mild to severe, which allows for monitoring of symptom fluctuation [47]. The ROME IV criteria for constipation are commonly used to define functional constipation and combine a detailed description of colonic and anorectal symptoms [48]. They are, however, not directly applicable in patients with AD-related gastroenteropathy.

The Diabetes Bowel Symptom Questionnaire is validated for assessment of GI symptoms, glycemic control, and quality of life in patients with DM, but has been used only sporadically [49]. Questionnaires addressing the broad spectrum of non-motor-symptoms in PD have been developed. These do not cover pan-enteric GI dysfunction in detail but are useful as screening tools [27].

3.3. Tests of Esophageal Motility

Within recent years, *high-resolution esophageal manometry* has been the method of choice for examining esophageal dysfunction in neurological disorders [50]. When an upper endoscopy with biopsies does not explain the underlying cause of symptoms such as dysphagia and regurgitation, esophageal manometry may be performed. The manometry catheter contains up to 36 pressure sensors distributed 1 cm apart. These sensors provide spatiotemporal, topographic maps of the propagating motor patterns by measuring amplitudes of contractile events within the regions of interest [51]. The clinical performance and interpretation of these data can be challenging. Therefore, when high-resolution esophageal manometry is used to assess AD, it is normally restricted to specialized centers [52]. Esophageal motor dysfunction is present in half of all patients with type 1 DM and dysphagia [53]. In addition, esophageal dysmotility is frequently seen in the α-synucleinopathies, most often as generally reduced peristalsis with ineffective swallows [31,33]. Absent or impaired esophageal activity is documented in POTS with conventional esophageal manometry and with high-resolution esophageal manometry in the Ehlers–Danlos Syndrome, hypermobility type [54,55].

The *modified barium swallowing test* can also be utilized in the diagnosis of these disorders. This examination permits the dynamic visualization of content movements through the upper GI system in real time with the use of videofluoroscopy [56]. The role of the modified barium swallowing test is not limited to the diagnose of dysmotility but can add to the understanding of the physiologic swallowing deficit, which can be useful to maximize the benefit of swallowing therapy [57]. Unfortunately, this examination suffers a highly variable inter- and intra-rater reliability, requires considerable resources, and is associated to radiation exposure as well as aspiration risks [56,58]. The modified barium swallowing test demonstrated slower initiation of airway closure in patients with PD [57]. The test is utilized in the diagnostics of esophageal dysmotility in other causes of autonomic dysfunction as well but the literature on this area is still scarce [59].

3.4. Gastric Emptying Tests

Assessment of gastric emptying time is indicated when patients with an autonomic disorder suffer from nausea, early satiety, lack of appetite, vomiting, postprandial pain, unpredictable absorption of orally administered medication, or large postprandial blood glucose fluctuations in DM. Various assessment techniques exist, and the choice of method primarily depends on its availability at each center performing the procedure.

Gastric emptying scintigraphy is the gold standard for measuring gastric emptying time. An ingested, standardized radiolabeled meal is followed by sequential gamma camera images at minimum 0, 1, 2, and 4 h after meal ingestion [60,61]. The region of interest is drawn manually on each image, and the percentage of activity remaining in the stomach at each time-point expresses gastric emptying [62]. The advantage of this technique is its effective and non-invasive character that does not interfere with normal gastric motility. However, exposure to radiation, high cost, and limited availability are major drawbacks for all scintigraphic measurements. Scintigraphy has shown delayed or rapid gastric emptying time in patients with DM, and delayed gastric emptying time in patients with multiple system atrophy and PD [8,63]. In patients with POTS gastric emptying time is more frequently rapid than delayed [64].

Gastric emptying breath test is a simple, inexpensive, non-invasive, and radiation-free technique to measure gastric emptying time. A solid meal containing the non-radioactive isotope ^{13}C is ingested and rapidly absorbed when it enters the small intestine. Gastric emptying is the rate-limiting step in the metabolic pathway for $^{13}CO_2$; and after metabolization in the liver, $^{13}CO_2$ is exhaled through the respiratory tract, whereby the accumulation of $^{13}CO_2$ in the breath samples indirectly reflects gastric emptying time [65]. Gastric emptying time measures from the gastric emptying breath test are reproducible and correlate with findings from gastric emptying scintigraphy in patients with DM [21,66]. The disadvantage of this technique is the multiple steps required from ingestion to exhalation, which may make the test less accurate. Normal lung and liver function are also a prerequisite. Patients with multiple system atrophy have significantly prolonged gastric emptying time when investigated with gastric emptying breath test [67]. Unfortunately, a recent meta-analysis showed that gastric emptying time obtained with gastric emptying scintigraphy and gastric emptying breath test correlate poorly in patients with PD, and the validity of the test is questioned in this disease [68].

3.5. Assessment of Gastric and Small Intestinal Motility

Antropyloroduodenal manometry can distinguish abnormal from normal motility patterns within the distal stomach, pylorus, and duodenum. The method is performed only at a few and highly specialized centers and usually as a supplement to gastric emptying tests. Specific motility patterns can be demonstrated in both fasting and postprandial states. However, different disorders may share common dysmotility patterns. Antropyloroduodenal manometry is in general seen as a valuable diagnostic tool and can guide treatment in various motility disorders [69]. The method has been used in patients with DM, but the clinical evidence is otherwise sparse in gastroenteropathy related to AD [69,70].

Usually, water-perfused or solid-state catheters are used with pressure sensors spaced 5–10 cm in the duodenal region and 0.5–1 cm in the antral and pyloric region. The recording period is often 6 h and includes the ingestion of a meal. However, ambulatory recording can be performed over 24 h, which may reduce variability among individuals but increases the risk of catheter displacement [71]. The method is reproducible and the interobserver agreement is comparable to that of other commonly used methods [69,72]. Normative values are available [73]. However, it may be unpleasant for the patients to carry the catheter, and expertise is needed to perform the investigations and to analyze data. Application of the high-resolution esophageal manometry catheter in the antropyloroduodenal region can demonstrate more detailed motility patterns than antropyloroduodenal manometry, but these catheters are expensive and more sensitive to external noise, such as cough and movements [74].

3.6. Tests of Small Intestinal and Colonic Transit

Assessment of small intestinal or colonic transit times is mainly indicated in patients with abdominal bloating and pain or in patients with symptoms of constipation. It may also be relevant in patients where symptoms of constipation or diarrhea coexist in order to obtain information on the underlying physiology and aid the choice of treatment, see Section 6.

Scintigraphy is established for measuring transit times through the small bowel, colon, and whole gut [75]. The basic principles are similar to those of gastric emptying scintigraphy. However, for small bowel transit time gamma images are continued for 6 h after ingestion, and single images at 24, 48, and 72 h are used to determine colonic transit time [62]. Only a few normative data with a wide normal range are available for small bowel transit time and the interpretation is potentially affected by abnormal gastric or colonic motility. Lack of standardization in clinical practice and time-consuming protocols are drawbacks for intestinal scintigraphy in general [61]. Thus, the method has only gained limited use in AD-related gastroenteropathies [76].

Radio-opaque markers are the most commonly used method for assessment of whole gut transit time, which in clinical practice can be seen as an approximation of colonic transit time. The method is simple, repeatable, well-tolerated, inexpensive, and easy to perform. In addition, good correlation has been demonstrated for colonic transit time measured with radio-opaque markers, Wireless Motility Capsule, and scintigraphy [77,78]. Usually, the markers are taken on a single day and visualized by an X-ray on day 5. If quantitative data are needed, a capsule containing 10 markers is ingested on 6 consecutive days with an abdominal X-ray on day 7 [79,80]. Estimation of segmental colonic transit times also requires ingestion of radio-opaque markers at consecutive days, and patient compliance has to be optimal. Other limitations are the radiation exposure and the lack of method standardization between centers, which challenges comparison of the results [61]. Assessment with radio-opaque markers in patients with PD, multiple system atrophy and DM showed significantly prolonged colonic transit time, especially within the left and rectosigmoid colon [5,27,81,82].

Hydrogen and methane breath tests can quantify orocecal transit time as a combined measure of gastric and small intestinal transit. The test is usually used as a supplement to assessment of colonic transit time with radiopaque markers and mainly in patients with bloating, abdominal discomfort, or diarrhea. When in contact with colonic bacteria, ingested non-absorbable carbohydrates undergo fermentation and release gases, such as hydrogen and methane, which are excreted through respiration within 3 min. Orocecal transit time is defined as the time interval between oral intake of carbohydrates (often 10 g lactulose) and a registered peak in expired gases by gas chromatography. The hydrogen and methane breath tests are simple, non-invasive, inexpensive, and without exposure to radiation. However, the correlation between the hydrogen breath test and scintigraphy is variable [83,84]. In addition, several other sources of error exist. The natural osmotic activity of lactulose potentially accelerates small intestinal transit and decelerates gastric emptying. The presence of SIBO may complicate the interpretation of orocecal transit time [61]. In both DM and PD, orocecal transit time was significantly prolonged compared with healthy controls when using the hydrogen breath test [85,86].

3.7. Assessment of Small Intestinal Bacterial Overgrowth

Patients with intestinal dysmotility, and among these patients with AD-related gastroenteropathy, are predisposed to SIBO [24,87]. The prevalence of SIBO depends on the choice of diagnostic method [32,88]. Assessment of this condition is primarily needed when abdominal discomfort, bloating, and diarrhea are present in patients with AD. The most valid method for diagnosing SIBO is a luminal, jejunal aspirate for culture retrieved by endoscopy, but this method is invasive, subject to contamination, and may underestimate the intraluminal amount of microbiota. In addition to their use for assessment of orocecal transit time, *hydrogen and methane breath tests* are frequently used as an indirect and non-invasive method to detect SIBO. When SIBO is present, an early peak of expired hydrogen or methane gas is recognized due to fermentation within the small intestine [32]. A North American consensus provides a practical guide to a standardized performance and interpretation of breath tests, and these tests are widely used in clinical practice [89]. However, recent studies have questioned the utility of breath tests for diagnosing SIBO [90]. Simultaneously performed scintigraphy and breath test showed that rapid orocecal transit time and hereby early colonic fermentation with production of hydrogen or methane gas could erroneously be interpreted as SIBO [91]. Jejunal aspirates for culture did not correlate well with the breath test, and in general methods for diagnosing SIBO lack sensitivity, specificity, reproducibility, and standardization [90].

3.8. Tests of Anorectal Motility

High-resolution anorectal manometry and *high-definition anorectal manometry* are increasingly used in clinical practice to evaluate continence and regulation of defecation, primarily in patients with either difficult evacuation of stools or fecal incontinence who do not respond to standard treatment modalities [92]. A consensus guideline for standardization of the methods was recently published [93]. Compared with conventional manometry, additional pressure sensors are closely incorporated within either a solid-state or a water-perfused catheter (often ≥8 sensors). A high-definition rigid catheter containing 256 pressure sensors arranged in a circumferential grid has also been developed [92,94]. In combination with anorectal sensibility tests or other diagnostic investigations, contractions in the distal rectum and anal canal in response to various stimuli may establish a diagnosis and direct different treatment modalities [93]. Normative values based on large datasets exist for both high-resolution and high-definition anorectal manometry [95,96]. Limitations to both techniques are their fragility and costs. Moreover, data analysis is challenging, limiting their use to investigation at specialized centers. High-resolution anorectal manometry has been used to evaluate anorectal dysfunction in PD, especially revealing dystonic contractions in the external anal sphincter as a pathophysiological mechanism for unsuccessful attempts of defecation [97,98]. Reduced anorectal sensibility and internal sphincter dysfunction contribute to fecal incontinence in patients with DM [35].

3.9. Whole Gut Assessment

When pan-enteric dysmotility is suspected, often due to combined upper and lower GI symptoms, *the Wireless Motility Capsule* (Smartpill Monitoring System; Medtronic) is considered the method of choice. An ingested capsule measures pH, intraluminal pressure, and temperature while it passes through the GI tract and transmits this information to a wireless receiver [99]. Accurate measures of the total and regional transit times are provided by using specific pH changes as a surrogate for GI physiological landmarks and temperature to verify expulsion, as seen in Figure 2 [36,99]. The advantages of this test are the availability of substantive normative data and its ambulatory, non-invasive, and radiation-free character [100,101]. Results from the wireless motility capsule correlate with established methods for measuring regional and whole gut transit times [102–104]. Lack of information on segmental colonic transit times is a drawback for the wireless motility capsule investigation. In addition, it only provides information on localized intestinal pressure changes rather than detecting a peristaltic wave, whereas external noise, such as a cough and body movements, can be misinterpreted as bowel movements. The SmartBar, ingested along with the wireless motility capsule, has a high sugar content, which may induce hyperglycemia and by this a slower gastric emptying in patients with DM [105]. Evidence suggests multi-segmental dysmotility in the GI system of both patients with POTS and DM, and a recent study showed that test results led to treatment changes in 73% of patients with DM [6,106]. In patients with PD, multi-segmental delayed transit times determined by the wireless motility capsule can also guide treatment [107]. Hence, evaluation of the entire GI tract with only one examination seems like a reasonable choice in AD-related gastroenteropathy [6,36,108].

Pan-enteric assessment methods, such as the wireless motility capsule, are not widely available. Thus, the initial assessment of motility-disturbances is commonly performed by combining a gastric emptying test (for example the gastric emptying scintigraphy), a breath test for SIBO (for example the hydrogen and methane breath tests) and a test of colonic transit time (for example the radio-opaque markers). Furthermore, guided by symptoms and objective motility findings, it may be relevant to perform one of the mentioned manometric investigations. The influence of the assessment methods on management will be reviewed briefly in Section 6.

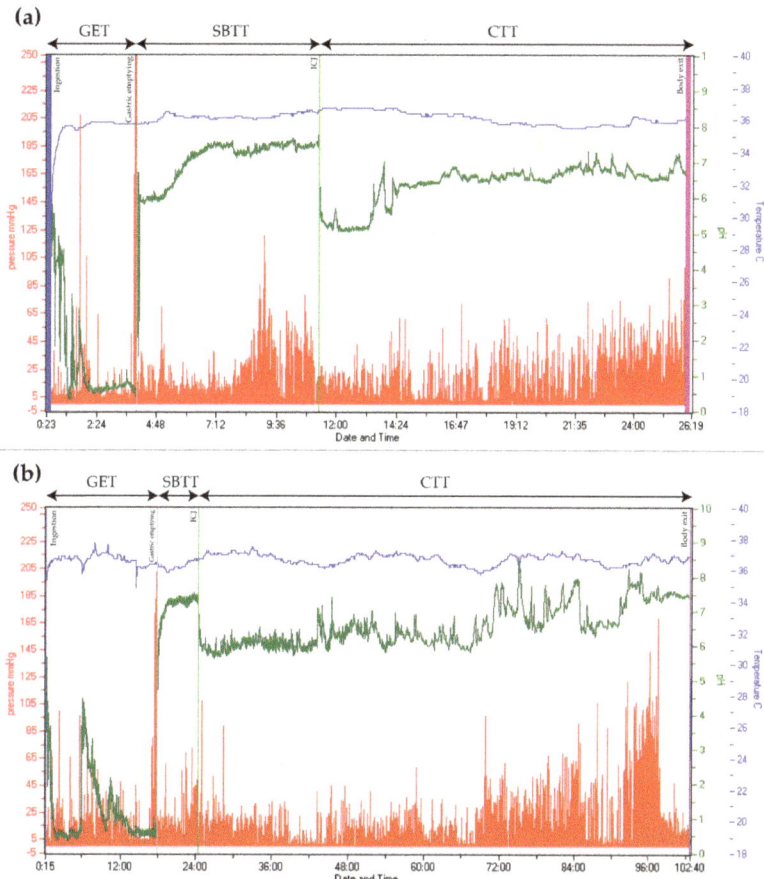

Figure 2. Wireless Motility Capsule recordings from two patients with type 2 diabetes. Time is displayed on the x-axis, pressure on the left y-axis (red), pH on the right y-axis (green), and temperature on the right y-axis (blue). (**a**) Normal transit times. (**b**) Delayed gastric emptying time (18 h) and colonic transit time (78 h). (GET = Gastric emptying time. SBTT = Small bowel transit time. CTT = Colonic transit time. ICJ = Ileocolic junction).

4. Emerging Methods for Assessment of Gastroenteropathy

4.1. Whole Gut Assessment

The *electromagnetic 3D-Transit* system (3D-Transit, Motilis Medica SA, Lausanne, Switzerland) is an ambulatory, minimally invasive, and capsule-based technique, which presents similarities to the wireless motility capsule by providing information on regional and whole gut transit times. As the only available technique, the 3D-Transit system can also be used to assess segmental colonic transit times and simultaneously provide a detailed assessment of contraction patterns in a precise anatomical location [109]. A detector plate worn in a belt around the abdomen detects the electromagnetic field emitted by an ingested electromagnetic capsule. The electromagnetic field is converted into space-time coordinates, with three spatial coordinates (x, y, and z) representing the three-dimensional capsule position within the GI system, and two orientational coordinates (ϕ, θ) representing the angular rotation of the capsule in two directions. An accelerometer within the detector plate and a thoracic belt detect postural changes and breathing artefacts to be filtered out in the data analysis [109,110]. Propagation of luminal content within the GI tract is expressed by the change in orientation of the capsules and capsule movement velocity. The characteristic contraction frequency in each GI segment is determined by angular rotations of the capsule providing information about anatomical landmarks [111,112]. The 3D-Transit system can track three capsules simultaneously without interference, and the measures of transit times are found to be valid, reproducible, and comparable to transit times measured with radio-opaque markers [110]. Normative data on healthy subjects are available and comparable to normative data on transit times from the wireless motility capsule [100,113,114]. The main drawbacks of using this pan-enteric, diagnostic tool is the time-consuming and challenging data analysis, no CE-marking, and no availability outside research settings [112].

3D-Transit has been applied to assess transit times and contraction patterns in various GI disorders and among these in patients with gastroenteropathy related to AD [112]. Patients with type 1 DM are shown to have prolonged gastric emptying time, colonic transit time, and whole gut transit time mainly due to an increased number of retrograde movements within the right colon [115]. Furthermore, widespread prolonged transit times, especially through the small intestine and right colon, and fewer antegrade mass movements have been found in PD [116].

4.2. Tests of Colorectal Contractions

High-resolution colonic manometry provides the most precise and detailed description of motor patterns within the colon and has essentially contributed to the understanding of normal colonic physiology [117]. The catheters used are either water-perfused, solid-state, or fiber-optic, with sensors spaced 1–3 cm apart to increase the resolution. The contractile activity is presented by spatiotemporal, color-graded, typographical maps, which allows detection of pressure amplitudes and movements in both antegrade and retrograde directions [118]. On the other hand, high-resolution colonic manometry is time-consuming and lacks standardization in respect to the type of catheter, number of sensors, distance between sensors, composition of ingested meals, use of anesthetics, and length of measurements. The technique involves colonoscopy for placement of the catheter and therefore a need for bowel preparation, which can affect colonic motor activity [118]. Data analysis requires an experienced investigator. However, a recently published consensus statement labelling colonic motor activity provides a common ground for future data analysis [119]. High-resolution colonic manometry is still primarily used for research but is a promising clinical tool for assessment of colonic motor activity, also in patients with gastroenteropathy and AD.

4.3. Imaging

4.3.1. Computed Tomography (CT)

In clinical practice, X-ray is the standard test to identify severe fecal retention, but an objective volume estimation technique to be used as a surrogate for the colonic function is lacking. Due to the increased prevalence of constipation in autonomic disorders, combined with alterations in the intestinal tissue, organ sizes may change [5,120,121].

A recent study defined the colonic and small intestinal volumes from CT scans in patients with type 1 DM, finding an increased volume [122]. Additionally, an increased intestinal volume was seen in the transverse colonic and rectosigmoid segments of patients with PD, representing the combination of slow transit constipation and outlet obstruction [5]. CT scans are widely available in all hospitals and often performed in clinical practice. However, ionizing radiation used in CT scans limits their use, especially in pediatric patients and pregnant women [123]. The data analysis in CT-extracted intestinal volumes is time-consuming and currently not applicable in a clinical setting. Colonic volumes from a CT scan are presented in Figure 3.

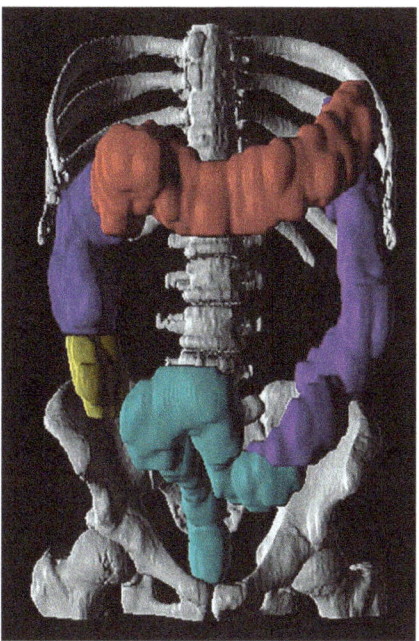

Figure 3. Example of colonic volumes from a computed tomography scan. Yellow: cecum, blue: ascending colon, red: transversal colon, purple: descending colon and turquoise: rectosigmoid colon. Used with permission from M. Klinge, Dissertation, January 2020.

4.3.2. Ultrasound Imaging

Ultrasound imaging is a useful radiation-free option for showing various diameters of the gut. However, the limitations of ultrasound imaging include difficulty in examining the deep abdominal loops, and a skilled radiologist is needed to obtain a sufficient result [123]. Ultrasound imaging is only sparsely used in gastroenteropathy related to AD [124].

4.3.3. Magnetic Resonance Imaging (MRI)

Visualization of the GI tract with *MRI* has advanced significantly during the past decade. MRI techniques provide morpho-functional information while being feasible and non-invasive [125,126]. MRI has been applied in patients with DM or PD, primarily for assessment of gastric motility [127–130]. At present, MRI holds promise for assessment of gastric function in terms of accommodation, motility indexes, gastric emptying velocity, and volumetric strain, while simultaneously describing the anatomy of the organ [127,131,132]. Gastric contraction waves and measurement of gastric volume obtained with MRI are seen in Figure 4. The small intestine is an especially challenging organ for imaging methods. However, MRI allows imaging of the small bowel wall, small intestinal lumen, and the surroundings in one scan without ionizing radiation. Enteral contrast agents can be added for better delineation of the intestinal wall [123]. Furthermore, colonic and rectosigmoid volumes can be assessed.

While promising, MRI examinations of GI volumes are not yet used in clinical practice because they are relatively expensive and require highly trained examiners.

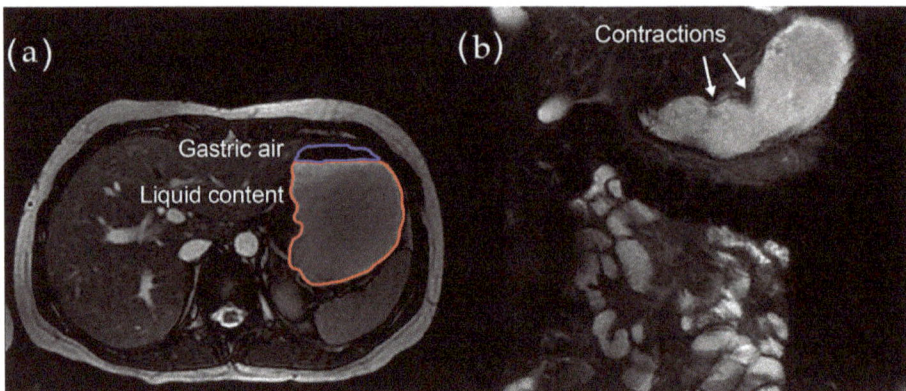

Figure 4. Magnetic resonance imaging of the stomach. (**a**) Gastric air volume and liquid content volume obtained in the segmentation process. (**b**) Contraction waves observed and quantified in the coronal plane.

4.3.4. ^{11}C-Donepezil Positron Emission Tomography/Computed Tomography (PET/CT)

[11]C-donepezil PET/CT scan visualizes the cholinergic innervation of the GI tract in vivo and may potentially fill the need for a future method to assess the severity of GI autonomic neuropathy [33]. The radioactive tracer (^{11}C-donepezil) is injected, and standardized uptake values in the internal organs are recorded. The scan is performed without bowel preparation in near-normal conditions. The validity of this imaging method to detect intestinal parasympathetic denervation is confirmed by a significantly decreased ^{11}C-donepezil intestinal signal in patients after truncal vagotomy [133]. Patients with early PD have a significant signal loss of ^{11}C-donepezil within the intestine as the result of cholinergic denervation [134]. This intestinal denervation corresponds well with the degree of α-synuclein in parasympathetic neurons in PD [33,135]. Parasympathetic intestinal denervation indicated by reduced ^{11}C-donepezil uptake is also found in patients with DM [122]. This is presented in Figure 5. The disadvantages of the method are that it is only performed in very few centers and requires comprehensive data analysis.

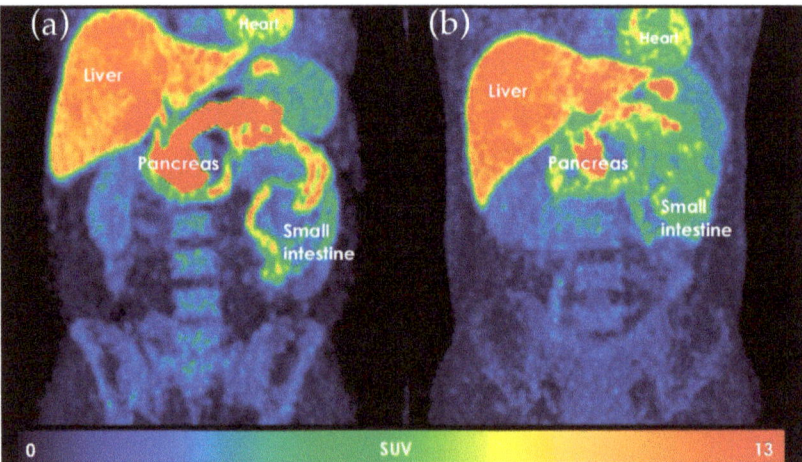

Figure 5. ^{11}C-donepezil positron emission tomography images. (**a**) Healthy control. (**b**) Patient with diabetes mellitus. Notice the difference in the standard value uptake in the pancreas and the small intestine. The picture is used with permission from Klinge, et al., 2020.

4.4. Gut Biopsies

Another way to diagnose GI autonomic neuropathy is to analyze intestinal biopsies. The optimal way to quantify enteric neurons is by obtaining whole-mount preparations to visualize both the submucosal plexus and the myenteric plexus by immunohistochemical neuronal markers [136]. Furthermore, it is possible to analyze the density of enteric neurons in formalin-fixed, paraffin-embedded biopsies, but the validity of this method remains debated. This is partly due to a lack of normative data and standardized quantitative methods for counting the neurons and the absence of a clear-cut definition of a ganglion [137]. Another limitation is that neurons are almost entirely drawn from the submucosa, unless full-wall biopsies are taken. Neurons of the enteric nervous system can partly be visualized by light microscope when stained with neuronal markers like neuron-specific enolase and synaptophysin. In addition, mast cells and ICC in enteric biopsies can be visualized and counted microscopically by staining with C-kit/CD117 [16,138] A new approach is non-invasive mapping of full-thickness segments of the gut and identification and quantification of ganglia of the enteric nervous system by a technique named *optical coherence microscopy* [139].

In a recent study, jejunal full-thickness biopsies were collected from patients suffering from severe gut dysmotility, either by laparoscopy or by conventional abdominal laparotomy. By quantifying the inter-ganglionic distance between neighboring myenteric ganglia and the number of neurons per ganglion in the myenteric and submucosal plexus, the authors showed that patients with enteric dysmotility had significantly fewer myenteric and submucosal neurons [140]. The methodology has been refined, and a new technique has utilized the evaluation of standard submucosal biopsies. The submucosa is microdissected and fixed for later immunofluorescence staining to characterize the morphometry of the plexus and the enteric glial cell. Immunohistochemically, the neurons of the enteric nervous system are visualized by a light microscope using standard protocols of staining [138]. Similarly, mucosal biopsies from the stomach of patients with DM have been used for quantifying gastric mucosal nerve fiber length and volume density [141]. Finally, α-synucleinopathies immunostaining of colonic submucosal biopsies has shown aggregation of α-synuclein in the enteric nervous system and holds promise as an early diagnostic marker for PD [24,142].

Taken together, several newly established techniques have been developed in which the submucosa and related plexuses are isolated from the mucosa in endoscopically obtained surface biopsies and can be used to evaluate the enteric nervous system in health and disease [143,144]. At present, the methods are almost entirely for research purposes. A morphological analysis of a submucosal biopsy is presented in Figure 6.

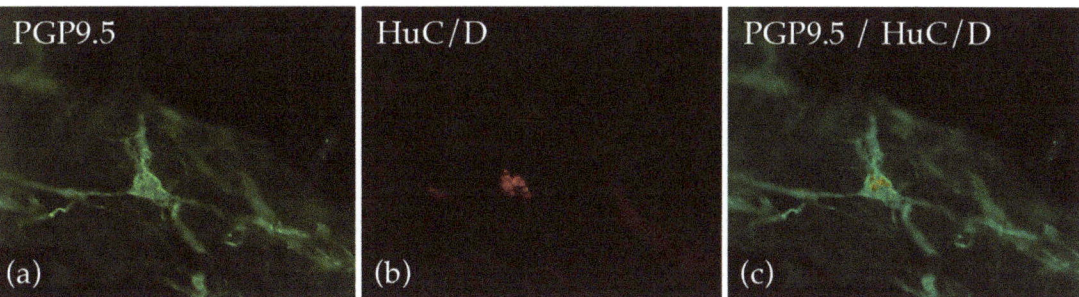

Figure 6. Morphological analysis on human submucosal plexi from colonic standard submucosal biopsies. The used primary antibodies encounter two general pan-neuronal markers, i.e.: (**a**) PGP9.5 recognizing perikarya and nerve fibers and (**b**) HuC/D detecting only neuronal cell bodies for quantitative analysis. (**c**) The two neuronal markers, PGP9.5 and HuC/D, used simultaneously. Giancola, Brock and de Giorgio, unpublished data.

4.5. Assessment of the Human Gut Microbiota

The human gut microbiota consists of trillions of symbiotic bacterial, viral, and fungal microorganisms [145]. New techniques for assessment of the human gut microbiome have facilitated large-scale analysis of the microbial community. Genetic analysis is based on sequence divergences of small subunit ribosomal RNA (16S rRNA). It can provide information on microbial diversity, qualitative and quantitative information on bacterial species, and changes in gut microbiota related to disease [146].

Studies have demonstrated that gut microbiota participate in many aspects of human physiology including the development of the immune system, energy metabolism, and activity of the nervous system [147]. Neurological diseases such as PD present a different gut microbiota composition than encountered in healthy controls [148,149]. Studies show an association between PD and the abundance of certain microbiota. However, it is not yet known whether it is the microbiota or the microbiota-derived metabolites that has an impact on the disease [150]. Microbial metabolites such as short chain fatty acids, which are considered neuro-reactive, are produced by the microbiota, and may enter the systemic circulation. Studies have shown that PD patients have lower levels of fecal short chain fatty acids, which may have a protective effect against the development of PD [151]. Further studies are required to determine the role between the presence or absence of specific microbiota and microbiota-derived metabolites.

Patients with type 1 DM have a less diverse and less stable gut microbiome than healthy controls [152,153]. Findings have not been conclusive, but most studies have found reduced diversity of the intestinal bacterial community and an increased proportion of Bacteroides [154]. Studies have also focused on the intestinal epithelial barrier which prevents food antigens and bacteria from leaving the gut lumen and entering the body leading to a systemic immune response. Disruption and increased permeability of the intestinal barrier have been shown in intestinal autoimmune diseases as well as type 1 DM [155,156]. Preclinical studies support the hypothesis that specific features of the microbiota give rise to impaired intestinal permeability [157], which further influences T cell autoimmunity and B-lymphocytes. This may lead to beta-cell destruction and type 1 DM. However, it has not been confirmed whether alterations in gut microbiota and increased gut permeability are causally related to the pathophysiology or merely a consequence of disease.

Microbiome analysis on the human gut microbiota has significantly improved our knowledge of gut microbiota composition and diversity. An understanding of the human gut microbial diversity in different types of disorders might provide insight into the clinical application in diagnosis and treatments of disease. However, a significant association between microbial patterns and disease initiation or progression has yet to be unveiled.

The above mentioned established and emerging methods for assessment of gut function are summarized in Table 1.

Table 1. Established and emerging methods for assessment of gastroenteropathy in autonomic disorders.

Investigation	Measurement	Primary Dysmotility Parameters	Advantages/Limitations							
			Minimally invasive	Radiation free	Standardized	Inexpensive	High Availability	Ambulatory assessment	Simple data analysis	High reliability
Established Assessment Methods										
Esophageal manometry	Esophageal contractility patterns	Reduced peristalsis and uncoordinated contractions	No	Yes	Yes	No	No	No	No	Yes
Gastric emptying scintigraphy	Gastric emptying time	Delayed gastric emptying time	Yes	No	Yes	No	Yes	No	No	Yes
^{13}C-octanoic acid breath test	Gastric emptying time	Delayed gastric emptying time	Yes	Yes	Yes	Yes	No	No	Yes	No
Antropyloroduodenal manometry	Antropyloroduodenal contractility patterns	Postprandial antral hypomotility and duodenal dysmotility in diabetes	No	Yes	No	No	No	No/Yes	No	Yes
Intestinal scintigraphy	Small intestinal and colonic transit times	Prolonged intestinal transit times	Yes	No	No	No	No	No	No	Yes
Radio-opaque markers	Small intestinal and colonic transit times	Prolonged whole gut and regional transit times	Yes	No	No	Yes	Yes	Yes	Yes	No
Hydrogen and methane breath test	Orocecal transit time and detection of small intestinal bacterial overgrowth	Prolonged orocecal transit time and increased frequency of small intestinal bacterial overgrowth	Yes	Yes	Yes	Yes	Yes	No	Yes	No
Anorectal manometry	Anorectal contractility patterns	1. Dystonic external anal sphincter during defecation in Parkinson's disease 2. Dysfunction of the internal anal sphincter in diabetes 3. Recto-anal dyscoordination	Yes	Yes	No	No	No	No	No	Yes
Wireless motility capsule	1. Whole gut and regional transit times 2. Motility patterns	Delayed whole gut- and regional transit times	Yes	Yes	Yes	No	No	Yes	Yes	Yes
Emerging Assessment Methods										
Colonic Manometry	Colonic contractility patterns	Colonic dysmotility	No	Yes	No	No	No	No	No	Yes
3D-Transit capsule	Whole gut and regional transit times	Delayed whole gut- and regional transit times	Yes	Yes	No	No	No	Yes	No	Yes
Computed tomography imaging	Small intestinal and colonic volume	Increased colonic volume	Yes	No	No	Yes	Yes	No	No	Yes
Magnetic resonance imaging	1. Whole gut and regional transit times 2. Whole gut contractility 3. Organ volumes	Delayed gastric emptying and increased intestinal volume	Yes	Yes	No	No	Yes	No	No	Yes
^{11}C-donepezil positron emission tomography/computed tomography imaging	Whole gut cholinergic innervation	Intestinal parasympathetic denervation	Yes	No	No	No	No	No	No	Yes
Submucosal biopsies	Quantification of enteric neurons	1. Reduced number of neurons in diabetes 2. Aggregation of α-synuclein in Parkinson's disease	No	Yes	No	No	No	No	No	No
Microbiota	Gut microbiota composition	1. Less stable and diverse in diabetes 2. Altered in Parkinson's disease	Yes	Yes	No	No	No	Yes	No	No

5. Assessment of Autonomic Neuropathy Outside the Gut

Since no commercially available in-vivo diagnostic test of enteric neuropathy exists and the described tests of GI physiological function all have significant limitations, some patients with symptoms of autonomic GI dysfunction may benefit from assessment of extraintestinal autonomic function in support of a diagnosis.

Diagnostic tests of cardiac autonomic neuropathy may serve as a surrogate for autonomic neuropathy within the GI system, but associations between autonomic neuropathy in the two different visceral systems remain incompletely understood. Reduced heart rate variability is associated with hyposensitivity of the esophagus and with hyposensitivity and stretch of the rectum in patients with DM [34,124,158]. However, results are ambiguous regarding associations between GI transit times and cardiac derived autonomic parameters such as heart rate variability or cardiac vagal tone [46]. Cardiac parasympathetic dysfunction can be verified by demonstrating decreased heart rate variability during rest, deep breathing, and the Valsalva maneuver [159]. Heart rate changes to deep breathing are simple to perform and have the highest specificity with vagal afferents and efferents mediating the response [160]. The efferent cardiovascular adrenergic function can be assessed by looking at blood pressure changes during the Valsalva maneuver, during orthostatic stress (active standing or tilt table testing), in response to isometric exercise, and a cold pressor test [161–163]. Twenty-four hour blood pressure measurement may detect non-dipping or reverse dipping conditions and postprandial hypotension. The prognostic role of non-dipping and reverse dipping is well-documented, but associations with GI function are unknown [164,165].

Further autonomic testing may be relevant in some patients to recognize AD. A commonly used questionnaire is the COMPASS-31, consisting of 31 questions formed into six symptom domains [38], which may be helpful to screen for AD-related symptoms and add to the assessment of GI autonomic impairment. Autonomic symptoms reflect the organ or function that is affected; however, in general, they are unspecific and will often require objective assessment with various tests [20,166–168]. Additionally, *The Quantitative Sweat Measurement System* (Q-Sweat) evaluates the postganglionic sympathetic cholinergic sudomotor function in the upper and lower extremities by measuring sweat collections in response to locally administered acetylcholine [169]. In combination with skin biopsies and quantitative sensory testing, the Q-Sweat contributes to the diagnosis of small-fiber polyneuropathy [14]. Normal values are based on published normative data [160]. Serum pancreatic polypeptide is an indirect measure of vagal influence on the GI tract [170,171], but its utility remains to be determined [172].

With no available standard diagnostic test of pan-enteric autonomic neuropathy, extraintestinal autonomic neuropathy may be used as proxy in clinical practice to verify AD outside the GI tract. However, acknowledgement of subjective GI symptoms and assessment of the physiological function of each GI segment remains the primary focus to aid diagnostics and guide treatment in patients with GI symptoms and suspected AD.

6. Assessment-Guided Treatment

Management of AD-related gastroenteropathy is challenging and treatment response is often unsatisfactory. The poor correlation between GI symptoms and objective findings underlines the need for objective measures to guide treatment.

The risk of malnutrition, electrolyte disturbances, weight loss, and dehydration is increased in patients with gastroparesis and enteropathy. Small and soft meals, preferably low in fat and fiber content, are recommended to ease gastric emptying and optimize the intestinal nutritional uptake in patients with gastroparesis or constipation [173]. Contrary, an increased fiber intake is shown to reduce symptoms of constipation and optimize medication absorption in PD [174]. To preserve a sufficient nutritional state, a feeding tube may be necessary for selected patients with weight loss.

Improvement of glycemic control and variability is important in patients with DM to reduce the risk of dysmotility due to hyper- or hypoglycemia. Continuous subcutaneous insulin infusion, and by this an optimized glycemic regulation, may diminish GI symptoms; however, the magnitude of this effect is uncertain [175].

Pharmacologic treatment with prokinetic drugs is widely used when upper GI symptoms combined with an objectively measured delayed GE or prolonged intestinal transit times are detected. The dopamine receptor antagonists (metoclopramide and domperidone), the motilin receptor agonist (erythromycin), and the selective 5-HT$_4$ receptor agonist (prucalopride) are commonly used in clinical practice [176]. However, prokinetic treatment has major limitations, especially the risk of extrapyramidal side effects including potentially irreversible tardive dyskinesia (metoclopramide), drug-induced arrhythmias (domperidone), and lack of evidence for long-term effectiveness [177,178]. In addition, metoclopramide is contraindicated in PD due to its extrapyramidal side effects [24]. Ghrelin receptor agonists (relamorelin and ulimorelin) may be a future treatment of gastroparesis, but solid evidence remains absent [175]. Immunotherapy in autoimmune autonomic ganglionopathy which can comprise gastroparesis is well indicated [179].

In medical refractory cases of gastroparesis, gastric electrical stimulation is the most used surgical option, but disagreement in randomized studies remains. Especially in diabetic gastroparesis, studies have shown significant symptom relief, maintained for over 10 years, and a reduction in days of hospitalization [180,181]. Other surgical interventions used for treating dysmotility within the upper GI tract comprise pyloric botulinum toxin injection, pyloroplasty, pyloromyotomy, gastrectomy, and gastric per-oral endoscopic myotomy (G-POEM). In general, surgical interventions rest on poor evidence, and patients should be carefully selected. A non-invasive neuromodulation technique, called transcutaneous vagus nerve stimulation, is investigated as a potential add-on treatment of GI symptoms in patients with DM and AD [182].

When SIBO is objectively verified, patients are treated with antibiotics to eradicate bacterial overgrowth, which provides significant symptom relief and enhances medication absorption. Either non-systemic antibiotics (rifaximin) or systemic antibiotics (ciprofloxacin or metronidazole) can be used [32]. However, the predisposing motility disturbance causes frequent recurrence [183]. The anti-diarrheal, peripherally acting u-opioid receptor agonist, loperamide, reduces intestinal peristalsis and can be effective in treating diarrhea and fecal incontinence. Moreover, octreotide, ondansetron, and bile-binding resins are used in selected patients with severe diarrhea [184]. When paralytic ileus occurs, neostigmine may be used in selected cases.

Prolonged colonic transit time indicates treatment with oral laxatives or suppositories following the general guidelines of treating chronic constipation [24]. If ordinary treatment fails, this may be combined with prucalopride due to its additional prokinetic effects [176]. When constipation coexists with abdominal pain and autonomic neuropathy, simple and adjuvant analgesics such as tricyclic antidepressants may be attempted. The balance between the relatively low analgesic effect and the frequent side effects must always be considered. The cholinesterase-inhibitor pyridostigmine is frequently used in patients with combined orthostatic hypotension and constipation [18]. Patients with comorbid mast cell activation syndrome may achieve symptomatic improvement when treated with mast cell stabilizers, such as anti-histamine and cromolyn sodium [16].

When obstructed defecation is verified with anorectal manometry, it is usually treated with rectal suppositories or mini-enema. Confirmed dyssynergic defecation in PD may be treated with injections of botulinum neurotoxin [24].

7. Conclusions

Pan-enteric dysmotility is common in patients with AD despite variation in the underlying pathophysiological changes within the nervous system. With no available standard method for direct assessment of GI autonomic neuropathy, the primary diagnostic approach is physiological, multi-segmental motility testing, and in some patients additional generalized tests of autonomic neuropathy.

Established assessment methods are commercially available for investigation of transit times throughout the entire GI tract and for contraction patterns in the esophageal, gastroduodenal, and anal regions. As the only commercially available method, the wireless motility capsule provides pan-enteric transit times and pressure patterns in one investigation. However, the established methods all present limitations, especially with regards to radiation exposure, lack of standardization, need for multiple tests to evaluate the entire GI tract, and a complicated practical performance or data interpretation, which may restrict the use to specialized centers.

Within recent years, several emerging assessment methods have been developed, potentially overcoming some of the above limitations and definitely providing more detailed knowledge on contractility patterns within specific GI segments. The 3D-Transit system, CT scans, and MRI scans hold promise for a multi-segmental and detailed evaluation of the whole GI tract within a single investigation. In the future, the diagnosis of enteric autonomic neuropathy may be established with ^{11}C-donepezil PET/CT scans or gut biopsies. Optimized future diagnostic tools and improved knowledge on motility disturbances in gastroenteropathy related to AD will hopefully improve the treatment of these severely ill patients.

Author Contributions: Conceptualization, D.S.K. and K.K.; writing—original draft preparation, D.S.K., A.J.T., M.W.K., K.L.H., D.B., H.H.A.K., and C.B.; writing—review and editing, K.K., A.J.T., P.B., A.M.D., and C.B.; project administration, D.S.K.; funding acquisition, K.K. All authors have read and agreed to the published version of the manuscript.

Funding: This research was supported by an educational grant from Coloplast, Denmark.

Acknowledgments: Figure 1 was created with BioRender.com accessed on 24 February 2021. Anne-Marie Wegeberg and Esben Bolvig Mark, from the Department of Gastroenterology and Hepatology at Aalborg University Hospital, provided data for Figures 3 and 5, respectively.

Conflicts of Interest: The authors declare no conflict of interest. The funders had no role in the writing of the manuscript or in the decision to publish the results.

References

1. Benarroch, E.E. Physiology and Pathophysiology of the Autonomic Nervous System. *Continuum* **2020**, *26*, 12–24. [CrossRef]
2. Mathias, C.J.B.R. *Autonomic Failure. A Textbook of Clinical Disorders of the Autonomic Nervous System*, 5th ed.; University Press: Oxford, UK, 2013.
3. Chung, K.A.; Pfeiffer, R.F. Gastrointestinal dysfunction in the synucleinopathies. *Clin. Auton. Res.* **2020**. [CrossRef]
4. Müller, T.; Erdmann, C.; Bremen, D.; Schmidt, W.E.; Muhlack, S.; Woitalla, D.; Goetze, O. Impact of gastric emptying on levodopa pharmacokinetics in Parkinson disease patients. *Clin. Neuropharmacol.* **2006**, *29*, 61–67. [CrossRef]
5. Knudsen, K.; Fedorova, T.D.; Bekker, A.C.; Iversen, P.; Østergaard, K.; Krogh, K.; Borghammer, P. Objective Colonic Dysfunction is Far more Prevalent than Subjective Constipation in Parkinson's Disease: A Colon Transit and Volume Study. *J. Park. Dis.* **2017**, *7*, 359–367. [CrossRef] [PubMed]
6. Rouphael, C.; Arora, Z.; Thota, P.N.; Lopez, R.; Santisi, J.; Funk, C.; Cline, M. Role of wireless motility capsule in the assessment and management of gastrointestinal dysmotility in patients with diabetes mellitus. *Neurogastroenterol. Motil.* **2017**, *29*. [CrossRef]
7. Gustafsson, R.J.; Littorin, B.; Berntorp, K.; Frid, A.; Thorsson, O.; Olsson, R.; Ekberg, O.; Ohlsson, B. Esophageal dysmotility is more common than gastroparesis in diabetes mellitus and is associated with retinopathy. *Rev. Diabet. Stud.* **2011**, *8*, 268–275. [CrossRef] [PubMed]
8. Bharucha, A.E.; Camilleri, M.; Forstrom, L.A.; Zinsmeister, A.R. Relationship between clinical features and gastric emptying disturbances in diabetes mellitus. *Clin. Endocrinol.* **2009**, *70*, 415–420. [CrossRef]
9. Karemaker, J.M. An introduction into autonomic nervous function. *Physiol. Meas.* **2017**, *38*, R89–R118. [CrossRef] [PubMed]
10. Costa, M.; Brookes, S.J. The enteric nervous system. *Am. J. Gastroenterol.* **1994**, *89*, S129–S137. [CrossRef]
11. Meldgaard, T.; Olesen, S.S.; Farmer, A.D.; Krogh, K.; Wendel, A.A.; Brock, B.; Drewes, A.M.; Brock, C. Diabetic Enteropathy: From Molecule to Mechanism-Based Treatment. *J. Diabetes Res.* **2018**, *2018*, 3827301. [CrossRef]
12. Gibbons, C.H.; Freeman, R. Treatment-induced neuropathy of diabetes: An acute, iatrogenic complication of diabetes. *Brain* **2015**, *138*, 43–52. [CrossRef] [PubMed]
13. Coon, E.A.; Cutsforth-Gregory, J.K.; Benarroch, E.E. Neuropathology of autonomic dysfunction in synucleinopathies. *Mov. Disord.* **2018**, *33*, 349–358. [CrossRef]
14. Terkelsen, A.J.; Karlsson, P.; Lauria, G.; Freeman, R.; Finnerup, N.B.; Jensen, T.S. The diagnostic challenge of small fibre neuropathy: Clinical presentations, evaluations, and causes. *Lancet Neurol.* **2017**, *16*, 934–944. [CrossRef]

15. Benarroch, E.E. Postural tachycardia syndrome: A heterogeneous and multifactorial disorder. *Mayo Clin. Proc.* **2012**, *87*, 1214–1225. [CrossRef]

16. Weinstock, L.B.; Pace, L.A.; Rezaie, A.; Afrin, L.B.; Molderings, G.J. Mast Cell Activation Syndrome: A Primer for the Gastroenterologist. *Dig. Dis. Sci.* **2020**. [CrossRef] [PubMed]

17. Beckers, A.B.; Keszthelyi, D.; Fikree, A.; Vork, L.; Masclee, A.; Farmer, A.D.; Aziz, Q. Gastrointestinal disorders in joint hypermobility syndrome/Ehlers-Danlos syndrome hypermobility type: A review for the gastroenterologist. *Neurogastroenterol. Motil.* **2017**, *29*. [CrossRef] [PubMed]

18. Benarroch, E.E. The clinical approach to autonomic failure in neurological disorders. *Nat. Rev. Neurol.* **2014**, *10*, 396–407. [CrossRef] [PubMed]

19. Soedamah-Muthu, S.S.; Chaturvedi, N.; Witte, D.R.; Stevens, L.K.; Porta, M.; Fuller, J.H. Relationship between risk factors and mortality in type 1 diabetic patients in Europe: The EURODIAB Prospective Complications Study (PCS). *Diabetes Care* **2008**, *31*, 1360–1366. [CrossRef]

20. Spallone, V. Update on the Impact, Diagnosis and Management of Cardiovascular Autonomic Neuropathy in Diabetes: What Is Defined, What Is New, and What Is Unmet. *Diabetes Metab J.* **2019**, *43*, 3–30. [CrossRef]

21. Bharucha, A.E.; Kudva, Y.C.; Prichard, D.O. Diabetic Gastroparesis. *Endocr. Rev.* **2019**, *40*, 1318–1352. [CrossRef]

22. Bytzer, P.; Talley, N.J.; Leemon, M.; Young, L.J.; Jones, M.P.; Horowitz, M. Prevalence of gastrointestinal symptoms associated with diabetes mellitus: A population-based survey of 15,000 adults. *Arch. Int. Med.* **2001**, *161*, 1989–1996. [CrossRef] [PubMed]

23. Talley, N.J.; Young, L.; Bytzer, P.; Hammer, J.; Leemon, M.; Jones, M.; Horowitz, M. Impact of chronic gastrointestinal symptoms in diabetes mellitus on health-related quality of life. *Am. J. Gastroenterol.* **2001**, *96*, 71–76. [CrossRef]

24. Fasano, A.; Visanji, N.P.; Liu, L.W.; Lang, A.E.; Pfeiffer, R.F. Gastrointestinal dysfunction in Parkinson's disease. *Lancet Neurol.* **2015**, *14*, 625–639. [CrossRef]

25. Bytzer, P.; Talley, N.J.; Hammer, J.; Young, L.J.; Jones, M.P.; Horowitz, M. GI symptoms in diabetes mellitus are associated with both poor glycemic control and diabetic complications. *Am. J. Gastroenterol.* **2002**, *97*, 604–611. [CrossRef] [PubMed]

26. Feldman, M.; Schiller, L.R. Disorders of gastrointestinal motility associated with diabetes mellitus. *Ann. Intern. Med.* **1983**, *98*, 378–384. [CrossRef] [PubMed]

27. Knudsen, K.; Krogh, K.; Østergaard, K.; Borghammer, P. Constipation in parkinson's disease: Subjective symptoms, objective markers, and new perspectives. *Mov. Disord.* **2017**, *32*, 94–105. [CrossRef]

28. Verbaan, D.; Marinus, J.; Visser, M.; van Rooden, S.M.; Stiggelbout, A.M.; van Hilten, J.J. Patient-reported autonomic symptoms in Parkinson disease. *Neurology* **2007**, *69*, 333–341. [CrossRef]

29. Wang, L.B.; Culbertson, C.J.; Deb, A.; Morgenshtern, K.; Huang, H.; Hohler, A.D. Gastrointestinal dysfunction in postural tachycardia syndrome. *J. Neurol. Sci.* **2015**, *359*, 193–196. [CrossRef] [PubMed]

30. DiBaise, J.K.; Harris, L.A.; Goodman, B. Postural Tachycardia Syndrome (POTS) and the GI Tract: A Primer for the Gastroenterologist. *Am. J. Gastroenterol.* **2018**, *113*, 1458–1467. [CrossRef]

31. Claus, I.; Suttrup, J.; Muhle, P.; Suntrup-Krueger, S.; Siemer, M.L.; Lenze, F.; Dziewas, R.; Warnecke, T. Subtle Esophageal Motility Alterations in Parkinsonian Syndromes: Synucleinopathies vs. Tauopathies. *Mov. Disord. Clin. Pract.* **2018**, *5*, 406–412. [CrossRef]

32. Rao, S.S.C.; Bhagatwala, J. Small Intestinal Bacterial Overgrowth: Clinical Features and Therapeutic Management. *Clin. Transl. Gastroenterol.* **2019**, *10*, e00078. [CrossRef] [PubMed]

33. Knudsen, K.; Borghammer, P. Imaging the Autonomic Nervous System in Parkinson's Disease. *Curr. Neurol. Neurosci. Rep.* **2018**, *18*, 79. [CrossRef]

34. Brock, C.; Søfteland, E.; Gunterberg, V.; Frøkjær, J.B.; Lelic, D.; Brock, B.; Dimcevski, G.; Gregersen, H.; Simrén, M.; Drewes, A.M. Diabetic autonomic neuropathy affects symptom generation and brain-gut axis. *Diabetes Care* **2013**, *36*, 3698–3705. [CrossRef]

35. Azpiroz, F.; Malagelada, C. Diabetic neuropathy in the gut: Pathogenesis and diagnosis. *Diabetologia* **2016**, *59*, 404–408. [CrossRef]

36. Farmer, A.D.; Pedersen, A.G.; Brock, B.; Jakobsen, P.E.; Karmisholt, J.; Mohammed, S.D.; Scott, S.M.; Drewes, A.M.; Brock, C. Type 1 diabetic patients with peripheral neuropathy have pan-enteric prolongation of gastrointestinal transit times and an altered caecal pH profile. *Diabetologia* **2017**, *60*, 709–718. [CrossRef] [PubMed]

37. Pavelić, A.; Krbot Skorić, M.; Crnošija, L.; Habek, M. Postprandial hypotension in neurological disorders: Systematic review and meta-analysis. *Clin. Auton. Res.* **2017**, *27*, 263–271. [CrossRef] [PubMed]

38. Sletten, D.M.; Suarez, G.A.; Low, P.A.; Mandrekar, J.; Singer, W. COMPASS 31: A refined and abbreviated Composite Autonomic Symptom Score. *Mayo Clin. Proc.* **2012**, *87*, 1196–1201. [CrossRef]

39. Rentz, A.M.; Kahrilas, P.; Stanghellini, V.; Tack, J.; Talley, N.J.; de la Loge, C.; Trudeau, E.; Dubois, D.; Revicki, D.A. Development and psychometric evaluation of the patient assessment of upper gastrointestinal symptom severity index (PAGI-SYM) in patients with upper gastrointestinal disorders. *Qual. Life Res.* **2004**, *13*, 1737–1749. [CrossRef] [PubMed]

40. Revicki, D.A.; Rentz, A.M.; Dubois, D.; Kahrilas, P.; Stanghellini, V.; Talley, N.J.; Tack, J. Gastroparesis Cardinal Symptom Index (GCSI): Development and validation of a patient reported assessment of severity of gastroparesis symptoms. *Qual. Life Res. Int. J. Qual. Life Asp. Treat. Care Rehabil.* **2004**, *13*, 833–844. [CrossRef]

41. Nilsson, M.; Poulsen, J.L.; Brock, C.; Sandberg, T.H.; Gram, M.; Frokjaer, J.B.; Krogh, K.; Drewes, A.M. Opioid-induced bowel dysfunction in healthy volunteers assessed with questionnaires and MRI. *Eur. J. Gastroenterol. Hepatol.* **2016**, *28*, 514–524. [CrossRef]

42. Jones, K.L.; Russo, A.; Stevens, J.E.; Wishart, J.M.; Berry, M.K.; Horowitz, M. Predictors of delayed gastric emptying in diabetes. *Diabetes Care* **2001**, *24*, 1264–1269. [CrossRef]

43. Cassilly, D.W.; Wang, Y.R.; Friedenberg, F.K.; Nelson, D.B.; Maurer, A.H.; Parkman, H.P. Symptoms of gastroparesis: Use of the gastroparesis cardinal symptom index in symptomatic patients referred for gastric emptying scintigraphy. *Digestion* **2008**, *78*, 144–151. [CrossRef]

44. Kulich, K.R.; Madisch, A.; Pacini, F.; Piqué, J.M.; Regula, J.; Van Rensburg, C.J.; Ujszászy, L.; Carlsson, J.; Halling, K.; Wiklund, I.K. Reliability and validity of the Gastrointestinal Symptom Rating Scale (GSRS) and Quality of Life in Reflux and Dyspepsia (QOLRAD) questionnaire in dyspepsia: A six-country study. *Health Qual. Life Outcomes* **2008**, *6*, 12. [CrossRef] [PubMed]

45. Revicki, D.A.; Wood, M.; Wiklund, I.; Crawley, J. Reliability and validity of the Gastrointestinal Symptom Rating Scale in patients with gastroesophageal reflux disease. *Qual. Life Res.* **1998**, *7*, 75–83. [CrossRef] [PubMed]

46. Wegeberg, A.L.; Brock, C.; Ejskjaer, N.; Karmisholt, J.S.; Jakobsen, P.E.; Drewes, A.M.; Brock, B.; Farmer, A.D. Gastrointestinal symptoms and cardiac vagal tone in type 1 diabetes correlates with gut transit times and motility index. *Neurogastroenterol. Motil.* **2020**, e13885. [CrossRef]

47. Agachan, F.; Chen, T.; Pfeifer, J.; Reissman, P.; Wexner, S.D. A constipation scoring system to simplify evaluation and management of constipated patients. *Dis. Colon Rectum* **1996**, *39*, 681–685. [CrossRef] [PubMed]

48. Simren, M.; Palsson, O.S.; Whitehead, W.E. Update on Rome IV Criteria for Colorectal Disorders: Implications for Clinical Practice. *Curr. Gastroenterol. Rep.* **2017**, *19*, 15. [CrossRef]

49. Quan, C.; Talley, N.J.; Cross, S.; Jones, M.; Hammer, J.; Giles, N.; Horowitz, M. Development and validation of the Diabetes Bowel Symptom Questionnaire. *Aliment. Pharmacol. Ther.* **2003**, *17*, 1179–1187. [CrossRef] [PubMed]

50. Kahrilas, P.J.; Bredenoord, A.J.; Fox, M.; Gyawali, C.P.; Roman, S.; Smout, A.J.; Pandolfino, J.E. The Chicago Classification of esophageal motility disorders, v3.0. *Neurogastroenterol. Motil.* **2015**, *27*, 160–174. [CrossRef]

51. Dhawan, I.; O'Connell, B.; Patel, A.; Schey, R.; Parkman, H.P.; Friedenberg, F. Utility of Esophageal High-Resolution Manometry in Clinical Practice: First, Do HRM. *Dig. Dis. Sci.* **2018**, *63*, 3178–3186. [CrossRef]

52. Yadlapati, R. High-resolution esophageal manometry: Interpretation in clinical practice. *Curr. Opin. Gastroenterol.* **2017**, *33*, 301–309. [CrossRef]

53. George, N.S.; Rangan, V.; Geng, Z.; Khan, F.; Kichler, A.; Gabbard, S.; Ganocy, S.; Fass, R. Distribution of Esophageal Motor Disorders in Diabetic Patients With Dysphagia. *J. Clin. Gastroenterol.* **2017**, *51*, 890–895. [CrossRef]

54. Huang, R.J.; Chun, C.L.; Friday, K.; Triadafilopoulos, G. Manometric abnormalities in the postural orthostatic tachycardia syndrome: A case series. *Dig. Dis. Sci.* **2013**, *58*, 3207–3211. [CrossRef]

55. Fikree, A.; Aziz, Q.; Sifrim, D. Mechanisms underlying reflux symptoms and dysphagia in patients with joint hypermobility syndrome, with and without postural tachycardia syndrome. *Neurogastroenterol. Motil.* **2017**, *29*. [CrossRef]

56. Martin-Harris, B.; Canon, C.L.; Bonilha, H.S.; Murray, J.; Davidson, K.; Lefton-Greif, M.A. Best Practices in Modified Barium Swallow Studies. *Am. J. Speech Lang. Pathol.* **2020**, *29*, 1078–1093. [CrossRef]

57. Schiffer, B.L.; Kendall, K. Changes in Timing of Swallow Events in Parkinson's Disease. *Ann. Otol. Rhinol. Laryngol.* **2019**, *128*, 22–27. [CrossRef] [PubMed]

58. Lee, J.W.; Randall, D.R.; Evangelista, L.M.; Kuhn, M.A.; Belafsky, P.C. Subjective Assessment of Videofluoroscopic Swallow Studies. *Otolaryngol. Head Neck Surg.* **2017**, *156*, 901–905. [CrossRef] [PubMed]

59. Alomari, M.; Hitawala, A.; Chadalavada, P.; Covut, F.; Al Momani, L.; Khazaaleh, S.; Gosai, F.; Al Ashi, S.; Abushahin, A.; Schneider, A. Prevalence and Predictors of Gastrointestinal Dysmotility in Patients with Hypermobile Ehlers-Danlos Syndrome: A Tertiary Care Center Experience. *Cureus* **2020**, *12*, e7881. [CrossRef] [PubMed]

60. Abell, T.L.; Camilleri, M.; Donohoe, K.; Hasler, W.L.; Lin, H.C.; Maurer, A.H.; McCallum, R.W.; Nowak, T.; Nusynowitz, M.L.; Parkman, H.P.; et al. Consensus recommendations for gastric emptying scintigraphy: A joint report of the American Neurogastroenterology and Motility Society and the Society of Nuclear Medicine. *Am. J. Gastroenterol.* **2008**, *103*, 753–763. [CrossRef]

61. Rao, S.S.; Camilleri, M.; Hasler, W.L.; Maurer, A.H.; Parkman, H.P.; Saad, R.; Scott, M.S.; Simren, M.; Soffer, E.; Szarka, L. Evaluation of gastrointestinal transit in clinical practice: Position paper of the American and European Neurogastroenterology and Motility Societies. *Neurogastroenterol. Motil.* **2011**, *23*, 8–23. [CrossRef]

62. Madsen, J.L. Scintigraphic assessment of gastrointestinal motility: A brief review of techniques and data interpretation. *Clin. Physiol. Funct. Imaging* **2014**, *34*, 243–253. [CrossRef]

63. Thomaides, T.; Karapanayiotides, T.; Zoukos, Y.; Haeropoulos, C.; Kerezoudi, E.; Demacopoulos, N.; Floodas, G.; Papageorgiou, E.; Armakola, F.; Thomopoulos, Y.; et al. Gastric emptying after semi-solid food in multiple system atrophy and Parkinson disease. *J. Neurol.* **2005**, *252*, 1055–1059. [CrossRef] [PubMed]

64. Loavenbruck, A.; Iturrino, J.; Singer, W.; Sletten, D.M.; Low, P.A.; Zinsmeister, A.R.; Bharucha, A.E. Disturbances of gastrointestinal transit and autonomic functions in postural orthostatic tachycardia syndrome. *Neurogastroenterol. Motil.* **2015**, *27*, 92–98. [CrossRef] [PubMed]

65. Ghoos, Y.F.; Maes, B.D.; Geypens, B.J.; Mys, G.; Hiele, M.I.; Rutgeerts, P.J.; Vantrappen, G. Measurement of gastric emptying rate of solids by means of a carbon-labeled octanoic acid breath test. *Gastroenterology* **1993**, *104*, 1640–1647. [CrossRef]

66. Zahn, A.; Langhans, C.D.; Hoffner, S.; Haberkorn, U.; Rating, D.; Haass, M.; Enck, P.; Stremmel, W.; Ruhl, A. Measurement of gastric emptying by 13C-octanoic acid breath test versus scintigraphy in diabetics. *Z. Gastroenterol.* **2003**, *41*, 383–390. [CrossRef] [PubMed]
67. Tanaka, Y.; Kato, T.; Nishida, H.; Yamada, M.; Koumura, A.; Sakurai, T.; Hayashi, Y.; Kimura, A.; Hozumi, I.; Araki, H.; et al. Is there delayed gastric emptying in patients with multiple system atrophy? An analysis using the (13)C-acetate breath test. *J. Neurol.* **2012**, *259*, 1448–1452. [CrossRef]
68. Knudsen, K.; Szwebs, M.; Hansen, A.K.; Borghammer, P. Gastric emptying in Parkinson's disease-A mini-review. *Parkinsonism. Relat. Disord.* **2018**, *55*, 18–25. [CrossRef] [PubMed]
69. Camilleri, M.; Bharucha, A.E.; di Lorenzo, C.; Hasler, W.L.; Prather, C.M.; Rao, S.S.; Wald, A. American Neurogastroenterology and Motility Society consensus statement on intraluminal measurement of gastrointestinal and colonic motility in clinical practice. *Neurogastroenterol. Motil.* **2008**, *20*, 1269–1282. [CrossRef]
70. Samsom, M.; Jebbink, R.J.; Akkermans, L.M.; van Berge-Henegouwen, G.P.; Smout, A.J. Abnormalities of antroduodenal motility in type I diabetes. *Diabetes Care* **1996**, *19*, 21–27. [CrossRef]
71. Patcharatrakul, T.; Gonlachanvit, S. Technique of functional and motility test: How to perform antroduodenal manometry. *J. Neurogastroenterol. Motil.* **2013**, *19*, 395–404. [CrossRef]
72. Penning, C.; Gielkens, H.A.; Hemelaar, M.; Lamers, C.B.; Masclee, A.A. Reproducibility of antroduodenal motility during prolonged ambulatory recording. *Neurogastroenterol. Motil.* **2001**, *13*, 133–141. [CrossRef] [PubMed]
73. Bortolotti, M.; Annese, V.; Coccia, G. Twenty-four hour ambulatory antroduodenal manometry in normal subjects (co-operative study). *Neurogastroenterol. Motil.* **2000**, *12*, 231–238. [CrossRef]
74. Desipio, J.; Friedenberg, F.K.; Korimilli, A.; Richter, J.E.; Parkman, H.P.; Fisher, R.S. High-resolution solid-state manometry of the antropyloroduodenal region. *Neurogastroenterol. Motil.* **2007**, *19*, 188–195. [CrossRef] [PubMed]
75. Bonapace, E.S.; Maurer, A.H.; Davidoff, S.; Krevsky, B.; Fisher, R.S.; Parkman, H.P. Whole gut transit scintigraphy in the clinical evaluation of patients with upper and lower gastrointestinal symptoms. *Am. J. Gastroenterol.* **2000**, *95*, 2838–2847. [CrossRef]
76. Maleki, D.; Camilleri, M.; Burton, D.D.; Rath-Harvey, D.M.; Oenning, L.; Pemberton, J.H.; Low, P.A. Pilot study of pathophysiology of constipation among community diabetics. *Dig. Dis. Sci.* **1998**, *43*, 2373–2378. [CrossRef]
77. Camilleri, M.; Thorne, N.K.; Ringel, Y.; Hasler, W.L.; Kuo, B.; Esfandyari, T.; Gupta, A.; Scott, S.M.; McCallum, R.W.; Parkman, H.P.; et al. Wireless pH-motility capsule for colonic transit: Prospective comparison with radiopaque markers in chronic constipation. *Neurogastroenterol. Motil.* **2010**, *22*, 874–882, e233. [CrossRef] [PubMed]
78. van der Sijp, J.R.; Kamm, M.A.; Nightingale, J.M.; Britton, K.E.; Mather, S.J.; Morris, G.P.; Akkermans, L.M.; Lennard-Jones, J.E. Radioisotope determination of regional colonic transit in severe constipation: Comparison with radio opaque markers. *Gut* **1993**, *34*, 402–408. [CrossRef]
79. Abrahamsson, H.; Antov, S.; Bosaeus, I. Gastrointestinal and colonic segmental transit time evaluated by a single abdominal X-ray in healthy subjects and constipated patients. *Scand. J. Gastroenterol. Suppl.* **1988**, *152*, 72–80. [CrossRef]
80. Metcalf, A.M.; Phillips, S.F.; Zinsmeister, A.R.; MacCarty, R.L.; Beart, R.W.; Wolff, B.G. Simplified assessment of segmental colonic transit. *Gastroenterology* **1987**, *92*, 40–47. [CrossRef]
81. Sakakibara, R.; Odaka, T.; Uchiyama, T.; Liu, R.; Asahina, M.; Yamaguchi, K.; Yamaguchi, T.; Yamanishi, T.; Hattori, T. Colonic transit time, sphincter EMG, and rectoanal videomanometry in multiple system atrophy. *Mov. Disord.* **2004**, *19*, 924–929. [CrossRef] [PubMed]
82. Jung, H.K.; Kim, D.Y.; Moon, I.H.; Hong, Y.S. Colonic transit time in diabetic patients–comparison with healthy subjects and the effect of autonomic neuropathy. *Yonsei Med. J.* **2003**, *44*, 265–272. [CrossRef]
83. Miller, M.A.; Parkman, H.P.; Urbain, J.L.; Brown, K.L.; Donahue, D.J.; Knight, L.C.; Maurer, A.H.; Fisher, R.S. Comparison of scintigraphy and lactulose breath hydrogen test for assessment of orocecal transit: Lactulose accelerates small bowel transit. *Dig. Dis. Sci.* **1997**, *42*, 10–18. [CrossRef]
84. Simrén, M.; Stotzer, P.O. Use and abuse of hydrogen breath tests. *Gut* **2006**, *55*, 297–303. [CrossRef]
85. Faria, M.; Pavin, E.J.; Parisi, M.C.; Lorena, S.L.; Brunetto, S.Q.; Ramos, C.D.; Pavan, C.R.; Mesquita, M.A. Delayed small intestinal transit in patients with long-standing type 1 diabetes mellitus: Investigation of the relationships with clinical features, gastric emptying, psychological distress, and nutritional parameters. *Diabetes Technol. Ther.* **2013**, *15*, 32–38. [CrossRef] [PubMed]
86. Davies, K.N.; King, D.; Billington, D.; Barrett, J.A. Intestinal permeability and orocaecal transit time in elderly patients with Parkinson's disease. *Postgrad. Med. J.* **1996**, *72*, 164–167. [CrossRef] [PubMed]
87. Gabrielli, M.; Bonazzi, P.; Scarpellini, E.; Bendia, E.; Lauritano, E.C.; Fasano, A.; Ceravolo, M.G.; Capecci, M.; Rita Bentivoglio, A.; Provinciali, L.; et al. Prevalence of small intestinal bacterial overgrowth in Parkinson's disease. *Mov. Disord.* **2011**, *26*, 889–892. [CrossRef] [PubMed]
88. Jacobs, C.; Coss Adame, E.; Attaluri, A.; Valestin, J.; Rao, S.S. Dysmotility and proton pump inhibitor use are independent risk factors for small intestinal bacterial and/or fungal overgrowth. *Aliment. Pharmacol. Ther.* **2013**, *37*, 1103–1111. [CrossRef]
89. Rezaie, A.; Buresi, M.; Lembo, A.; Lin, H.; McCallum, R.; Rao, S.; Schmulson, M.; Valdovinos, M.; Zakko, S.; Pimentel, M. Hydrogen and Methane-Based Breath Testing in Gastrointestinal Disorders: The North American Consensus. *Am. J. Gastroenterol.* **2017**, *112*, 775–784. [CrossRef]
90. Di Stefano, M.; Quigley, E.M.M. The diagnosis of small intestinal bacterial overgrowth: Two steps forward, one step backwards? *Neurogastroenterol. Motil.* **2018**, *30*, e13494. [CrossRef]

91. Yu, D.; Cheeseman, F.; Vanner, S. Combined oro-caecal scintigraphy and lactulose hydrogen breath testing demonstrate that breath testing detects oro-caecal transit, not small intestinal bacterial overgrowth in patients with IBS. *Gut* **2011**, *60*, 334–340. [CrossRef]
92. Scott, S.M.; Carrington, E.V. The London Classification: Improving Characterization and Classification of Anorectal Function with Anorectal Manometry. *Curr. Gastroenterol. Rep.* **2020**, *22*, 55. [CrossRef]
93. Carrington, E.V.; Heinrich, H.; Knowles, C.H.; Fox, M.; Rao, S.; Altomare, D.F.; Bharucha, A.E.; Burgell, R.; Chey, W.D.; Chiarioni, G.; et al. The international anorectal physiology working group (IAPWG) recommendations: Standardized testing protocol and the London classification for disorders of anorectal function. *Neurogastroenterol. Motil.* **2020**, *32*, e13679. [CrossRef]
94. Lee, T.H.; Bharucha, A.E. How to Perform and Interpret a High-resolution Anorectal Manometry Test. *J. Neurogastroenterol. Motil.* **2016**, *22*, 46–59. [CrossRef]
95. Oblizajek, N.R.; Gandhi, S.; Sharma, M.; Chakraborty, S.; Muthyala, A.; Prichard, D.; Feuerhak, K.; Bharucha, A.E. Anorectal pressures measured with high-resolution manometry in healthy people-Normal values and asymptomatic pelvic floor dysfunction. *Neurogastroenterol. Motil.* **2019**, *31*, e13597. [CrossRef] [PubMed]
96. Li, Y.; Yang, X.; Xu, C.; Zhang, Y.; Zhang, X. Normal values and pressure morphology for three-dimensional high-resolution anorectal manometry of asymptomatic adults: A study in 110 subjects. *Int. J. Colorectal Dis.* **2013**, *28*, 1161–1168. [CrossRef] [PubMed]
97. De Pablo-Fernández, E.; Passananti, V.; Zárate-López, N.; Emmanuel, A.; Warner, T. Colonic transit, high-resolution anorectal manometry and MRI defecography study of constipation in Parkinson's disease. *Parkinsonism Relat. Disord.* **2019**, *66*, 195–201. [CrossRef] [PubMed]
98. Yu, T.; Wang, Y.; Wu, G.; Xu, Q.; Tang, Y.; Lin, L. High-resolution Anorectal Manometry in Parkinson Disease With Defecation Disorder: A Comparison With Functional Defecation Disorder. *J. Clin. Gastroenterol.* **2016**, *50*, 566–571. [CrossRef]
99. Sarosiek, I.; Selover, K.H.; Katz, L.A.; Semler, J.R.; Wilding, G.E.; Lackner, J.M.; Sitrin, M.D.; Kuo, B.; Chey, W.D.; Hasler, W.L.; et al. The assessment of regional gut transit times in healthy controls and patients with gastroparesis using wireless motility technology. *Aliment. Pharmacol. Ther.* **2010**, *31*, 313–322. [CrossRef]
100. Wang, Y.T.; Mohammed, S.D.; Farmer, A.D.; Wang, D.; Zarate, N.; Hobson, A.R.; Hellstrom, P.M.; Semler, J.R.; Kuo, B.; Rao, S.S.; et al. Regional gastrointestinal transit and pH studied in 215 healthy volunteers using the wireless motility capsule: Influence of age, gender, study country and testing protocol. *Aliment. Pharmacol. Ther.* **2015**, *42*, 761–772. [CrossRef]
101. Farmer, A.D.; Wegeberg, A.L.; Brock, B.; Hobson, A.R.; Mohammed, S.D.; Scott, S.M.; Bruckner-Holt, C.E.; Semler, J.R.; Hasler, W.L.; Hellstrom, P.M.; et al. Regional gastrointestinal contractility parameters using the wireless motility capsule: Inter-observer reproducibility and influence of age, gender and study country. *Aliment. Pharmacol. Ther.* **2018**, *47*, 391–400. [CrossRef]
102. Maqbool, S.; Parkman, H.P.; Friedenberg, F.K. Wireless capsule motility: Comparison of the SmartPill GI monitoring system with scintigraphy for measuring whole gut transit. *Dig. Dis. Sci.* **2009**, *54*, 2167–2174. [CrossRef]
103. Kuo, B.; McCallum, R.W.; Koch, K.L.; Sitrin, M.D.; Wo, J.M.; Chey, W.D.; Hasler, W.L.; Lackner, J.M.; Katz, L.A.; Semler, J.R.; et al. Comparison of gastric emptying of a nondigestible capsule to a radio-labelled meal in healthy and gastroparetic subjects. *Aliment. Pharmacol. Ther.* **2008**, *27*, 186–196. [CrossRef] [PubMed]
104. Rao, S.S.; Kuo, B.; McCallum, R.W.; Chey, W.D.; DiBaise, J.K.; Hasler, W.L.; Koch, K.L.; Lackner, J.M.; Miller, C.; Saad, R.; et al. Investigation of colonic and whole-gut transit with wireless motility capsule and radiopaque markers in constipation. *Clin. Gastroenterol. Hepatol.* **2009**, *7*, 537–544. [CrossRef] [PubMed]
105. Fraser, R.J.; Horowitz, M.; Maddox, A.F.; Harding, P.E.; Chatterton, B.E.; Dent, J. Hyperglycaemia slows gastric emptying in type 1 (insulin-dependent) diabetes mellitus. *Diabetologia* **1990**, *33*, 675–680. [CrossRef] [PubMed]
106. Zhou, W.; Zikos, T.A.; Clarke, J.O.; Nguyen, L.A.; Triadafilopoulos, G.; Neshatian, L. Regional Gastrointestinal Transit and Contractility Patterns Vary in Postural Orthostatic Tachycardia Syndrome (POTS). *Dig. Dis. Sci.* **2021**. [CrossRef] [PubMed]
107. Su, A.; Gandhy, R.; Barlow, C.; Triadafilopoulos, G. Utility of the wireless motility capsule and lactulose breath testing in the evaluation of patients with Parkinson's disease who present with functional gastrointestinal symptoms. *BMJ Open Gastroenterol.* **2017**, *4*, e000132. [CrossRef] [PubMed]
108. Coleski, R.; Wilding, G.E.; Semler, J.R.; Hasler, W.L. Blunting of Colon Contractions in Diabetics with Gastroparesis Quantified by Wireless Motility Capsule Methods. *PLoS ONE* **2015**, *10*, e0141183. [CrossRef]
109. Mark, E.B.; Poulsen, J.L.; Haase, A.M.; Espersen, M.; Gregersen, T.; Schlageter, V.; Scott, S.M.; Krogh, K.; Drewes, A.M. Ambulatory assessment of colonic motility using the electromagnetic capsule tracking system. *Neurogastroenterol. Motil.* **2019**, *31*, e13451. [CrossRef]
110. Haase, A.M.; Gregersen, T.; Schlageter, V.; Scott, M.S.; Demierre, M.; Kucera, P.; Dahlerup, J.F.; Krogh, K. Pilot study trialling a new ambulatory method for the clinical assessment of regional gastrointestinal transit using multiple electromagnetic capsules. *Neurogastroenterol. Motil.* **2014**, *26*, 1783–1791. [CrossRef]
111. Worsoe, J.; Fynne, L.; Gregersen, T.; Schlageter, V.; Christensen, L.A.; Dahlerup, J.F.; Rijkhoff, N.J.; Laurberg, S.; Krogh, K. Gastric transit and small intestinal transit time and motility assessed by a magnet tracking system. *BMC Gastroenterol.* **2011**, *11*, 145. [CrossRef]
112. Brinck, C.E.; Mark, E.B.; Winther Klinge, M.; Ejerskov, C.; Sutter, N.; Schlageter, V.; Scott, S.M.; Mohr Drewes, A.; Krogh, K. Magnetic tracking of gastrointestinal motility. *Physiol. Meas.* **2020**. [CrossRef]

113. Sutter, N.; Klinge, M.W.; Mark, E.B.; Nandhra, G.; Haase, A.M.; Poulsen, J.; Knudsen, K.; Borghammer, P.; Schlageter, V.; Birch, M.; et al. Normative values for gastric motility assessed with the 3D-transit electromagnetic tracking system. *Neurogastroenterol. Motil.* **2020**, e13829. [CrossRef] [PubMed]

114. Nandhra, G.K.; Mark, E.B.; Di Tanna, G.L.; Haase, A.M.; Poulsen, J.; Christodoulides, S.; Kung, V.; Klinge, M.W.; Knudsen, K.; Borghammer, P.; et al. Normative values for region-specific colonic and gastrointestinal transit times in 111 healthy volunteers using the 3D-Transit electromagnet tracking system: Influence of age, gender, and body mass index. *Neurogastroenterol. Motil.* **2020**, *32*, e13734. [CrossRef] [PubMed]

115. Klinge, M.W.; Haase, A.M.; Mark, E.B.; Sutter, N.; Fynne, L.V.; Drewes, A.M.; Schlageter, V.; Lund, S.; Borghammer, P.; Krogh, K. Colonic motility in patients with type 1 diabetes and gastrointestinal symptoms. *Neurogastroenterol. Motil.* **2020**, e13948. [CrossRef] [PubMed]

116. Knudsen, K.; Haase, A.M.; Fedorova, T.D.; Bekker, A.C.; Ostergaard, K.; Krogh, K.; Borghammer, P. Gastrointestinal Transit Time in Parkinson's Disease Using a Magnetic Tracking System. *J. Park. Dis.* **2017**, *7*, 471–479. [CrossRef] [PubMed]

117. Dinning, P.G.; Carrington, E.V.; Scott, S.M. The use of colonic and anorectal high-resolution manometry and its place in clinical work and in research. *Neurogastroenterol. Motil.* **2015**, *27*, 1693–1708. [CrossRef]

118. Dinning, P.G. A new understanding of the physiology and pathophysiology of colonic motility? *Neurogastroenterol. Motil.* **2018**, *30*, e13395. [CrossRef]

119. Corsetti, M.; Costa, M.; Bassotti, G.; Bharucha, A.E.; Borrelli, O.; Dinning, P.; Di Lorenzo, C.; Huizinga, J.D.; Jimenez, M.; Rao, S.; et al. First translational consensus on terminology and definitions of colonic motility in animals and humans studied by manometric and other techniques. *Nat. Rev. Gastroenterol. Hepatol.* **2019**, *16*, 559–579. [CrossRef]

120. Campbell-Thompson, M.L.; Kaddis, J.S.; Wasserfall, C.; Haller, M.J.; Pugliese, A.; Schatz, D.A.; Shuster, J.J.; Atkinson, M.A. The influence of type 1 diabetes on pancreatic weight. *Diabetologia* **2016**, *59*, 217–221. [CrossRef]

121. Zhao, J.; Yang, J.; Gregersen, H. Biomechanical and morphometric intestinal remodelling during experimental diabetes in rats. *Diabetologia* **2003**, *46*, 1688–1697. [CrossRef] [PubMed]

122. Klinge, M.W.; Borghammer, P.; Lund, S.; Fedorova, T.; Knudsen, K.; Haase, A.M.; Christiansen, J.J.; Krogh, K. Enteric cholinergic neuropathy in patients with diabetes: Non-invasive assessment with positron emission tomography. *Neurogastroenterol. Motil.* **2020**, *32*, e13731. [CrossRef]

123. Masselli, G.; Gualdi, G. MR imaging of the small bowel. *Radiology* **2012**, *264*, 333–348. [CrossRef] [PubMed]

124. Frøkjaer, J.B.; Brock, C.; Brun, J.; Simren, M.; Dimcevski, G.; Funch-Jensen, P.; Drewes, A.M.; Gregersen, H. Esophageal distension parameters as potential biomarkers of impaired gastrointestinal function in diabetes patients. *Neurogastroenterol. Motil.* **2012**, *24*, e1016–e1544. [CrossRef] [PubMed]

125. Banerjee, S.; Pal, A.; Fox, M. Volume and position change of the stomach during gastric accommodation and emptying: A detailed three-dimensional morphological analysis based on MRI. *Neurogastroenterol. Motil.* **2020**, *32*, e13865. [CrossRef]

126. Menys, A.; Keszthelyi, D.; Fitzke, H.; Fikree, A.; Atkinson, D.; Aziz, Q.; Taylor, S.A. A magnetic resonance imaging study of gastric motor function in patients with dyspepsia associated with Ehlers-Danlos Syndrome-Hypermobility Type: A feasibility study. *Neurogastroenterol. Motil.* **2017**, *29*. [CrossRef]

127. Lehmann, R.; Borovicka, J.; Kunz, P.; Crelier, G.; Boesiger, P.; Fried, M.; Schwizer, W.; Spinas, G.A. Evaluation of delayed gastric emptying in diabetic patients with autonomic neuropathy by a new magnetic resonance imaging technique and radio-opaque markers. *Diabetes Care* **1996**, *19*, 1075–1082. [CrossRef] [PubMed]

128. Carbone, S.F.; Tanganelli, I.; Capodivento, S.; Ricci, V.; Volterrani, L. Magnetic resonance imaging in the evaluation of the gastric emptying and antral motion: Feasibility and reproducibility of a fast not invasive technique. *Eur. J. Radiol.* **2010**, *75*, 212–214. [CrossRef]

129. Cho, J.; Lee, Y.J.; Kim, Y.H.; Shin, C.M.; Kim, J.M.; Chang, W.; Park, J.H. Quantitative MRI evaluation of gastric motility in patients with Parkinson's disease: Correlation of dyspeptic symptoms with volumetry and motility indices. *PLoS ONE* **2019**, *14*, e0216396. [CrossRef]

130. Unger, M.M.; Hattemer, K.; Möller, J.C.; Schmittinger, K.; Mankel, K.; Eggert, K.; Strauch, K.; Tebbe, J.J.; Keil, B.; Oertel, W.H.; et al. Real-time visualization of altered gastric motility by magnetic resonance imaging in patients with Parkinson's disease. *Mov. Disord.* **2010**, *25*, 623–628. [CrossRef]

131. Froehlich, J.M.; Patak, M.A.; von Weymarn, C.; Juli, C.F.; Zollikofer, C.L.; Wentz, K.U. Small bowel motility assessment with magnetic resonance imaging. *J. Magn Reson. Imaging* **2005**, *21*, 370–375. [CrossRef]

132. Ajaj, W.; Goehde, S.C.; Papanikolaou, N.; Holtmann, G.; Ruehm, S.G.; Debatin, J.F.; Lauenstein, T.C. Real time high resolution magnetic resonance imaging for the assessment of gastric motility disorders. *Gut* **2004**, *53*, 1256–1261. [CrossRef] [PubMed]

133. Fedorova, T.D.; Knudsen, K.; Hartmann, B.; Holst, J.J.; Viborg Mortensen, F.; Krogh, K.; Borghammer, P. In vivo positron emission tomography imaging of decreased parasympathetic innervation in the gut of vagotomized patients. *Neurogastroenterol. Motil.* **2020**, *32*, e13759. [CrossRef]

134. Fedorova, T.D.; Seidelin, L.B.; Knudsen, K.; Schacht, A.C.; Geday, J.; Pavese, N.; Brooks, D.J.; Borghammer, P. Decreased intestinal acetylcholinesterase in early Parkinson disease: An (11)C-donepezil PET study. *Neurology* **2017**, *88*, 775–781. [CrossRef] [PubMed]

135. Gjerløff, T.; Fedorova, T.; Knudsen, K.; Munk, O.L.; Nahimi, A.; Jacobsen, S.; Danielsen, E.H.; Terkelsen, A.J.; Hansen, J.; Pavese, N.; et al. Imaging acetylcholinesterase density in peripheral organs in Parkinson's disease with 11C-donepezil PET. *Brain* **2015**, *138*, 653–663. [CrossRef] [PubMed]

136. Knowles, C.H.; Lindberg, G.; Panza, E.; De Giorgio, R. New perspectives in the diagnosis and management of enteric neuropathies. *Nat. Rev. Gastroenterol. Hepatol.* **2013**, *10*, 206–218. [CrossRef] [PubMed]

137. Swaminathan, M.; Kapur, R.P. Counting myenteric ganglion cells in histologic sections: An empirical approach. *Hum. Pathol.* **2010**, *41*, 1097–1108. [CrossRef]

138. Ippolito, C.; Segnani, C.; De Giorgio, R.; Blandizzi, C.; Mattii, L.; Castagna, M.; Moscato, S.; Dolfi, A.; Bernardini, N. Quantitative evaluation of myenteric ganglion cells in normal human left colon: Implications for histopathological analysis. *Cell Tissue Res.* **2009**, *336*, 191–201. [CrossRef]

139. Coron, E.; Auksorius, E.; Pieretti, A.; Mahé, M.M.; Liu, L.; Steiger, C.; Bromberg, Y.; Bouma, B.; Tearney, G.; Neunlist, M.; et al. Full-field optical coherence microscopy is a novel technique for imaging enteric ganglia in the gastrointestinal tract. *Neurogastroenterol. Motil.* **2012**, *24*, e611–e621. [CrossRef]

140. Boschetti, E.; Malagelada, C.; Accarino, A.; Malagelada, J.R.; Cogliandro, R.F.; Gori, A.; Bonora, E.; Giancola, F.; Bianco, F.; Tugnoli, V.; et al. Enteric neuron density correlates with clinical features of severe gut dysmotility. *Am. J. Physiol. Gastrointest. Liver. Physiol.* **2019**, *317*, G793–G801. [CrossRef]

141. Selim, M.M.; Wendelschafer-Crabb, G.; Redmon, J.B.; Khoruts, A.; Hodges, J.S.; Koch, K.; Walk, D.; Kennedy, W.R. Gastric mucosal nerve density: A biomarker for diabetic autonomic neuropathy? *Neurology* **2010**, *75*, 973–981. [CrossRef]

142. Sprenger, F.S.; Stefanova, N.; Gelpi, E.; Seppi, K.; Navarro-Otano, J.; Offner, F.; Vilas, D.; Valldeoriola, F.; Pont-Sunyer, C.; Aldecoa, I.; et al. Enteric nervous system α-synuclein immunoreactivity in idiopathic REM sleep behavior disorder. *Neurology* **2015**, *85*, 1761–1768. [CrossRef]

143. Lebouvier, T.; Neunlist, M.; Bruley des Varannes, S.; Coron, E.; Drouard, A.; N'Guyen, J.M.; Chaumette, T.; Tasselli, M.; Paillusson, S.; Flamand, M.; et al. Colonic biopsies to assess the neuropathology of Parkinson's disease and its relationship with symptoms. *PLoS ONE* **2010**, *5*, e12728. [CrossRef]

144. Giancola, F.; Fracassi, F.; Gallucci, A.; Sadeghinezhad, J.; Polidoro, G.; Zini, E.; Asti, M.; Chiocchetti, R. Quantification of nitrergic neurons in the myenteric plexus of gastric antrum and ileum of healthy and diabetic dogs. *Auton. Neurosci.* **2016**, *197*, 25–33. [CrossRef]

145. Blum, H.E. The human microbiome. *Adv. Med. Sci.* **2017**, *62*, 414–420. [CrossRef] [PubMed]

146. Fraher, M.H.; O'Toole, P.W.; Quigley, E.M. Techniques used to characterize the gut microbiota: A guide for the clinician. *Nat. Rev. Gastroenterol. Hepatol.* **2012**, *9*, 312–322. [CrossRef] [PubMed]

147. Marchesi, J.R.; Adams, D.H.; Fava, F.; Hermes, G.D.; Hirschfield, G.M.; Hold, G.; Quraishi, M.N.; Kinross, J.; Smidt, H.; Tuohy, K.M.; et al. The gut microbiota and host health: A new clinical frontier. *Gut* **2016**, *65*, 330–339. [CrossRef]

148. Hasegawa, S.; Goto, S.; Tsuji, H.; Okuno, T.; Asahara, T.; Nomoto, K.; Shibata, A.; Fujisawa, Y.; Minato, T.; Okamoto, A.; et al. Intestinal Dysbiosis and Lowered Serum Lipopolysaccharide-Binding Protein in Parkinson's Disease. *PLoS ONE* **2015**, *10*, e0142164. [CrossRef]

149. Keshavarzian, A.; Green, S.J.; Engen, P.A.; Voigt, R.M.; Naqib, A.; Forsyth, C.B.; Mutlu, E.; Shannon, K.M. Colonic bacterial composition in Parkinson's disease. *Mov. Disord.* **2015**, *30*, 1351–1360. [CrossRef]

150. Sampson, T.R.; Debelius, J.W.; Thron, T.; Janssen, S.; Shastri, G.G.; Ilhan, Z.E.; Challis, C.; Schretter, C.E.; Rocha, S.; Gradinaru, V.; et al. Gut Microbiota Regulate Motor Deficits and Neuroinflammation in a Model of Parkinson's Disease. *Cell* **2016**, *167*, 1469–1480.e12. [CrossRef] [PubMed]

151. Unger, M.M.; Spiegel, J.; Dillmann, K.U.; Grundmann, D.; Philippeit, H.; Bürmann, J.; Faßbender, K.; Schwiertz, A.; Schäfer, K.H. Short chain fatty acids and gut microbiota differ between patients with Parkinson's disease and age-matched controls. *Parkinsonism Relat. Disord.* **2016**, *32*, 66–72. [CrossRef]

152. Brown, C.T.; Davis-Richardson, A.G.; Giongo, A.; Gano, K.A.; Crabb, D.B.; Mukherjee, N.; Casella, G.; Drew, J.C.; Ilonen, J.; Knip, M.; et al. Gut microbiome metagenomics analysis suggests a functional model for the development of autoimmunity for type 1 diabetes. *PLoS ONE* **2011**, *6*, e25792. [CrossRef]

153. Giongo, A.; Gano, K.A.; Crabb, D.B.; Mukherjee, N.; Novelo, L.L.; Casella, G.; Drew, J.C.; Ilonen, J.; Knip, M.; Hyöty, H.; et al. Toward defining the autoimmune microbiome for type 1 diabetes. *ISME J.* **2011**, *5*, 82–91. [CrossRef]

154. Siljander, H.; Honkanen, J.; Knip, M. Microbiome and type 1 diabetes. *EBioMedicine* **2019**, *46*, 512–521. [CrossRef]

155. Miranda, M.C.G.; Oliveira, R.P.; Torres, L.; Aguiar, S.L.F.; Pinheiro-Rosa, N.; Lemos, L.; Guimarães, M.A.; Reis, D.; Silveira, T.; Ferreira, Ê.; et al. Frontline Science: Abnormalities in the gut mucosa of non-obese diabetic mice precede the onset of type 1 diabetes. *J. Leukoc. Biol.* **2019**, *106*, 513–529. [CrossRef]

156. Vaarala, O.; Atkinson, M.A.; Neu, J. The "perfect storm" for type 1 diabetes: The complex interplay between intestinal microbiota, gut permeability, and mucosal immunity. *Diabetes* **2008**, *57*, 2555–2562. [CrossRef]

157. Cani, P.D. Microbiota and metabolites in metabolic diseases. *Nat. Rev. Endocrinol.* **2019**, *15*, 69–70. [CrossRef]

158. Softeland, E.; Brock, C.; Frokjaer, J.B.; Brogger, J.; Madacsy, L.; Gilja, O.H.; Arendt-Nielsen, L.; Simren, M.; Drewes, A.M.; Dimcevski, G. Association between visceral, cardiac and sensorimotor polyneuropathies in diabetes mellitus. *J. Diabetes Complicat.* **2014**, *28*, 370–377. [CrossRef] [PubMed]

159. Pop-Busui, R.; Boulton, A.J.; Feldman, E.L.; Bril, V.; Freeman, R.; Malik, R.A.; Sosenko, J.M.; Ziegler, D. Diabetic Neuropathy: A Position Statement by the American Diabetes Association. *Diabetes Care* **2017**, *40*, 136–154. [CrossRef] [PubMed]

160. Low, P.A.; Denq, J.C.; Opfer-Gehrking, T.L.; Dyck, P.J.; O'Brien, P.C.; Slezak, J.M. Effect of age and gender on sudomotor and cardiovagal function and blood pressure response to tilt in normal subjects. *Muscle Nerve* **1997**, *20*, 1561–1568. [CrossRef]

161. Sandroni, P.; Benarroch, E.E.; Low, P.A. Pharmacological dissection of components of the Valsalva maneuver in adrenergic failure. *J. Appl. Physiol.* **1991**, *71*, 1563–1567. [CrossRef]
162. Benarroch, E.E.; Opfer-Gehrking, T.L.; Low, P.A. Use of the photoplethysmographic technique to analyze the Valsalva maneuver in normal man. *Muscle Nerve* **1991**, *14*, 1165–1172. [CrossRef]
163. Freeman, R.; Chapleau, M.W. Testing the autonomic nervous system. *Handb. Clin. Neurol.* **2013**, *115*, 115–136. [CrossRef]
164. Spallone, V. Blood Pressure Variability and Autonomic Dysfunction. *Curr. Diabetes Rep.* **2018**, *18*, 137. [CrossRef]
165. Freeman, R.; Wieling, W.; Axelrod, F.B.; Benditt, D.G.; Benarroch, E.; Biaggioni, I.; Cheshire, W.P.; Chelimsky, T.; Cortelli, P.; Gibbons, C.H.; et al. Consensus statement on the definition of orthostatic hypotension, neurally mediated syncope and the postural tachycardia syndrome. *Clin. Auton. Res.* **2011**, *21*, 69–72. [CrossRef]
166. Cheshire, W.P., Jr. Autonomic History, Examination, and Laboratory Evaluation. *Continuum* **2020**, *26*, 25–43. [CrossRef] [PubMed]
167. Freeman, R. Autonomic Peripheral Neuropathy. *Continuum* **2020**, *26*, 58–71. [CrossRef]
168. Spallone, V.; Ziegler, D.; Freeman, R.; Bernardi, L.; Frontoni, S.; Pop-Busui, R.; Stevens, M.; Kempler, P.; Hilsted, J.; Tesfaye, S.; et al. Cardiovascular autonomic neuropathy in diabetes: Clinical impact, assessment, diagnosis, and management. *Diabetes Metab Res. Rev.* **2011**, *27*, 639–653. [CrossRef] [PubMed]
169. Sletten, D.M.; Weigand, S.D.; Low, P.A. Relationship of Q-sweat to quantitative sudomotor axon reflex test (QSART) volumes. *Muscle Nerve* **2010**, *41*, 240–246. [CrossRef] [PubMed]
170. Schwartz, T.W. Pancreatic polypeptide: A unique model for vagal control of endocrine systems. *J. Auton. Nerv. Syst.* **1983**, *9*, 99–111. [CrossRef]
171. Knudsen, K.; Hartmann, B.; Fedorova, T.D.; Østergaard, K.; Krogh, K.; Møller, N.; Holst, J.J.; Borghammer, P. Pancreatic Polypeptide in Parkinson's Disease: A Potential Marker of Parasympathetic Denervation. *J. Park. Dis.* **2017**, *7*, 645–652. [CrossRef]
172. Desai, A.; Low, P.A.; Camilleri, M.; Singer, W.; Burton, D.; Chakraborty, S.; Bharucha, A.E. Utility of the plasma pancreatic polypeptide response to modified sham feeding in diabetic gastroenteropathy and non-ulcer dyspepsia. *Neurogastroenterol. Motil.* **2020**, *32*, e13744. [CrossRef]
173. Parkman, H.P.; Yates, K.P.; Hasler, W.L.; Nguyan, L.; Pasricha, P.J.; Snape, W.J.; Farrugia, G.; Calles, J.; Koch, K.L.; Abell, T.L.; et al. Dietary intake and nutritional deficiencies in patients with diabetic or idiopathic gastroparesis. *Gastroenterology* **2011**, *141*, 486–498, 498.e481–487. [CrossRef]
174. Astarloa, R.; Mena, M.A.; Sánchez, V.; de la Vega, L.; de Yébenes, J.G. Clinical and pharmacokinetic effects of a diet rich in insoluble fiber on Parkinson disease. *Clin. Neuropharmacol.* **1992**, *15*, 375–380. [CrossRef]
175. Jalleh, R.; Marathe, C.S.; Rayner, C.K.; Jones, K.L.; Horowitz, M. Diabetic Gastroparesis and Glycaemic Control. *Curr. Diabetes Rep.* **2019**, *19*, 153. [CrossRef]
176. Acosta, A.; Camilleri, M. Prokinetics in gastroparesis. *Gastroenterol. Clin. N. Am.* **2015**, *44*, 97–111. [CrossRef] [PubMed]
177. Giudicessi, J.R.; Ackerman, M.J.; Camilleri, M. Cardiovascular safety of prokinetic agents: A focus on drug-induced arrhythmias. *Neurogastroenterol. Motil.* **2018**, *30*, e13302. [CrossRef]
178. Kumar, M.; Chapman, A.; Javed, S.; Alam, U.; Malik, R.A.; Azmi, S. The Investigation and Treatment of Diabetic Gastroparesis. *Clin. Ther.* **2018**, *40*, 850–861. [CrossRef] [PubMed]
179. Iodice, V.; Kimpinski, K.; Vernino, S.; Sandroni, P.; Low, P.A. Immunotherapy for autoimmune autonomic ganglionopathy. *Auton. Neurosci.* **2009**, *146*, 22–25. [CrossRef] [PubMed]
180. McCallum, R.W.; Lin, Z.; Forster, J.; Roeser, K.; Hou, Q.; Sarosiek, I. Gastric electrical stimulation improves outcomes of patients with gastroparesis for up to 10 years. *Clin. Gastroenterol. Hepatol.* **2011**, *9*, 314–319.e1. [CrossRef]
181. Klinge, M.W.; Rask, P.; Mortensen, L.S.; Lassen, K.; Ejskjaer, N.; Ehlers, L.H.; Krogh, K. Early Assessment of Cost-effectiveness of Gastric Electrical Stimulation for Diabetic Nausea and Vomiting. *J. Neurogastroenterol. Motil.* **2017**, *23*, 541–549. [CrossRef]
182. Okdahl, T.; Bertoli, D.; Brock, B.; Krogh, K.; Krag Knop, F.; Brock, C.; Drewes, A.M. Study protocol for a multicentre, randomised, parallel group, sham-controlled clinical trial investigating the effect of transcutaneous vagal nerve stimulation on gastrointestinal symptoms in people with diabetes complicated with diabetic autonomic neuropathy: The DAN-VNS Study. *BMJ Open* **2021**, *11*, e038677. [CrossRef] [PubMed]
183. Lauritano, E.C.; Gabrielli, M.; Scarpellini, E.; Lupascu, A.; Novi, M.; Sottili, S.; Vitale, G.; Cesario, V.; Serricchio, M.; Cammarota, G.; et al. Small intestinal bacterial overgrowth recurrence after antibiotic therapy. *Am. J. Gastroenterol.* **2008**, *103*, 2031–2035. [CrossRef] [PubMed]
184. Selby, A.; Reichenbach, Z.W.; Piech, G.; Friedenberg, F.K. Pathophysiology, Differential Diagnosis, and Treatment of Diabetic Diarrhea. *Dig. Dis. Sci.* **2019**, *64*, 3385–3393. [CrossRef] [PubMed]

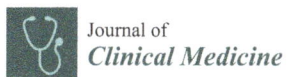

Journal of
Clinical Medicine

MDPI

Article

Validation of the Monitoring Efficacy of Neurogenic Bowel Treatment on Response (MENTOR) Tool in a Japanese Rehabilitation Setting

Masashi Nomi [1,*], Atsushi Sengoku [1], Klaus Krogh [2], Anton Emmanuel [3] and Albert Bohn Christiansen [4]

[1] Department of Urology, Hyogo Prefectural Central Rehabilitation Hospital, Hyogo 651-2181, Japan; a_sengoku@hwc.or.jp
[2] Department of Hepatology and Gastroenterology, Aarhus University Hospital, 8000 Aarhus, Denmark; klaukrog@rm.dk
[3] GI Physiology Unit, University College Hospital, London NW1 2BU, UK; anton.emmanuel@nhs.net
[4] Medical Affairs, Coloplast A/S, 2970 Humlebaek, Denmark; dkalbc@coloplast.com
* Correspondence: m_nomi@hwc.or.jp; Tel.: +81-78-927-2727

Citation: Nomi, M.; Sengoku, A.; Krogh, K.; Emmanuel, A.; Christiansen, A.B. Validation of the Monitoring Efficacy of Neurogenic Bowel Treatment on Response (MENTOR) Tool in a Japanese Rehabilitation Setting. *J. Clin. Med.* **2021**, *10*, 934. https://doi.org/10.3390/jcm10050934

Academic Editor: Romain Coriat

Received: 9 December 2020
Accepted: 18 February 2021
Published: 1 March 2021

Publisher's Note: MDPI stays neutral with regard to jurisdictional claims in published maps and institutional affiliations.

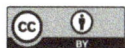

Copyright: © 2021 by the authors. Licensee MDPI, Basel, Switzerland. This article is an open access article distributed under the terms and conditions of the Creative Commons Attribution (CC BY) license (https://creativecommons.org/licenses/by/4.0/).

Abstract: Study design: Prospective observational study. Objective: To validate the Monitoring Efficacy of NBD Treatment On Response (MENTOR) tool in individuals with a spinal cord injury (SCI) or spina bifida, suffering from neurogenic bowel dysfunction (NBD) in a rehabilitation center in Japan. Methods: First, the MENTOR tool was translated from English to Japanese using a validated translation process. Second, the MENTOR tool was validated in a rehabilitation clinic in Japan. Participants completed the MENTOR tool prior to a consultation with an expert physician. According to the results of the tool, each participant was allocated to one of three categories regarding change in treatment: "adequately treated," "further discussion," and "recommended change." The results of the MENTOR tool were compared with the treatment decision made by an expert physician, who was blinded to the results of the MENTOR tool. Results: A total of 60 participants completed the MENTOR tool. There was an acceptable concordance between individuals allocated as respectively, being adequately treated (100%) and recommended change in treatment (61%) and the physicians' decision on treatment. The concordance was lower for individuals allocated as requiring further discussion (48%). Conclusions: In this study the MENTOR tool was successfully validated in a Japanese rehab setting. The tool will help identify individuals with SCI that need further treatment of their NBD symptoms.

Keywords: neurogenic bowel; spinal cord injury; treatment assessment

1. Introduction

Symptoms of constipation and fecal incontinence often occur in individuals with central nervous system injury or disease [1,2]. Such symptoms are categorized as neurogenic bowel dysfunction (NBD) and have a profound negative impact on quality of life and social integration [3]. NBD is also associated with increased health service costs [4]. However, with optimal bowel management, NBD has been shown to improve [5–7], hence it is important to identify and treat those individuals suffering from NBD. Though several options for management of NBD exist, it has been found that NBD was a problem among 78% of individuals with spinal cord injury (SCI) and 71% had not modified any aspect of their bowel routine for more than 5 years [8]. In Japan, there are only a few specialists in NBD and guidelines on how to treat NBD were only recently published [9], making it even more difficult to identify and treat Japanese individuals who suffer from NBD [10,11].

A recently published study reviewed currently available scores for assessment of NBD in individuals with SCI [12]. However, none of these scores have yet been globally validated or accepted. The International Standards to document remaining Autonomic

Function after Spinal Cord Injury (ISAFSCI) is a measure that can be used by physicians to assess the remaining autonomic function after SCI, but it is used to assess all autonomic functions and not only the bowel function [13]. The international basic bowel function data set was developed to standardize the collection of information on NBD in daily practice, but it is a static and not a dynamic measure [14]. The NBD score is a symptom-based score developed for assessment of NBD symptoms specifically in individuals with SCI [15]. Though an increase in the NBD score has been shown to correlate with a decreased quality of life, the score does not include patients' subjective impression of their symptoms [15]. Recently, a new measure capable of reflecting change, called the Monitoring Efficacy of NBD Treatment On Response (MENTOR) tool, was developed with the objective to assess the severity of NBD in individuals with SCI by combining the NBD score with special attention symptoms (SAS), which are the elements of comorbidity that may be linked to poor bowel management [16], and patients' perception of satisfaction with their bowel function [16]. The MENTOR tool has already been validated for use in rehabilitation clinics and gastroenterology clinics in the USA and Europe where the MENTOR tool showed good correspondence with the decisions made by expert physicians [16]. However, it has not yet been validated in Japan or any other Asian country.

2. Experimental Section

In this prospective observational study, the MENTOR tool was validated in a Japanese setting. The study was approved by the Hyogo Prefectural Central Rehabilitation Hospital Ethics Committee reference number 1917.

All patients filled out an ICF prior to participating, with assistance from an onsite nurse.

2.1. The MENTOR Tool

The MENTOR tool consists of three components. The first component is bowel/defecation symptoms assessed by the validated NBD score. The NBD score comprises ten items which showed good reproducibility and validity, and which allow stratification into four tiers of severity, and which are significantly associated with impact on QOL [15]. Based on odds ratios for associations between items and impact on QOL, each has a corresponding number of points in the NBD score. The second component is SAS listed in Table 1. The third component is the patient's perception of satisfaction with their bowel function which includes the following options; satisfied, acceptable, dissatisfied, and very dissatisfied.

Table 1. Special attention symptoms of neurogenic bowel dysfunction.

Special Attention Symptoms
1. Intense pain in abdomen or rectum.
2. New or increased rectal bleeding.
3. Hospitalization due to bowel problems.
4. Loss of independence or change in circumstances that potentially impacts bowel care or bowel function.
5. Episode of autonomic dysreflexia related to bowel problems.

After completing all three components of the MENTOR tool, patients were assigned to one of three zones; a green, a yellow, or a red zone. As illustrated in Figure 1, the combination of an NBD score and patient satisfaction allocates the patients to one of the three zones in the MENTOR grid. Further, if an individual reports any of the listed SAS they will be moved one grid square up and to the right, effactually escalating their treatment recommendation. The green zone represents adequate treatment of individuals, the yellow zone reflects suboptimal treatment and a need of further discussions with the individual and the possibility of change in treatment and/or further monitoring and the red zone suggests inadequate treatment and a need for further examination and most likely, change in current treatment.

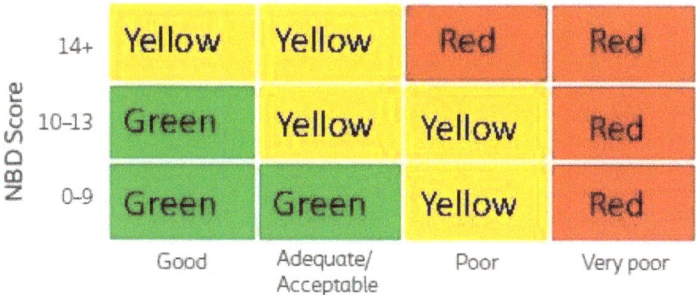

Figure 1. The MENTOR (Monitoring Efficacy of NBD Treatment On Response) grid to determine treatment assessment outcome. Green "Monitor", Yellow "Discuss" and Red "Act".

2.2. Translation of the MENTOR Tool into Japanese

To ensure that the tool was correctly translated into Japanese a thorough translation process was performed. First, the MENTOR tool was double forward translated from English to Japanese by two bilingual residents of Japan who were professionally qualified in translating. Second, the two translated versions of the tool were compared and merged into a single Japanese version. Third, a backward translation from Japanese to English was performed and this version was compared with the original English version of the MENTOR tool to identify and resolve any discrepancies between the two versions. Finally, the edited Japanese version of the MENTOR was reviewed by a panel of expert clinicians before proofreading and formatting were performed.

2.3. Validation of the MENTOR Tool in a Japanese Setting

The validation of the MENTOR tool was performed in one rehabilitation clinic in the Hyogo prefecture of Japan. All adults ≥18 years with a confirmed diagnosis of non-congenital SCI of more than 3 months or a confirmed diagnosis of spina bifida were eligible for inclusion if they also had a confirmed diagnosis of NBD, with use of a minimum of one method for managing their bowel function.

Of these, individuals with a scheduled consultation at the rehabilitation clinic in the period January 2020 to July 2020, were invited to participate in the study. Participants received a self-completion questionnaire comprising the MENTOR tool prior to their consultation with a physician.

To assess the ease of use of the MENTOR tool a clinician registered the time it took for each individual to complete the questionnaire and after completion each individual was asked whether the questionnaire was easy to understand (yes/no answer). Further, the clinician verified that all items of the questionnaire were completed.

After completion of the MENTOR tool, the scheduled consultation with the physician took place as per usual and the physician was not informed on the results of the MENTOR tool. At the end of the consultation, the physician registered one of the three following outcomes: (1) no treatment change, (2) discussion but no treatment change, or (3) recommendation of change in treatment due to inadequate current treatment in the physician template.

2.4. Statistical Analysis

All data including data from the MENTOR tool and the outcome registered by the physician were entered into a predetermined and locked Excel file. All data were analyzed using Excel including means with standard deviations for normally distributed data and proportions. The results of the MENTOR tool and the decisions made by a physician were compared by calculating the concordance of the results of the MENTOR tool with the decision made by the expert physician.

3. Results

A total of 57 individuals with SCI and 3 with spina bifida were included from one rehabilitation clinic located in the Hyogo prefecture, Japan. Of these, most were males (n = 55), and the mean age was 46.9 years (Standard deviation [SD] 14.2).

According to the MENTOR tool, 15 patients (25%) were allocated to the green zone indicating they received adequate treatment, 27 (45%) were allocated to the yellow zone indicating that they received suboptimal treatment, and 18 (30%) were allocated to the red zone indicating that they received inadequate treatment (Figure 2). The MENTOR tool was reported by patients to be easy to understand in 97%, and it took a mean of 4.1 min (range 1–14 min) to complete.

Distribution of MENTOR outcomes

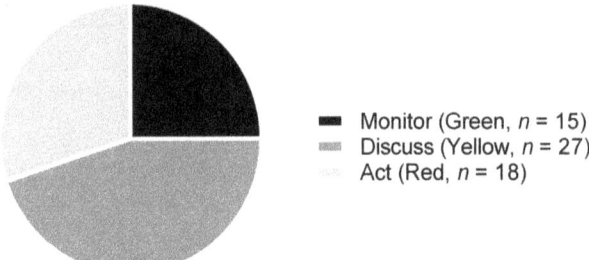

Figure 2. Distribution of MENTOR outcome in Hyogo Prefectural Central Rehabilitation Hospital (n = 60). Green "Monitor", Yellow "Discuss," and Red "Act".

When comparing the results of the MENTOR tool with the decision made by the physician, agreement was obtained in 65% of all cases (Figure 3, Table 2). There was 100% concordance with the physicians' decision for individuals in the green zone of the MENTOR grid, 61% concordance for individuals in the red zone, and only 48% concordance for individuals in the yellow zone. Notably, of the 27 individuals in the yellow zone, 24 (89%) were not recommended change in treatment by the physician at the rehabilitation clinic.

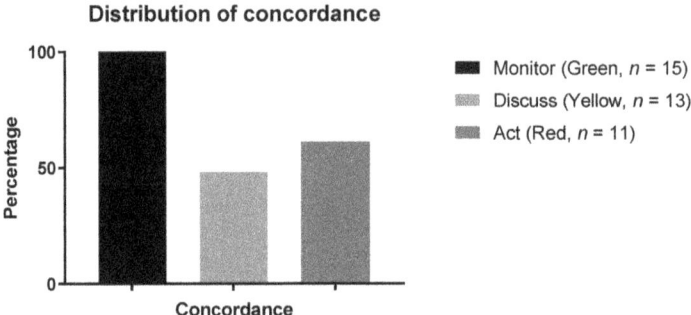

Figure 3. Distribution of concordance between MENTOR and clinician treatment assessment decision (n = 60), total concordance (n = 39).

Table 2. MENTOR results and agreement with physician.

	N	%
Total participants	60	100
Participants allocated to the three zones:		
Green zone	15	25
Yellow zone	27	45
Red zone	18	30
Concordance according to the three zones:		
Green zone	15	100
Yellow zone	13	48
Red zone	11	61
Green + Red zone	26	79
Total concordance (Green + Yellow + Red zone)	39	65
Recommendation of change in treatment in the Yellow zone: [1]		
Yellow + Change in treatment	3	11
Yellow + No change in treatment	24	89
Total participants recommended change in treatment	11	18

[1] Recommendation made by the physician.

When looking at the three specific components of the MENTOR tool, we observed an association between each of the three components and recommendation of change in treatment (Figure 4). Overall, a total of 13 participants (22%) were recommended change in treatment by the physician. For the NBD score, only 2 of 26 (8%) individuals with an NBD score of less than 14 were recommended change in their treatment, while 11 of 34 (32%) individuals with an NBD score of more than 14 were recommended change in their treatment (Figure 4A). For the SAS component, 6 of 48 (13%) individuals with no SAS were recommended change in their treatment, which increased to 5 of 12 (42%) individuals with one SAS and 3 of 4 (75%) individuals with more than one SAS (Figure 4B). For the patient satisfaction component, the proportion of individuals who were recommended change in their treatment increased with dissatisfaction of their bowel function (Figure 4C). No individuals who reported that they were satisfied with their bowel function were recommended change in their treatment (0 of 14 individuals) while 6 of 36 (17%) individuals who reported their bowel function was acceptable, 4 of 9 (44%) individuals who reported they were dissatisfied with their bowel function, and 1 of 1 (100%) individual who reported he/she was very dissatisfied with the bowel function, were recommended change in their treatment.

A

NBD score (cut-off 14) vs change of treatment offered

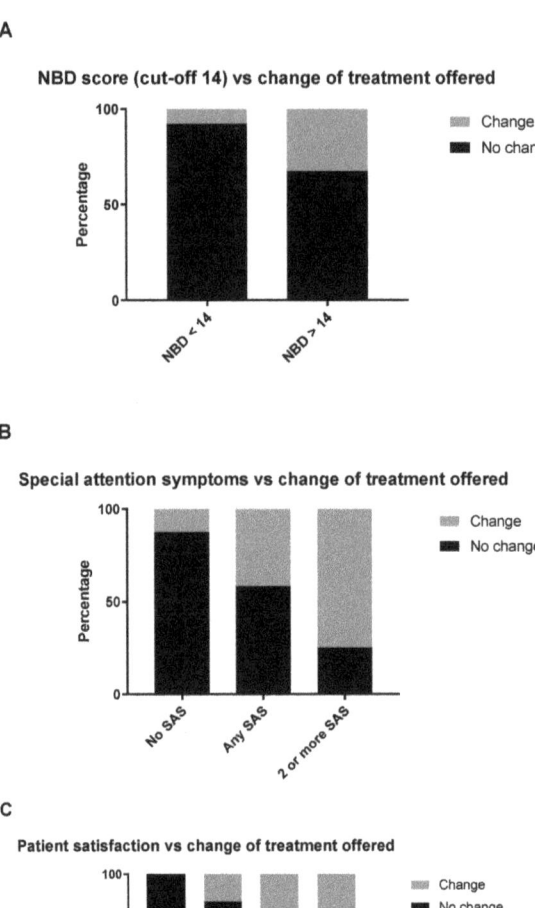

Figure 4. (A) Severe neurogenic bowel dysfunction (NBD) score associates with treatment change. (B) Linear association of special attention symptoms (SAS) and treatment change. (C) Inverse association between patient satisfaction and treatment change.

4. Discussion

In this observational study the MENTOR tool was validated in a Japanese setting. We found that NBD patients' subjective experience of treatment adequacy assessed by the MENTOR tool corresponded well to the independent decision made by the clinicians. The MENTOR tool was easy to understand and complete.

While there was acceptable concordance between individuals assigned to the green and red zone and the physicians' decision (as shown in the combined data in Table 2), there was only 48% concordance between individuals assigned to the intermediate yellow zone and the physicians' decision. Most of these individuals were not recommended any treatment change by the physician (24 of 27 individuals, 89%) though allocation to the yellow zone could indicate that they only had a suboptimal treatment. This could be explained by patients having a tendency not to address their symptoms at the consultation because they are unaware of the severity of their symptoms or that they are embarrassed by their symptoms [17]. Nevertheless, it is important to identify this group of patients as studies have reported that suboptimal care of bowel management has a negative impact on the quality of life [4]. Our results indicate that the MENTOR tool could help identify this group of patients.

When comparing the Japanese validation with the International validation of the MENTOR tool in rehabilitation clinics, we found an overall consistency between results e.g., the concordance of individuals allocated to respectively the green and red zone were 100% and 61% in our Japanese validation study and 86% and 68% in the international validation study [16]. This suggests that the MENTOR tool is also applicable in rehabilitation clinics in Japan. Notably, in the International validation study, the MENTOR tool was also validated by two NBD experts at two gastroenterology clinics [16]. Interestingly, there was more than 90% agreement between the results of the MENTOR tool and decisions made by the expert physicians in NBD [16]. This supports the hypothesis that the MENTOR tool is even more comparable to decisions made by the expert physicians in NBD. In countries like Japan where there are fewer experts in NBD, use of the MENTOR tool seems particularly important, as this may help identify those patients who need input from an expert in NBD.

Importantly, one study found that the severity of NBD symptoms increased significantly over time in individuals with SCI [18], which implicates that there is a need of lifelong follow-up on the severity of NBD in these patients. Indeed, the MENTOR tool would be an easy way to consistently monitor the need of further treatment of NBD. As some patients may not have follow-up visits at a gastroenterology clinic or a rehabilitation center the tool could also help physicians and caregivers in non-hospital settings to become aware of the worsening of NBD symptoms in individuals with SCI and a potential requirement of further management [19].

When patients who need further treatment of NBD are identified with the MENTOR tool, it is imperative that physicians choose the right treatment. Recently, Paralyzed Veterans of America published a clinical practice guideline for healthcare providers on how to manage NBD in adults after SCI [7]. The practical guide thoroughly describes all treatment options of NBD, indications of each treatment, and current evidence of efficacy of treatments [7]. In most countries including Japan, a stepwise approach to NBD treatment starting from the least invasive method is recommended [7,20,21]. Conservative bowel management (CBM) is first-line treatment for most patients with neurogenic bowel dysfunction. CBM includes diet and fluid management, a scheduled bowel routine, physical activity, and oral and rectal medications [7,21]. In patients with insufficient results of CBM, transanal irrigation (TAI) is most often recommended [7,21]. During TAI, feces evacuates from the bowel by introducing water into the colon and rectum through the anus [21]. If treatment with CBM and TAI fails, functional electrical stimulation of the sacral nerve or antegrade colonic irrigation either through appendicostomy or percutaneous endoscopic colostomy may be considered [7,21]. Colostomy is often considered as the last treatment option due to its invasive nature. However, colostomy is successful in a large proportion of patients and associated with a reduced bowel management time and improved quality of life [21]. Implementation of the MENTOR tool can help clinicians assess and identify when the patient should revise their current treatment following the stepwise approach.

This is the first time the MENTOR tool was translated into a non-European language. However, the NBD score, which is one of the components in the MENTOR tool, has already been translated into several languages spoken outside Europe and the USA including Japanese, Arabic, Mandarin, and Turkish [10,22,23]. In our study, 97% of participants reported that the Japanese version of the MENTOR tool was easy to understand and complete indicating that the translation of the MENTOR tool into Japanese was successful.

While it may seem paradoxical to describe the score as readily understood by patients when it contains terms like "autonomic dysreflexia" it is important to note that a key part of training of SCI patients is to help them recognize the alarm features to be aware of. As such, spinally injured individuals in a rehabilitation setting will generally have a good understanding of the features of dysreflexia.

Some limitations apply to our study. No information was given on whether specific components of the MENTOR tool e.g., the SAS, were the reason of allocation of individuals into the yellow zone. Due to lack of this information, it is not possible to explain the reason why only a few individuals in the yellow zone were recommended change in treatment by the physician. The tool was only validated in one rehabilitation clinic in the Hyogo prefecture of Japan why it may not be generalizable to other prefectures of Japan. However, a total of 60 patients participated in our study, making it the second largest study group that have validated the MENTOR tool [16].

5. Conclusions

We conclude that the MENTOR tool is applicable in a Japanese rehab setting. The MENTOR tool will help identify individuals with SCI who are unaware of the severity of their NBD symptoms and thereby facilitate the discussion with the physician and possibly lead to an improvement treatment.

Further studies to identify whether it can improve symptoms, reduce hospitalizations, urinary tract infections, and other comorbidities in the longer term would be interesting to pursue.

Author Contributions: Conceptualization; M.N., A.S., K.K., and A.B.C.; methodology, M.N., A.S., K.K., and A.B.C.; validation M.N., A.S., K.K., A.E., and A.B.C.; formal analysis, M.N., A.S., K.K., and A.B.C.; investigation, M.N. and A.S; resources, M.N., A.S., K.K., A.E., and A.B.C.; data curation, M.N., A.S., K.K., A.E., and A.B.C.; writing—original draft preparation M.N., A.S., K.K., A.E., and A.B.C.; writing—review and editing, M.N., A.S., K.K., A.E., and A.B.C.; visualization, M.N., A.S., K.K., A.E., and A.B.C.; supervision, A.B.C.; project administration, A.B.C.; funding acquisition, A.B.C. All authors have read and agreed to the published version of the manuscript.

Funding: This study was supported by Coloplast A/S, Denmark and Coloplast K.K., Japan for translation and expenses for project administration.

Institutional Review Board Statement: The study was conducted according to the guidelines of the Declaration of Helsinki, and approved by the Hyogo Rehabilitation Central Hospital Ethics Committee (protocol code 1917: date of approval 27 January 2020).

Informed Consent Statement: Informed consent was obtained from all subjects involved in the study.

Data Availability Statement: The data that support the findings are available from the corresponding author (M. N.) upon reasonable request.

Acknowledgments: The authors want to thank the following people for their contribution to the project: Anne-Sofie Halling-Sønderby from Herlev and Gentofte Hospital (Copenhagen, Denmark). Anne-Sofie contributed to data analysis, interpreting results, writing the report and creating the reference list.

Conflicts of Interest: Klaus Krogh and Anton Emmanuel are members of Coloplast A/S Global Bowel Advisory Board and Albert Bohn Christiansen is employed as a Medical Specialist at Coloplast A/S. The funder had a role in the project management and data analyses of the project.

References

1. Stone, J.M.; Nino-Murcia, M.; Wolfe, V.A.; Perkash, I. Chronic gastrointestinal problems in spinal cord injury patients: A prospective analysis. *Am. J. Gastroenterol.* **1990**, *85*, 1114–1119.
2. Hinds, J.P.; Eidelman, B.H.; Wald, A. Prevalence of bowel dysfunction in multiple sclerosis. A population survey. *Gastroenterology* **1990**, *98*, 1538–1542. [CrossRef]
3. Glickman, S.; Kamm, M.A. Bowel dysfunction in spinal-cord-injury patients. *Lancet* **1996**, *347*, 1651–1653. [CrossRef]
4. Emmanuel, A.; Kumar, G.; Christensen, P.; Mealing, S.; Størling, Z.M.; Andersen, F.; Kirshblum, S. Long-Term Cost-Effectiveness of Transanal Irrigation in Patients with Neurogenic Bowel Dysfunction. *PLoS ONE* **2016**, *11*, e0159394. [CrossRef] [PubMed]

5. Krogh, K.; Nielsen, J.; Djurhuus, J.C.; Mosdal, C.; Sabroe, S.; Laurberg, S. Colorectal function in patients with spinal cord lesions. *Dis. Colon Rectum* **1997**, *40*, 1233–1239. [CrossRef] [PubMed]
6. Preziosi, G.; Emmanuel, A. Neurogenic bowel dysfunction: Pathophysiology, clinical manifestations and treatment. *Expert. Rev. Gastroenterol. Hepatol.* **2009**, *3*, 417–423. [CrossRef] [PubMed]
7. Coggrave, M.; Norton, C.; Wilson-Barnett, J. Management of neurogenic bowel dysfunction in the community after spinal cord injury: A postal survey in the United Kingdom. *Spinal Cord.* **2009**, *47*, 323–330. [CrossRef] [PubMed]
8. Inskip, J.A.; Lucci, V.M.; McGrath, M.S.; Willms, R.; Claydon, V.E. A Community Perspective on Bowel Management and Quality of Life after Spinal Cord Injury: The Influence of Autonomic Dysreflexia. *J. Neurotrauma* **2018**, *35*, 1091–1105. [CrossRef]
9. Available online: https://www.jascol.jp/member_news/2020/files/20200331.pdf?v=2 (accessed on 15 December 2020).
10. Katoh, S.; Sengoku, A.; Nomi, M.; Noto, S. A Web based Survey on Neurogenic Bowel Dysfunction in Japan. *JJASCoL* **2017**, *30*, 44–48.
11. Sengoku, A.; Noto, S.; Nomi, M.; Emmanuel, A.; Murata, T.; Mimura, T. Cost-Effectiveness Analysis of Transanal Irrigation for Managing Neurogenic Bowel Dysfunction in Japan. *J. Health Econ. Outcomes Res.* **2018**, *6*, 37–52. [CrossRef] [PubMed]
12. Tate, D.G.; Wheeler, T.; Lane, G.I.; Forchheimer, M.; Anderson, K.D.; Biering-Sorensen, F.; Cameron, A.P.; Santacruz, B.G.; Jakeman, L.B.; Kennelly, M.J.; et al. Recommendations for evaluation of neurogenic bladder and bowel dysfunction after spinal cord injury and/or disease. *J. Spinal Cord Med.* **2020**, *43*, 141–164. [CrossRef] [PubMed]
13. Krassioukov, A.; Biering-Sørensen, F.; Donovan, W.; Kennelly, M.; Kirshblum, S.; Krogh, K.; Alexander, M.S.; Vogel, L.; Wecht, J. Autonomic Standards Committee of the American Spinal Injury Association/International Spinal Cord Society. International standards to document remaining autonomic function after spinal cord injury. *J. Spinal Cord Med.* **2012**, *35*, 201–210. [CrossRef] [PubMed]
14. Krogh, K.; Perkash, I.; Stiens, S.A.; Biering-Sørensen, F. International bowel function basic spinal cord injury data set. *Spinal Cord.* **2009**, *47*, 230–234. [CrossRef]
15. Krogh, K.; Christensen, P.; Sabroe, S.; Laurberg, S. Neurogenic bowel dysfunction score. *Spinal Cord.* **2006**, *44*, 625–631. [CrossRef]
16. Emmanuel, A.; Krogh, K.; Kirshblum, S.; Christensen, P.; Spinelli, M.; van Kuppevelt, D.; Abel, R.; Leder, D.; Santacruz, B.G.; Bain, K.; et al. Creation and validation of a new tool for the monitoring efficacy of neurogenic bowel dysfunction treatment on response: The MENTOR tool. *Spinal Cord.* **2020**, *58*, 795–802. [CrossRef]
17. Brown, H.W.; Rogers, R.G.; Wise, M.E. Barriers to seeking care for accidental bowel leakage: A qualitative study. *Int. Urogynecol. J.* **2017**, *28*, 543–551. [CrossRef]
18. Faaborg, P.M.; Christensen, P.; Finnerup, N.; Laurberg, S.; Krogh, K. The pattern of colorectal dysfunction changes with time since spinal cord injury. *Spinal Cord.* **2008**, *46*, 234–238. [CrossRef] [PubMed]
19. Nielsen, S.D.; Faaborg, P.M.; Finnerup, N.B.; Christensen, P.; Krogh, K. Ageing with neurogenic bowel dysfunction. *Spinal Cord.* **2017**, *55*, 769–773. [CrossRef]
20. Emmanuel, A.V.; Krogh, K.; Bazzocchi, G.; Leroi, A.M.; Bremers, A.; Leder, D.; Van Kuppevelt, D.; Mosiello, G.; Vogel, M.; Perrouin-Verbe, B.; et al. Consensus review of best practice of transanal irrigation in adults. *Spinal Cord.* **2013**, *51*, 732–738. [CrossRef] [PubMed]
21. Emmanuel, A. Neurogenic bowel dysfunction. *F1000Research* **2019**, *8*, 1800. [CrossRef] [PubMed]
22. Mallek, A.; Elleuch, M.H.; Ghroubi, S. Neurogenic bowel dysfunction (NBD) translation and linguistic validation to classical Arabic. *Prog. Urol.* **2016**, *26*, 553–557. [CrossRef] [PubMed]
23. Erdem, D.; Hava, D.; Keskinoğlu, P.; Bircan, Ç.; Peker, Ö.; Krogh, K.; Gülbahar, S. Reliability, validity and sensitivity to change of neurogenic bowel dysfunction score in patients with spinal cord injury. *Spinal Cord.* **2017**, *55*, 1084–1087. [CrossRef] [PubMed]

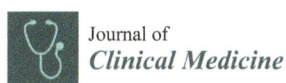

Journal of
Clinical Medicine

MDPI

Article

The Monitoring Efficacy of Neurogenic Bowel Dysfunction Treatment on Response (MENTOR) in a Non-Hospital Setting

Sofie Dagmar Studsgaard Slot [1], Simon Mark Dahl Baunwall [1], Anton Emmanuel [2], Peter Christensen [3] and Klaus Krogh [1,*]

[1] Department of Hepatology and Gastroenterology, Aarhus University Hospital of Aarhus, DK8200 Aarhus N, Denmark; sofie.studsgaard@hotmail.com (S.D.S.S.); SIMJOR@rm.dk (S.M.D.B.)
[2] GI Physiology Unit, University College Hospital, London NW1 2BU, UK; anton.emmanuel@nhs.net
[3] Department of Surgery, Aarhus University Hospital of Aarhus, DK8200 Aarhus N, Denmark; petchris@rm.dk
* Correspondence: klaukrog@rm.dk

Abstract: Background: Most patients with a spinal cord injury (SCI) suffer from neurogenic bowel dysfunction (NBD). In spite of well-established treatment algorithms, NBD is often insufficiently managed. The Monitoring Efficacy of Neurogenic bowel dysfunction Treatment On Response (MENTOR) has been validated in a hospital setting as a tool to support clinical decision making in individual patients. The objective of the present study was to describe clinical decisions recommended by the MENTOR (either "monitor", "discuss" or "act") and the use of the tool to monitor NBD in a non-hospital setting. Methods: A questionnaire describing background data, the MENTOR, ability to work and participation in various social activities was sent by mail to all members of The Danish Paraplegic Association. Results: Among 1316 members, 716 (54%) responded, 429 men (61%) and 278 women (39%), aged 18 to 92 (median 61) years. Based on MENTOR, the recommended clinical decision is to monitor treatment of NBD in 281 (44%), discuss change in treatment in 175 (27%) and act/change treatment in 181 (28%). A recommendation to discuss or change treatment was associated with increasing age of the respondent ($p = 0.016$) and with impaired ability to work or participate in social activities ($p < 0.0001$). Conclusion: A surprisingly high proportion of persons with SCI have an unmet need for improved bowel care. The MENTOR holds promise as a tool for evaluation of treatment of NBD in a non-hospital setting.

Keywords: SCI; MENTOR; NBD; constipation; fecal incontinence

Citation: Studsgaard Slot, S.D.; Baunwall, S.M.D.; Emmanuel, A.; Christensen, P.; Krogh, K. The Monitoring Efficacy of Neurogenic Bowel Dysfunction Treatment on Response (MENTOR) in a Non-Hospital Setting. *J. Clin. Med.* **2021**, *10*, 263. https://doi.org/10.3390/jcm10020263

Received: 22 December 2020
Accepted: 7 January 2021
Published: 12 January 2021

Publisher's Note: MDPI stays neutral with regard to jurisdictional claims in published maps and institutional affiliations.

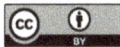

Copyright: © 2021 by the authors. Licensee MDPI, Basel, Switzerland. This article is an open access article distributed under the terms and conditions of the Creative Commons Attribution (CC BY) license (https://creativecommons.org/licenses/by/4.0/).

1. Introduction

The term neurogenic bowel dysfunction (NBD) covers gastrointestinal symptoms that complicate lesions or diseases in the central nervous system. NBD is normal among patients with spinal cord injury (SCI), multiple sclerosis, spina bifida or cauda equina syndrome. The most common symptoms are constipation and/or faecal incontinence, which affect more than 80% of SCI patients [1,2]. Symptoms of NBD restrict social activities and impair quality of life [1,2]. Especially, the loss of independence controlling or achieving defecation is burdensome [3,4]. Despite the consequences of NBD and existing stepwise treatment approaches, the management of NBD is usually not systematically evaluated. This may delay initiation of appropriate treatment [5–8].

Evaluation of NBD is usually based on patient reported symptoms. Several scores exist for assessment of either constipation or faecal incontinence. Unfortunately, most have not been validated for use in patients with neurological disorders and they do not cover the full spectrum of bowel symptoms experienced by such patients. The NBD score is a 10-item score developed and validated among persons with SCI [9]. It has been translated into more than 15 languages and remains the most cited score for description of NBD or as endpoint in clinical trials [9–11]. The NBD score correlates with the impact of NBD on the quality of life in persons with NBD, but it was not developed for clinical decision making in individual patients [12].

Monitoring Efficacy of Neurogenic bowel dysfunction Treatment On Response (MENTOR) is a tool to monitor treatment and determine progression of treatment for NBD. It combines three domains: the NBD score, special attention symptoms indicating insufficient treatment, and patient satisfaction with their bowel function. Thus, it offers a holistic outcome that has been shown to be both easy and reliable to use in clinical practice [5,13]. The MENTOR was developed in a hospital setting, and it has been validated among persons with SCI in four European countries and the USA [13]. At present, MENTOR has not been applied in a broader community-based group of people with NBD. Such data is warranted as it will provide valuable information about the need for improved treatment of people with SCI in general and inform whether systematic monitoring of the patient group is required. Most changes in treatment for NBD are decided at scheduled control visits at specialist clinics. If useful in a non-hospital setting, the MENTOR could prove valuable as a tool for patients and caregivers outside specialist clinics to identify who is in need for enhanced treatment of NBD and therefore should be referred to specialist centres.

The aim of the present study was to describe clinical decisions recommended by the MENTOR (either "monitor", "discuss" or "act") and the use of the tool to monitor NBD in a non-hospital setting.

2. Methods

In this cross-sectional survey, a questionnaire was sent by mail to all 1316 active members of the Danish Paraplegic Association. The Danish Paraplegic Associations is a patient organisation covering more than 35% of Danish persons with SCI from all regions of the country.

All members were mailed the questionnaire at the same time with instructions on how to return the responses by mail. Members who did not respond within 4 weeks were mailed a reminder with the questionnaire. Once the questionnaires were returned, all data were entered twice to minimise transcription errors.

The questionnaire included 29 items describing age; gender; time since spinal cord lesion; function of hand and legs; cutaneous sensibility; previous abdominal surgery; stoma; constipation; method of defecation; bowel habits; faecal incontinence; contact with healthcare providers; satisfaction with current bowel function; and impact of NBD on social activities, ability to work or quality of life. Included in the questionnaire were the NBD score and the MENTOR. Based on the respondent's description of motor and sensory function, the level of the SCI was described as either cervical or thoracic/lumbar and either sensory and motor complete or incomplete.

Special attention symptoms are symptoms that indicate insufficient management of NBD. Those symptoms were included in the questionnaire and have been described in detail previously [13].

According to MENTOR, all participants were grouped as either green, yellow or red. These groups indicate that symptoms should be monitored (green), a need for discussion of change in treatment (yellow) or a need to change treatment modality for NBD.

According to Danish legislation, questionnaire studies do not need approval from Ethics Committee.

3. Statistical Analysis

Statistical analysis was performed in GraphPad Software (Prism 8 8.4.3, GraphPad Software, Inc., San Diego, CA, USA). Results are given as median with range or proportions with confidence interval. For continuous normal data, we used Kruskal Wallis test across the three MENTOR groups, and for categorical data we used chi square test. In the grouping of MENTOR, we considered incomplete responses as no responses to limit potential reporting bias and provide the most conservative estimates. In specific analyses on each item separately, incomplete answers were omitted from the analysis. A *p*-value of less than 0.05 was considered statistically significant.

Among 1316 members of The Danish Paraplegic Association, 716 (54%) responded, 429 men (61%) and 278 women (39%), aged 18 to 92 (median 61) years. Time since the lesion was 2 to 90 (median 20) years. The level of lesion was cervical in 312 (47%) and thoracic or lumbar in 352 (53%). The lesion was sensory complete in 285 (41%) and motor complete in 356 (51%). A total of 79 respondents (11%) had a stoma and were excluded from the following analysis leaving a total 630 respondents. The respondent's contact to the healthcare system and the follow-up regarding bowel care are summarised in Table 1. In total, 366 (62%) had been seen for follow-up at specialist SCI centres within the last two years and 312 (52%) had discussed bowel care with a healthcare provider. However, 182 (30%) had not discussed methods for bowel care within the last five years.

Table 1. The respondent's contact to the healthcare system.

	When Have You Last Seen a Doctor/Nurse Because of SCI?	When Have You Last Discussed Your Bowel Function with a Doctor/Nurse?
Less than one year ago	166 (28%)	156 (26%)
1–2 years	200 (34%)	156 (26%)
>2–5 years	147 (25%)	113 (19%)
More than 5 years	63 (11%)	78 (13%)
Never	20 (3%)	105 (17%)
Missing values	34 (5%)	22 (3%)

SCI: Spinal cord injury.

3.1. Neurogenic Bowel Dysfunction Score

Responses to each of the 10 items in the NBD score are shown in Table 2. Median NBD score was 8 (range 0–34). Among respondents, 235 (38%) had no or very minor, 122 (20%) had minor, 141 (23%) had moderate and 123 (20%) had severe NBD.

Table 2. The response to the 10 items of the Neurogenic Bowel Dysfunction (NBD).

NBD Score	*n* (%)
1. How often do you defacate?	
Daily	335 (53.3%)
2–6 times per week	281 (44.7%)
Less than once per week	12 (1.9%)
2. How much times do you spend on each defaecation?	
Less than 30 min.	402 (64.1%)
31–60 min.	190 (30.3%)
More than an hour	35 (5.6%)
3. Do you experience uneasiness, sweating or headaches during or after defaecation?	
Yes	150 (23.9%)
No	478 (76.1%)
4. Do you take medication (tablets) to treat constipation?	
Yes	281 (45.0%)
No	344 (55.0%)
5. Do you take medication (drops or liquid) to treat constipation?	
Yes	170 (27.2%)
No	455 (72.8%)
6. How often do you use digital evacuation?	
Less than once per week (score 0)	329 (52.6%)
Once or more per week (score 6)	297 (47.4%)

Table 2. *Cont.*

NBD Score	*n* (%)
7. How often do you have involuntary defaecation?	
Daily	5 (0.8%)
1–6 times a week	19 (3.0%)
3–4 times a month	83 (13.3%)
A few times a year or less	518 (82.9%)
8. Do you take medication to treat faecal incontinence?	
Yes	23 (3.7%)
No	605 (96.3%)
9. Do you experience uncontrollable flatus?	
Yes	379 (60.4%)
No	248 (39.6%)
10. Do you have peri-anal skin problems?	
Yes	118 (19.0%)
No	508 (81.2%)

3.2. Satisfaction with Bowel Function

In total, 132 (21%) rated satisfaction with their bowel function within the past 4 weeks as good, 324 (53%) as acceptable, 136 (22%) as bad and 25 (4%) as very bad (Table 3).

Table 3. Distribution of responses according to the NBD score and patient satisfaction before adjusting for special attention symptoms.

NBD Score	Patient Satisfaction			
	Good	Acceptable	Poor	Very Poor
14 or more	9 (1.5%)	44 (7.1%)	51 (8.3%)	17 (2.8%)
10–13	27 (4.4%)	75 (12.2%)	36 (5.8%)	3 (0.5%)
0–9	96 (15.6%)	205 (33.3%)	49 (7.9%)	5 (0.8%)

Based on 617 respondents, 20 (3%) respondents had incomplete responses to calculate the NDB score or did not answer patient satisfaction. Percentages are of the total number of complete responses.

3.3. Special Attention Symptoms

Special attention symptoms were experienced by 224 (38%). These included intense pain in the abdomen or rectum (n = 116, 20%), new or increased bleeding from the anus (n = 92, 16%), hospitalisation due to bowel problems within the last year (n = 29, 5%), reduction in independence with regard to bowel care (n = 51, 9%) and episodes of autonomic dysreflexia related to bowel management (n = 87, 15%).

3.4. The MENTOR Tool

According to the MENTOR tool, the proposed clinical decision was to "monitor/control" (green) in 281 (44%), "discuss treatment options" (yellow) in 175 (27%) and "act/change treatment" in 181 (28%) (Table 3). Table 3 presents the MENTOR classification before adjusting for special attention symptoms. In total, 134 (21%) changed MENTOR group due to special attention symptoms, and across the MENTOR groups the median (IQR) number of special attention symptoms was 0 (0–0) for green, 0 (0–1) for yellow and 1 (1–2) red.

There was a significant association between the increasing need for change in treatment and age of the respondents (p = 0.016). There was no association between response to the MENTOR and time since SCI (p = 0.155), gender (p = 0.106), sensory completeness (p = 0.868) or motor completeness of the lesion (p = 0.263).

3.5. Effects of Neurogenic Bowel Dysfunction on Daily Life

Among respondents, 240 (38%) reported that NBD restricted various aspects of daily life (Figure 1). Thus, 36 (6%) reported that NBD prevented them from having income-generating work, 54 (9%) from volunteering in organizations or similar, 150 (24%) from social activities with family or friends, 54 (9%) from daily activities in or around the home (washing dishes, cleaning, shopping or similar), 115 (18%) from sports or other physical activity, 128 (20%) from cultural events (cinema, theatre, concerts, sporting events, zoo, circus or similar), 89 (14%) from nature experiences (a walk in the woods or to the beach, bird watching, star gazing or similar), 78 (12%) from shopping (groceries, clothing, electronics or similar) and 35 (6%) from other activities.

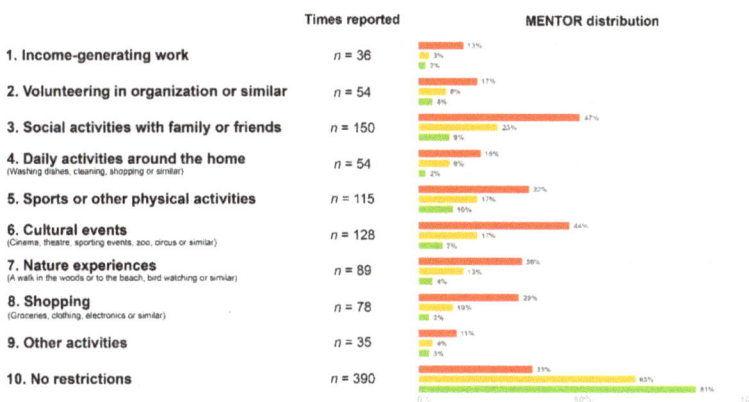

Figure 1. Daily restrictions experienced by the respondents and relative frequency according Monitoring Efficacy of Neurogenic bowel dysfunction Treatment on Response (MENTOR) group. Label: mentor frequencies are derived from the relative count divided by the total number of patients in each of the three MENTOR groups.

The recommendation from the MENTOR was associated with self-reported impairment of one or more aspects of daily life due to NBD ($p < 0.0001$) (Table 4). Among respondents reporting that NBD caused some restriction of daily life, the MENTOR would recommend "discuss treatment" (yellow) or "act/change treatment" (red) in 77% and "monitor/control" (green) in 23%. If respondents reported no restriction in daily activities, the MENTOR recommended "monitor/control" (green) or "discuss treatment" (yellow) in 85% and "act/change treatment" (red) in 15%. Among the respondents for whom the MENTOR recommended "monitor/control" (green), 81% reported no impairment of daily life because of NBD. Among those for whom MENTOR recommended "act/change treatment" (red), 67% reported some impairment in daily life due to NBD.

Table 4. Self-reported restriction in various aspects of daily life within the three MENTOR groups.

	Green $n = 281$	Yellow $n = 175$	Red $n = 181$
Income-generating work	6 (2.14%)	6 (3.43%)	24 (13.26%)
Volunteering in organization or similar	10 (3.56%)	14 (8%)	30 (16.57%)
Social activities with family or friends	24 (8.54%)	41 (23.43%)	85 (46.96%)
Daily activities around the home (washing dishes, cleaning, shopping or similar)	5 (1.78%)	16 (9.14%)	33 (18.23%)
Sports or other physical activities	28 (9.96%)	29 (16.57%)	58 (32.04%)
Cultural events (cinema, theatre, sporting events, zoo, circus or similar)	19 (6.76%)	29 (16.57%)	80 (44.2%)
Nature experiences (a walk in the woods or to the beach, bird watching or similar)	12 (4.27%)	22 (12.57%)	55 (30.39%)
Shopping (groceries, clothing, electronics or similar)	8 (2.85%)	18 (10.29%)	52 (28.73%)
Other activities	9 (3.2%)	7 (4%)	19 (10.5%)
No restrictions	228 (81.14%)	110 (62.86%)	59 (32.6%)

4. Discussion

The MENTOR was developed as an easy-to-use instrument for assessment of the need for change in bowel care in individuals with SCI [13]. It incorporates the commonly used 10-item NBD score; patient satisfaction with current treatment; and so called "special attention symptoms", which indicate unsatisfactory bowel management. Based on the MENTOR, the potential need for change in bowel care is classified as either "monitor", indicating that bowel care is sufficient; "discuss", indicating that there may be a need for change; and "act", indicating that bowel care is unsatisfactory and that there is a need for change. The grouping of responses into the three categories corresponds well with the opinion of experts in NBD [13]. The main finding of the present study was that 56% of non-hospitalised persons with SCI had a need for discussion or change of bowel management. This includes 28% who most likely had a serious need for change. The secondary finding was that results from the MENTOR were associated with restriction in various social activities caused by NBD. This further validates the MENTOR as a clinical tool and supports its future use in a non-hospital setting.

Diseases or lesions within the spinal cord disrupt normal bowel function. Anorectal sensation is reduced or lost, rectal evacuation at defecation is reduced and transit time through the colon is prolonged [14–16]. The resulting symptom complex is usually termed NBD. Most common symptoms of NBD are constipation and faecal incontinence [2,3]. Neurogenic bowel dysfunction severely restricts social activities and has a negative impact on quality of life. Within recent decades, several new treatment modalities have been introduced against NBD [17,18]. A detailed description of treatment algorithms for NBD is beyond the scope of the present paper. However, a stepwise treatment algorithm has been endorsed and described in detail in previous publications [5,19]. Unfortunately, the improvement in treatment options has not yet sufficiently changed clinical practice. Thus, most persons with NBD due to SCI have used the same method for bowel care in spite of 40% being dissatisfied with their bowel function. Insufficiently treated NBD is unfortunate because correct treatment is both cost-effective and improves the quality of life of the patient [20–22]. It is for this reason that the MENTOR instrument was developed, to identify individuals at need for change of method for bowel care.

Neurogenic bowel dysfunction is a clinical diagnosis. Thus, several symptom-based instruments for assessment of NBD have been developed and recently critically reviewed [17]. The most commonly used and best validated tool was found to be the NBD score, which includes 10 items describing various aspects of NBD [9]. Each item is weighted from its impact on quality of life. The score was developed among Danish persons with SCI, and it was later validated among patients with multiple sclerosis. Lately, it has been incorporated in the International SCI Bowel Function Data Set [19]. The NBD score was not created for decision making in individual patients. For this purpose, and to facilitate the progression through treatment, the MENTOR was developed.

The MENTOR includes three dimensions: the NBD score, patient satisfaction with current treatment of NBD and special attention symptoms. The latter are single symptoms or experiences that strongly indicate severe bowel dysfunction whether related to NBD or not. Interestingly, 38% of respondents reported one or more of such symptoms, the commonest being pain or bleeding from the rectum. These symptoms do not only indicate that treatment of NBD is insufficient, but they may also be alarm symptoms warning the clinician that other pathology could be present. Spinal cord injury mainly affects the colorectum and the anal canal. The effects of NBD are, however, not limited to these segments. Fynne et al. found that transit through the upper gastrointestinal tract was delayed in persons with SCI [23]. Moreover, constipation or anorectal digitation during bowel care may cause autonomic dysreflexia with very high blood pressure in persons with SCI above the sixth thoracic level [6,24]. Insufficient treatment of NBD increases the risk of urinary tract infections and causes hospitalization [18,20,25]. Hence, some of the special attention symptoms were included to cover consequences of NBD beyond bowel symptoms.

The awareness about NBD has increased dramatically in recent decades [3]. It is increasingly recognised that autonomic consequences of SCI should be considered equally with the impairment of motor function [17,19,26]. Most persons with SCI rate NBD among the three most bothersome consequences of SCI. Even though NBD is life-long, it is not a stable condition. Constipation and impairment of quality of life become more severe with time since injury [27–29]. This calls for life-long control of bowel function. We find that MENTOR qualifies for this purpose both among patients seen in hospital and in the community.

There are limitations to the present study. To ensure an acceptable response rate to our survey, we had to keep the mailed questionnaire short and simple. For this reason, we choose to compare the recommendations from the MENTOR with the self-reported impact on various aspects of daily life. These items were developed by members of the Danish Paraplegic Association but have not been validated. The inclusion of a validated score for quality of life would have been preferable. In the previous study on the MENTOR tool, the recommendations "monitor/control" (green) and "act/change treatment" (red) correlated well with the opinion of experienced experts. In the present study, there was a fair correlation between the same recommendations from the MENTOR and the self-reported impairment of daily life. Like in a previous publication, the middle group "discuss" (yellow) performed less well [13]. In our opinion this does not disqualify the MENTOR, because a recommendation of "discuss" will lead to a decision of monitoring or to act after the discussion with the patient. The majority of respondents (61%) were males. We do not know the exact male/female proportion among members of the Danish Paraplegic association, but there are significantly more male than female members. Hence, the gender distribution among respondents most likely reflects that of the association.

The present study was restricted to adult persons with NBD due to SCI. Several other groups of patients suffer from NBD too. Thus, NBD is reported by approximately 50% of patients with multiple sclerosis or spina bifida. The NBD score has proven useful in patients with NBD caused by multiple sclerosis [8,30]. Future studies will determine whether the MENTOR is applicable outside an SCI population. Healthcare systems are changing around the world, and electronic collection and remote monitoring of patients reported outcomes will without doubt become a part of clinical monitoring of future patients. The MENTOR is easily understandable and takes approximate 5 min to complete [13]. In the present study, we found it useful as part of a survey.

5. Conclusions

In conclusion, we found that 28% of non-hospitalised persons with SCI had bowel symptoms mandating a change in methods for bowel care and another 27% had a need for discussion of a potential change in treatment strategy. Moreover, recommendations from the MENTOR correlated with self-reported impairment of daily activities caused by NBD.

Author Contributions: Formal analysis, S.D.S.S. and S.M.D.B.; Supervision, K.K.; Writing original draft, S.D.S.S.; Writing review & editing, S.D.S.S., S.M.D.B., A.E., P.C. and K.K. All authors have read and agreed to the published version of the manuscript.

Funding: The study was supported by an educational grant from Coloplast, Denmark.

Informed Consent Statement: According to Danish legislation, questionnaire studies do not need approval from Ethics Committee.

Acknowledgments: The Danish Paraplegic Association (RYK) and Stig Langvad are thanked for their assistance.

Conflicts of Interest: The authors declare no conflict of interest. The funders had no role in the design of the study; in the collection, analyses, or interpretation of data; in the writing of the manuscript, or in the decision to publish the results.

References

1. Ebert, E. Gastrointestinal involvement in spinal cord injury: A clinical perspective. *J. Gastrointestin Liver Dis.* **2012**, *21*, 75–82. [PubMed]
2. Krogh, K.; Nielsen, J.; Djurhuus, J.C.; Mosdal, C.; Sabroe, S.; Laurberg, S. Colorectal function in patients with spinal cord lesions. *Dis. Colon Rectum.* **1997**, *40*, 1233–1239. [CrossRef] [PubMed]
3. Glickman, S.; Kamm, M.A. Bowel dysfunction in spinal-cord-injury patients. *Lancet* **1996**, *347*, 1651–1653. [CrossRef]
4. Pardee, C.; Bricker, D.; Rundquist, J.; MacRae, C.; Tebben, C. Characteristics of neurogenic bowel in spinal cord injury and perceived quality of life. *Rehabil. Nurs.* **2012**, *37*, 128–135. [CrossRef] [PubMed]
5. Emmanuel, A.V.; Krogh, K.; Bazzocchi, G.; Leroi, A.M.; Bremers, A.; Leder, D.; van Kuppevelt, D.; Mosiello, G.; Vogel, M.; Perrouin-Verbe, B.; et al. Consensus review of best practice of transanal irrigation in adults. *Spinal Cord* **2013**, *51*, 732–738. [CrossRef] [PubMed]
6. Inskip, J.A.; Lucci, V.M.; McGrath, M.S.; Willms, R.; Claydon, V.E. A Community Perspective on Bowel Management and Quality of Life after Spinal Cord Injury: The Influence of Autonomic Dysreflexia. *J. Neurotrauma.* **2018**, *35*, 1091–1105. [CrossRef] [PubMed]
7. Emmanuel, A. Managing neurogenic bowel dysfunction. *Clin. Rehabil.* **2010**, *24*, 483–488. [CrossRef]
8. Coggrave, M.; Norton, C. Management of faecal incontinence and constipation in adults with central neurological diseases. *Cochrane Database Syst. Rev.* **2013**. [CrossRef]
9. Krogh, K.; Christensen, P.; Sabroe, S.; Laurberg, S. Neurogenic bowel dysfunction score. *Spinal Cord* **2006**, *44*, 625–631. [CrossRef]
10. Mallek, A.; Elleuch, M.H.; Ghroubi, S. Neurogenic bowel dysfunction (NBD) translation and linguistic validation to classical Arabic. *Prog. Urol.* **2016**, *26*, 553–557. [CrossRef]
11. Erdem, D.; Hava, D.; Keskinoğlu, P.; Bircan, Ç.; Peker, Ö.; Krogh, K.; Gülbahar, S. Reliability, validity and sensitivity to change of neurogenic bowel dysfunction score in patients with spinal cord injury. *Spinal Cord* **2017**, *55*, 1084–1087. [CrossRef]
12. Krause, J.S.; Kjorsvig, J.M. Mortality after spinal cord injury: A four-year prospective study. *Arch. Phys. Med. Rehabil.* **1992**, *73*, 558–563. [CrossRef]
13. Emmanuel, A.; Krogh, K.; Kirshblum, S.; Christensen, P.; Spinelli, M.; van Kuppevelt, D.; Abel, R.; Leder, D.; Santacruz, B.G.; Bain, K.; et al. Creation and validation of a new tool for the monitoring efficacy of neurogenic bowel dysfunction treatment on response: The MENTOR tool. *Spinal Cord.* **2020**, *58*, 795–802. [CrossRef] [PubMed]
14. Krogh, K.; Mosdal, C.; Gregersen, H.; Laurberg, S. Rectal wall properties in patients with acute and chronic spinal cord lesions. *Dis. Colon Rectum.* **2002**, *45*, 641–649. [CrossRef]
15. Krogh, K.; Olsen, N.; Christensen, P.; Madsen, J.L.; Laurberg, S. Colorectal transport during defecation in patients with lesions of the sacral spinal cord. *Neurogastroenterol. Motil.* **2003**, *15*, 25–31. [CrossRef] [PubMed]
16. Rasmussen, M.M.; Krogh, K.; Clemmensen, D.; Bluhme, H.; Rawashdeh, Y.; Christensen, P. Colorectal transport during defecation in subjects with supraconal spinal cord injury. *Spinal Cord* **2013**, *51*, 683–687. [CrossRef] [PubMed]
17. Tate, D.G.; Wheeler, T.; Lane, G.I.; Forchheimer, M.; Anderson, K.D.; Biering-Sorensen, F.; Cameron, A.P.; Santacruz, B.G.; Jakeman, L.B.; Kennelly, M.J.; et al. Recommendations for evaluation of neurogenic bladder and bowel dysfunction after spinal cord injury and/or disease. *J. Spinal Cord Med.* **2020**, *43*, 141–164. [CrossRef]
18. Krassioukov, A.; Eng, J.J.; Claxton, G.; Sakakibara, B.M.; Shum, S. Neurogenic bowel management after spinal cord injury: A systematic review of the evidence. *Spinal Cord* **2010**, *48*, 718–733. [CrossRef]
19. Krogh, K.; Emmanuel, A.; Perrouin-Verbe, B.; Korsten, M.A.; Mulcahey, M.J.; Biering-Sørensen, F. International spinal cord injury bowel function basic data set (Version 2.0). *Spinal Cord* **2017**, *55*, 692–698. [CrossRef]
20. Christensen, P.; Bazzocchi, G.; Coggrave, M.; Abel, R.; Hultling, C.; Krogh, K.; Media, S.; Laurberg, S. A randomized, controlled trial of transanal irrigation versus conservative bowel management in spinal cord-injured patients. *Gastroenterology* **2006**, *131*, 738–747. [CrossRef]
21. Burns, A.S.; St-Germain, D.; Connolly, M.; Delparte, J.J.; Guindon, A.; Hitzig, S.L.; Craven, B.C. Phenomenological study of neurogenic bowel from the perspective of individuals living with spinal cord injury. *Arch. Phys. Med. Rehabil.* **2015**, *96*, 49–55. [CrossRef] [PubMed]
22. Emmanuel, A.; Kumar, G.; Christensen, P.; Mealing, S.; Størling, Z.M.; Andersen, F.; Kirshblum, S. Long-Term Cost-Effectiveness of Transanal Irrigation in Patients with Neurogenic Bowel Dysfunction. *PLoS ONE* **2016**, *11*, e0159394. [CrossRef] [PubMed]
23. Fynne, L.; Worsøe, J.; Gregersen, T.; Schlageter, V.; Laurberg, S.; Krogh, K. Gastric and small intestinal dysfunction in spinal cord injury patients. *Acta Neurol. Scand.* **2012**, *125*, 123–128. [CrossRef] [PubMed]
24. Faaborg, P.M.; Christensen, P.; Krassioukov, A.; Laurberg, S.; Frandsen, E.; Krogh, K. Autonomic dysreflexia during bowel evacuation procedures and bladder filling in subjects with spinal cord injury. *Spinal Cord* **2014**, *52*, 494–498. [CrossRef]
25. Coggrave, M.; Norton, C.; Wilson-Barnett, J. Management of neurogenic bowel dysfunction in the community after spinal cord injury: A postal survey in the United Kingdom. *Spinal Cord* **2009**, *47*, 323–330, quiz 331-323. [CrossRef]
26. Alexander, M.S.; Biering-Sorensen, F.; Bodner, D.; Brackett, N.L.; Cardenas, D.; Charlifue, S.; Creasey, G.; Dietz, V.; Ditunno, J.; Donovan, W.; et al. International standards to document remaining autonomic function after spinal cord injury. *Spinal Cord* **2009**, *47*, 36–43. [CrossRef]
27. Faaborg, P.M.; Christensen, P.; Finnerup, N.; Laurberg, S.; Krogh, K. The pattern of colorectal dysfunction changes with time since spinal cord injury. *Spinal Cord* **2008**, *46*, 234–238. [CrossRef]

28. Faaborg, P.M.; Christensen, P.; Rosenkilde, M.; Laurberg, S.; Krogh, K. Do gastrointestinal transit times and colonic dimensions change with time since spinal cord injury? *Spinal Cord* **2011**, *49*, 549–553. [CrossRef]

29. Nielsen, S.D.; Faaborg, P.M.; Finnerup, N.B.; Christensen, P.; Krogh, K. Ageing with neurogenic bowel dysfunction. *Spinal Cord* **2017**, *55*, 769–773. [CrossRef]

30. Burns, A.S.; St-Germain, D.; Connolly, M.; Delparte, J.J.; Guindon, A.; Hitzig, S.L.; Craven, B.C. Neurogenic bowel after spinal cord injury from the perspective of support providers: A phenomenological study. *Phys. Med. Rehabil. Clin.* **2015**, *7*, 407–416. [CrossRef]

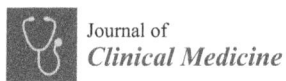

Journal of
Clinical Medicine

MDPI

Review

Pharmacological Management of Neurogenic Bowel Dysfunction after Spinal Cord Injury and Multiple Sclerosis: A Systematic Review and Clinical Implications

Jeffery S Johns [1],*, Klaus Krogh [2], Karen Ethans [3], Joanne Chi [4], Matthew Quérée [4,5], Janice J Eng [4,5] and Spinal Cord Injury Research Evidence Team [†]

[1]   Department of Physical Medicine and Rehabilitation, Vanderbilt University Medical Center, Nashville, TN 37232, USA
[2]   Department of Hepatology and Gastroenterology, Aarhus University Hospital, 8200 Aarhus, Denmark; klaus.krogh@clin.au.dk
[3]   Physical Medicine and Rehabilitation, University of Manitoba, Winnipeg Health Sciences Centre, Winnipeg, MB R3A 1R9, Canada; kethans@hsc.mb.ca
[4]   Department of Physical Therapy, University of British Columbia and Rehabilitation Research Program, GF Strong Rehab Centre, Vancouver, BC V5Z 2G9, Canada; joanne.chi.1999@gmail.com (J.C.); matthew.queree@ubc.ca (M.Q.); JANICE.ENG@UBC.CA (J.J.E.)
[5]   Spinal Cord Injury Research Evidence Team, Vancouver, BC V5Z 2G9, Canada
*   Correspondence: Jeff.Johns@Vanderbilt.edu; Tel.: +615-322-0738
[†]   The Spinal Cord Injury Research Evidence Team Executive consists of: Dalton Wolfe, Jane Hsieh, Dr. Bob Teasell, Dr. Eldon Loh, Shannon Sproule, Vanessa Noonan, Dr. Andrea Townson, Bill Miller, Ben Mortenson, Amanda McIntyre, Matthew Quérée and Janice J Eng. Their business is proving executive leadership for the SCIRE Project, reviewing the SCI literature, and writing the SCIRE chapters; scire.project@ubc.ca.

Citation: Johns, J.S; Krogh, K.; Ethans, K.; Chi, J.; Quérée, M.; Eng, J.J.; Pharmacological Management of Neurogenic Bowel Dysfunction after Spinal Cord Injury and Multiple Sclerosis: A Systematic Review and Clinical Implications. *J. Clin. Med.* **2021**, *10*, 882. https://doi.org/10.3390/jcm10040882

Academic Editor: Marilena Durazzo

Received: 27 January 2021
Accepted: 18 February 2021
Published: 22 February 2021

Publisher's Note: MDPI stays neutral with regard to jurisdictional claims in published maps and institutional affiliations.

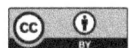

Copyright: © 2021 by the authors. Licensee MDPI, Basel, Switzerland. This article is an open access article distributed under the terms and conditions of the Creative Commons Attribution (CC BY) license (https://creativecommons.org/licenses/by/4.0/).

Abstract: Neurogenic bowel dysfunction (NBD) is a common problem for people with spinal cord injury (SCI) and multiple sclerosis (MS), which seriously impacts quality of life. Pharmacological management is an important component of conservative bowel management. The objective of this study was to first assemble a list of pharmacological agents (medications and medicated suppositories) used in current practice. Second, we systematically examined the current literature on pharmacological agents to manage neurogenic bowel dysfunction of individuals specifically with SCI or MS. We searched Medline, EMBASE and CINAHL databases up to June 2020. We used the GRADE System to provide a systematic approach for evaluating the evidence. Twenty-eight studies were included in the review. We found a stark discrepancy between the large number of agents currently prescribed and a very limited amount of literature. While there was a small amount of literature in SCI, there was little to no literature available for MS. There was low-quality evidence supporting rectal medications, which are a key component of conservative bowel care in SCI. Based on the findings of the literature and the clinical experience of the authors, we have provided clinical insights on proposed treatments and medications in the form of three case study examples on patients with SCI or MS.

Keywords: spinal cord injury; multiple sclerosis; neurogenic bowel dysfunction; pharmacological; systematic review

1. Introduction

Neurogenic bowel dysfunction (NBD) is a prevalent issue for people with neurological disorders; changes in bowel motility and sphincter control can present a major problem for people with spinal cord injury (SCI) and multiple sclerosis (MS). The reported prevalence of NBD varies, with most reports of constipation occurring in the range of 30–40% of people with chronic SCI. However, some studies have found the prevalence of constipation to be closer to 80%, and upwards of 75% of individuals with SCI experience fecal incontinence [1,2]. NBD is also prevalent in people with MS. A systematic review found the prevalence of constipation to range from 18–43%, and fecal incontinence occurs in 3–51% of people with MS, based on studies with over 100 patients [3]. In the general population, constipation and fecal incontinence have been reported to be 19.7% and 4.3% respectively, in a 70,000-plus population-based sample, with increasing prevalence in older age patients [4]. Thus, it is clear that bowel dysfunction is far more prevalent in people with SCI and MS and requires special attention.

Bowel dysfunction due to SCI or MS has a substantial negative impact on quality of life [5]. Even when a bowel program is in place to effectively manage NBD, it can be onerous and time-consuming and may take up to 1–2 h per session, repeated every day or alternate days. It can interfere significantly with a person's education, work, and social life and presents a major challenge to quality of life, independence, and community reintegration after SCI. Loss of bowel control is a source of anxiety and distress [6,7]. Treatment of bowel dysfunction rates highly for patients in both clinical and research domains of SCI and MS [8,9]. Regaining bowel function has been ranked similarly in priority to regaining walking after SCI [10].

The major symptoms of NBD are fecal incontinence and constipation. Fecal incontinence is the accidental passing of bowel movements, including solid stools, liquid stools, or mucus. This often occurs if muscles in the rectum and anus are not functioning to store and hold back a bowel movement due to muscle injury or nervous system damage, as well as a loss of rectal sensation [11]. Constipation is defined as a reduction in the frequency of stools, but a lack of a daily bowel movement is not necessarily equivalent to constipation as some people have as few as three bowel movements per week. Symptoms of constipation could include difficulty with stool passage, infrequent bowel movements or passage of hard stools [12].

Generally, people with higher and more severe injuries tend to have more significant bowel dysfunction, particularly constipation [13]; the studies by Liu [14,15] found that severity of NBD was significantly higher for people with higher American Spinal Cord Injury Association Impairment Scale (AIS) score classification and that people with AIS A SCI were at 12.8 times greater risk of severe NBD than those with AIS D.

There are two distinct patterns in the clinical presentation of bowel dysfunction in SCI: injury above the conus medullaris results in upper motor neuron (UMN) bowel syndrome, while injury at the conus medullaris and cauda equina results in lower motor neuron (LMN) bowel syndrome [2,16]. The upper motor neuron bowel, or hyperreflexic bowel, usually occurs with injuries above the sacral spinal cord and is characterized by loss of voluntary (cortical) control of the external anal sphincter, which remains involuntarily overactive, thereby promoting retention of stool. Transit time is prolonged throughout the colon. Fecal incontinence occurs concomitantly in many cases due to reduced or absent anorectal sensation and lack of voluntary control of the external anal sphincter muscle. Although there is the loss of supraspinal control, the nerve connections between the spinal cord and the colon remain intact; therefore, there is preserved reflex coordination and stool propulsion. Stool evacuation in these individuals occurs in response to stimulation of reflex activity, such as the presence of feces in the rectum, a suppository, enema, or digital rectal stimulation causing rectal distension.

The lower motor neuron bowel, or areflexic bowel, usually occurs with injuries at the sacral spinal cord or below and is characterized by the loss of centrally mediated (spinal cord) peristalsis and loss of reflex activity, resulting in slow stool propulsion and impaired reflex stool evacuation. Segmental colonic peristalsis occurs only due to the activity of the enteric nervous system, which is slower and less efficient without the centrally mediated peristalsis. The result is increased transit time through the distal colon and rectum with the production of drier and round-shaped stool. Lower motor neuron bowel syndrome is commonly associated with constipation. There is also a substantial risk for fecal incontinence due to the atonic external anal sphincter and lack of sensation and voluntary control over the external anal sphincter muscle.

In MS, the pattern of bowel dysfunction is similar to the pattern described for SCI. The neurological lesion is, however, less well defined in MS. The presence of bowel symptoms in MS is correlated to the expanded disability status scale [17], to the degree of spinal atrophy [18], and to disease duration, but not particularly with the type of MS [19]. The precise neuropathological mechanism in NBD and MS is not completely defined, but one study theorizes that at the cortical level, demyelination within the frontal lobe may affect a person's voluntary control over bowel movements [20]. Regardless, it has been noted that severe constipation is often one of the first presenting symptoms of MS [21].

A regular bowel program helps to ensure that evacuation occurs regularly– facilitating continence and reducing constipation. Prevention of constipation will reduce symptoms, such as abdominal pain and bloating and minimize the development of anorectal morbidities associated with NBD, including hemorrhoids, anal fissure, rectal abscess, and rectal prolapse.

A comprehensive bowel program will combine a number of interventions in an individualized routine and may include a specific diet to ensure adequate fiber and fluid, digital rectal stimulation, digital removal of stool, stimulation of the gastrocolic reflex, and use of oral or rectal (suppositories, enemas) medication. The different components of a bowel program are illustrated in Figure 1. Such a program will usually be performed on a daily or alternate day basis, depending on the needs of the individual. Undertaking physical activity, including standing and passive movements, may also help to reduce constipation. Some medications that are being used for other medical conditions or symptoms may also contribute to constipation. If these additional medications cannot be eliminated, stool softeners or oral laxatives may be used to modulate stool consistency and promote stool transit.

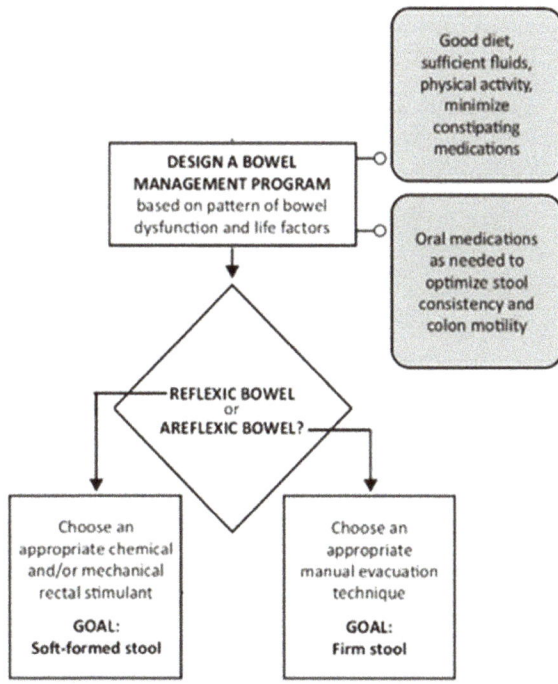

Figure 1. Designing a neurogenic bowel program. Reprinted (a portion of the original algorithm) from "Management of Neurogenic Bowel Dysfunction in Adults after Spinal Cord Injury: Clinical Practical Guidelines for Healthcare Providers (2020), with permission from Paralyzed Veterans of America.

Neurogenic bowel guidelines [22,23] recommend that a conservative bowel program should be developed initially in the rehabilitation phase following injury and that a comprehensive evaluation of bowel function and management is undertaken at least annually. The evaluation may include a patient history (including a detailed history of current bowel routine management, stool form, continence and time spent on evacuation, diet and fluid intake, relevant medical conditions and medications, the extent of care provision and home adaptations) and a detailed physical examination (including neurological examination to determine level and completeness of SCI as well as an abdominal and rectal examination). In some centers, comprehensive assessment tools, such as the International Spinal Cord Society (ISCoS) Bowel Data Set, are used to collect this information in a standardized manner.

A recent systematic review by Musco et al. [24] assessed the literature on all NBD treatments for adults, including both pharmacological and non-pharmacological approaches. From the results of the six studies included in the section on pharmacological treatments, there were statistically significant increases in weekly bowel movements and a decrease in colonic transit time with the use of 2 mg of prucalopride among individuals with SCI. However, there were no significant improvements in the duration of bowel care or the reduction of fecal incontinence and the need for digital evacuation of stool. In addition, the review found that mechanical evacuation (tap water enema) without oral stimulant laxatives was superior in bowel control (time required for evacuation) compared to irritant and stimulant-medication groups. Furthermore, from the six studies, only three included populations of individuals with SCI and none with MS, presenting a need for further investigation and clinical insights on the effectiveness of pharmacological management in NBD among both populations.

Hence, the objective of this investigation was to first assemble a list of current pharmacological agents (medications and medicated suppositories) used in current practice through the clinical expertise of our team, which included members from the United States, Europe, and Canada. Second, we systematically examined the current literature to determine the potential in managing NBD of individuals specifically with SCI or MS. We also reviewed literature outside of our designated populations of interest and with regards to other methods of bowel management to inform our approach and help us provide guidance for healthcare professionals as to when it is appropriate and timely to prescribe medication for NBD. Based on the findings of the literature and the clinical experience of the authors, we have provided clinical insights on proposed treatments and medications in the form of three case study examples on patients with SCI or MS.

2. Methods

2.1. List of Current Pharmacological Agents

We generated a list of current pharmacological agents (medications, medicated suppositories) prescribed for adults with NBD through a combination of clinical expertise from the United States, Canada and Europe and web-based searches on the drug monographs to define generic and trade names and common side effects.

2.2. Literature Search and Study Selection

We searched the electronic databases Ovid MEDLINE®, EMBASE, and CINAHL for relevant literature dated from 1980 through June 2020, using search terms related to adult bowel dysfunction (e.g., constipation, bowel/fecal incontinence), spinal cord injury (e.g., paraplegia, tetraplegia, spinal cord injury/dysfunction), Multiple Sclerosis (or MS), and the brand names/generic names of all medications used for bowel dysfunction suggested by the author team and the university health librarian. We also identified additional studies through hand-searching the reference lists of included studies and reviews. Studies on medications for colonoscopy preparation were excluded as they do not reflect treatments for daily bowel management.

Two reviewers independently assessed titles and abstracts of citations for inclusion and the quality of the studies, with disagreements resolved by a third person. Review articles were only included if it was a systematic review. All articles were limited to English only. Animal studies and articles describing the neurophysiology of bowel were excluded. Duplicate studies were identified and removed using RefWorks management software (Ex Libris, Ann Arbor, MI, USA).

2.3. Inclusion Criteria

Three principles guided study inclusion: (1) studies were included if the population of interest was people with SCI or MS, (2) if they measured any outcomes related to bowel or bowel-related dysfunction (e.g., using the NBD or Wexner scores, or reporting the number of occurrences of fecal incontinence or constipation, colonic transit time, or duration/frequency of bowel movements), and (3) if the independent variable or inquiry of interest was some form of medication (e.g., prucalopride) and/or medicated suppository (e.g., bisacodyl). We endeavored to include all research designs, but qualitative studies and case reports were excluded. Results published only in abstract form or in conference proceedings *could be included* if adequate details were available for quality assessment (e.g., risk of bias) and if the area of inquiry had relatively little published information. Mixed populations were acceptable if the sample consisted of at least 20% people with SCI or MS.

2.4. Data Extraction and Synthesis

We extracted information from included studies and constructed evidence tables showing the study characteristics, outcomes, adverse effects, and quality ratings/risk of bias for all included studies. We presented the studies using a hierarchy of evidence approach, where the best evidence is presented first in tables and is the focus of any results, point estimates, or conclusions. If no literature was found for a commonly used medication (e.g., oral laxative), then practice guidelines or meta-analyses were sought in non-NBD populations (e.g., individuals with idiopathic chronic constipation).

2.5. Validity Assessment (Risk of Bias)

We used the grading of recommendations, assessment, development, and evaluations (GRADE) system to provide a systematic approach for evaluating the evidence [25]. We assessed the internal validity (risk of bias) of trials, observational studies, and systematic reviews, which include an evaluation of randomization, allocation concealment, blinding, the similarity of compared groups at baseline, loss to follow-up, and the accounting for any statistical confounds.

A study with a high attrition rate (e.g., 15% or greater) or a low response rate (lower than 50%) was automatically rated as a high risk of bias. Systematic reviews were rated on the clarity of review question, specification of inclusion and exclusion criteria, use of multiple databases for searching, sufficient detail of included studies, adequate assessment of the risk of bias of included studies, and providing an adequate summary of primary studies. Observational studies were rated on non-biased selection, loss to follow-up, pre-specification of outcomes, well-described and adequate ascertainment techniques, statistical analysis of potential confounders, and adequate duration of follow-up.

3. Results

3.1. Current Bowel Oral Medication and Medicated Suppositories

Table 1 provides an overview of current medications identified by our expert clinicians. A number of oral medications were identified. Docusate sodium is a commonly used stool softener that draws water into the stool, making it easier to pass. Osmotic softeners, such as polyethylene glycol (PEG), are laxatives that increase the moisture in the stool to make it easier to pass and are usually taken once or twice per day or as needed. Stimulant laxatives activate contractions of the intestinal wall, thereby promoting transit. Commonly used oral stimulant laxatives include bisacodyl and sennosides. Prokinetic agents stimulate the contraction of the muscle cells of the gut and promote transit. Like stimulant laxatives, prokinetic agents are medications that increase digestive tract muscle activity to move the stool through digestion. Secretory drugs increase intestinal fluids, which then accelerate intestinal transit. Narcotic antagonists are used to treating opioid-induced constipation without blocking the effect of narcotics on pain.

Table 1. Current Medications used in neurogenic bowel dysfunction (NBD), including mechanism of action.

Generic Names	Examples of Trademark Names	Mechanism of Action
Oral Laxatives		
Polyethylene glycol (PEG)	Miralax, Movicol, Restorolax, Lax a Day	Osmotic laxative
Magnesium hydroxide	Milk of Magnesia	Osmotic laxative
Docusate sodium	Colace, Surfak	Osmotic laxative
Lactulose	Lactulose, Kristalose	Osmotic laxative
Bisacodyl	Dulcolax	Stimulant laxative
Sennosides	ExLax, Senokot	Stimulant laxative
Rectal Laxatives		
Polyethylene glycol (peg)	Glycolax (suppository)	Osmotic laxative
Sodium citrate	Microlax (micro enema; also includes sodium lauryl and sorbitol)	Osmotic laxative
Bisacodyl	Dulcolax (suppository), Magic Bullet (suppository)	Stimulant laxative
Sennosides	Senokot (suppository)	Stimulant laxative
Docusate sodium	Colace (glycerin suppository or micro enema), Surfak, Enemeez (mini enema)	Stool softener laxative
Prokinetic drugs		
Prucalopride	Resotran, Resolor	Oral serotonin HT4 agonist with prokinetic properties
Secretory		
Linaclotide	Linzess or Constella	Oral guanylate cyclase-c agonist, which increases intestinal secretions
Narcotic Antagonists		
Naloxegol	Movantik, Movantig	Oral opioid antagonist
Lubiprostone	Amitiza	Oral opioid antagonist
Methylnaltrexone bromide	Relistor	Oral or subcutaneous injection opioid antagonist

Medicated suppositories and enemas are also commonly prescribed for NBD. Stimulant suppositories contain medications (such as bisacodyl) that stimulate the bowel reflex. Suppositories are usually inserted 15–30 min before planned bowel emptying. The time to bowel movement is influenced by the type and route of administration. For example, oral bisacodyl may produce a bowel movement within 6–12 h, a rectal bisacodyl suppository within an hour and a rectal bisacodyl enema within 20 m. However, the medication used and even the base that the medication is dissolved in can affect how quickly the medication is absorbed. For example, bisacodyl is a water-soluble polyethylene glycol base (e.g., Magic Bullet) that allows shorter times to empty than bisacodyl in a vegetable oil base [26,27]. Lubricating suppositories contain non-medicated substances (such as glycerin), which hold water in the bowel to make the stool softer, so it is easier to expel.

3.2. Systematic Review

We initially found 1850 articles, and after duplicates were removed, we reviewed 1576 potentially relevant records through our searches for medications (including medicated suppositories and enemas) and NBD in SCI and MS. We assessed 62 articles for eligibility at the full-text level and ultimately included 28 studies that assessed the effects of medication on NBD in the MS ($n = 2$) and SCI population ($n = 26$).

3.3. Indication and Efficacy by Medication from the Systematic Review

Detailed abstraction tables are available in the online supplementary. A summary of the evidence is provided below.

3.4. Oral Laxatives

Oral laxatives are the first-line treatment for constipation; however, no studies were found testing them specifically in SCI and MS, so we resorted to previous reviews conducted on the effects of medications on constipation in the general population. Luthra et al. [28] conducted a network meta-analysis to compare the efficacy of different medications in people with chronic idiopathic constipation. They found 33 RCTs conducted with 17,214 patients and found that stimulant laxatives bisacodyl and sodium picosulfate was ranked first after 4 weeks, and prucalopride was ranked first after 12 weeks of treatment. Similarly, Alsalimy et al. [29] found that senna and lactulose were superior to placebo when studied in long-term care patients. Paré and Fedorak [30] reviewed the literature and found that both nonstimulant and stimulant laxatives provided better relief than a placebo, albeit with minor side effects. In another meta-analysis, Nelson et al. [31] tested the number needed to treat (NNT) chronic constipation and found that osmotic and stimulant laxatives had an NNT of 3, lubiprostone had an NNT of 4, and prucalopride and linaclotide both had an NNT of 6. Note, none of these studies examined the long-term efficacy of these medications.

Given the lack of evidence in NBD populations, the prescription of oral laxatives relies on the above evidence from the general population and expert opinion. Oral laxatives are applicable to both areflexic and reflexic bowel management. In an individual with constipation after MS and SCI, we recommend starting with a simple agent, such as magnesium hydroxide (Milk of Magnesia) or PEG, which may have fewer adverse effects. Start the night before the bowel routine (typically every other day, or 3X/week), then reassess this regimen's effectiveness after a few weeks. It should be evaluated whether the oral medications are moving the stools toward their ideal consistency (soft, formed, bulky) and have resulted in improved evacuation. If not effective, a stimulant laxative can be tried. If the patient is in earlier stages of their injury (e.g., undergoing inpatient rehabilitation), more frequent assessments (every few days) and changes may be required.

Oral medications may address constipation but may not necessarily treat fecal incontinence. This may be due to the less predictable timing of results following oral medications. The goal of treating incontinence in NBD is to trigger a bowel evacuation at a patient-preferred time, so the movement does not occur as an unexpected or unplanned event, thus becoming incontinence. While there are no studies specifically on oral medications and fecal incontinence in the MS and SCI populations, a systematic review in adults with symptoms of fecal incontinence [32] found that medications, such as lactulose and loperamide, seemed to perform better than a placebo on measures of bowel function, such as frequency, urgency, and reduction in diarrhea, though more participants experienced adverse effects (e.g., constipation, abdominal pain, diarrhea, headache, and nausea).

3.5. Prokinetic Drugs

When oral laxatives are not effective, prokinetic drugs may be an alternative. Evidence for prokinetic drug studies was found for prucalopride, metoclopramide and neostigmine in SCI (1 RCT for prucalopride, 2 RCTs and one observational study for neostigmine, and two observational studies for metoclopramide). Metoclopramide stimulates the muscles of the gastrointestinal tract through dopamine and acetylcholine receptors and is approved for use to treat nausea and vomiting associated with chemotherapy, gastroesophageal reflux disease or diabetic gastroparesis. Though metoclopramide has been shown to be an effective drug to stimulate a one-time increase in gastric emptying in SCI [33], its role in ongoing neurogenic bowel management has not been established. Similarly, intravenous or intramuscular neostigmine has been shown to induce bowel evaluation in SCI but has not been tested in routine bowel management [34,35]. It is possible that metoclopramide or neostigmine may have a potential role in one-time bowel preparation procedures, such as colonoscopy in SCI.

Given that metoclopramide and neostigmine are not used for current neurogenic bowel management, the rest of this section will focus on prucalopride, a prokinetic agent that acts with high selectivity on serotonin type 4 receptors to initiate peristalsis, colonic mass movements, and facilitates defecation [36]. A systematic review of the general population found ten phase III trials that supported its efficacy and safety of prucalopride for the treatment of chronic idiopathic constipation and four phase IV trials, including one, which demonstrated efficacy over 24 months [37]. Prucalopride is recommended for idiopathic constipation if patients are not responsive to laxatives as the drug can have a high-cost [37]. Currently, tablet formulations of prucalopride have been approved in many countries and their regulating agencies, including the US Food and Drug Administration, Health Canada, and the European Medicines Agency.

A low-level of evidence, comprised of one RCT, may support the use of prucalopride to treat NBD after SCI; however, while confidence intervals were presented, no formal statistics were undertaken, which limits the interpretability of this study. Individuals who were treated with prucalopride may have experienced dose-dependent improvements in bowel movement frequency and perception of treatment efficacy. The greatest efficacy was observed at 2 mg daily dose where patients reported a 0.6 increase (95% CI 0.2 to 1.2) in weekly bowel frequency, a 73 median effectiveness rating (0 = ineffective and 100 = extremely effective), and a 38.5 h median decrease in colonic transit time [38]. Although patients receiving prucalopride perceived a higher treatment efficacy than those receiving the placebo, bowel frequency remained unchanged following a 4-week regimen of daily 1 mg prucalopride [38].

These outcomes should also be interpreted with caution as 50% of the 2 mg prucalopride group withdrew from the study, which introduces substantial bias [38]. In Krogh et al.'s study [38], adverse events were reported by 6/7 in the placebo group and by 7/8 and 6/8 in the 1 and 2 mg groups, respectively. Individuals receiving 1mg prucalopride treatment experienced the following complications more frequently than the placebo group: flatulence, bradycardia, headache, and diarrhea. Among those receiving the 2 mg prucalopride treatment, the following adverse effects were more common than in the placebo group: bradycardia, headache, abdominal pain, and diarrhea [38]. The primary medication-related reactions cited for withdrawal within the 2 mg group were headaches in combination with either abdominal pain or diarrhea [38]. The brand name Resotran monograph states hypersensitivity to Resotran, renal impairment requiring dialysis, and intestinal perforation or obstruction as contraindications [39]. Krogh et al.'s study [38] recommends starting individuals with SCI on a 1 mg daily dose before transitioning them to a 2 mg daily dose. The authors speculate that this protocol could potentially reduce dose-dependent increases in adverse events observed in the study [38].

3.6. Potassium Channel Blocker

Fampridine is a potassium channel blocker that can enhance synaptic transmission, and it has been approved for use to improve walking for adults with MS, but in a case series, 1 out of 23 MS participants reported improvements in urinary and fecal incontinence after six months of use [40]. Two of the four RCTs in SCI showed improvements in the number of bowel movements [41,42], but this was a secondary outcome of these studies. Currently, the mechanism by which fampridine may facilitate bowel function is unclear. While fampridine is not currently used for bowel management in current practice, the possible improvements in bowel function are intriguing; the mixed results warrant the need to study the effect of fampridine on bowel function in future studies.

3.7. Suppositories and Enemas

Rectal medications are typically a key component of bowel care of SCI patients with reflexic bowel or upper motor neuron lesions [23]. Rectal medications (suppositories, enemas) chemically stimulate the anal sphincter reflex to evacuate stool, and thus, the presence of an intact reflex is usually required. Suppositories are solid forms of rectal medication, while enemas are liquid, which are more difficult to insert if a patient has poor dexterity. Thus, the suppository is often first-line, especially for an individual doing their own bowel care. Rectal medications treat the dual problem of constipation and fecal incontinence. As these medications control the timing and predictability of bowel movement, they can have substantial benefits on the management of fecal incontinence. A number of cross-sectional studies demonstrate that rectal medications are used to treat more severe cases of NBD as those using rectal medications were associated with cervical injuries [6], poorer quality of life [43], extended hospitalization [44], longer bowel care [6,45], and presence of fecal incontinence [6].

Despite the common usage of suppositories, there is relatively little research on their effectiveness in SCI or MS. The small number of prospective controlled trials that have been conducted support the usage of suppositories; time to flatus, defecation sessions and total bowel care time all decreased [26,27,46]. We found only one crossover trial comparing different types of suppositories in SCI [47] that showed no significant difference in total colonic transit time between docusate sodium and benzocaine mini-enemas and mineral oil enemas, though both had a significantly shorter colonic transit time than bisacodyl or glycerin suppositories.

Of the two variations of bisacodyl suppositories, polyethylene glycol-based (PGB) bisacodyl outperformed hydrogenated vegetable-oil-based (HVB) bisacodyl across multiple outcomes and studies. Individuals receiving PGB bisacodyl had flatus 12.8–15 m after administration [26,27], 20–32 min long defecation sessions [26,27] and a total bowel care times of 43–66 min [26,27,46]. These outcomes were 44.8–58.7% faster than when HVB bisacodyl was given to the same individuals to initiate bowel care. Stiens et al. [27] attributed this difference to PGB suppositories' more effective ability to readily dissolve from body heat, distribute bisacodyl on mucus membranes, and sustain reflex propulsion of stool. Despite the documented benefits of the PGB formulation, HVB bisacodyl suppositories are more commonly used, primarily due to the fact that the HVB version generally costs less and is easier to obtain.

When analyzed against docusate sodium and benzocaine mini-enemas in a repeated measures study with a randomized sequence of the agent, PGB bisacodyl produced comparable results [26]. The authors of this study also stated that a docusate sodium-benzocaine mini-enema was more difficult for those with limited dexterity as the serrated edge of the enema could cause anal mucosal perforation during insertion, and it required squeezing for administration [26]. In contrast, Dunn and Galka [48] demonstrated that individuals with SCI had significantly shorter evacuation times with docusate sodium-benzocaine enema than with bisacodyl. However, the type of base (HVB or PGB) of the bisacodyl suppository was not stated, which could alter these interpretations. This information was once again missing in Amir et al. [47], where bowel evacuation time was longer after bisacodyl than mineral oil enemas, docusate sodium-benzocaine enemas, or glycerin suppositories. Although in the same study, bisacodyl did reduce the difficulties of evacuations better than glycerin suppositories [47].

A bisacodyl suppository is typically used as a first-line rectal medication as it is relatively inexpensive, easier to handle than a full-sized enema, and has some evidence of its effect. The suppository is easy to insert even for individuals with impaired dexterity and does not require voluntary contraction of the external anal sphincter for retention [27]. The suppository acts as a contact irritant to enhance gastric motility, increase the fecal water content, and reduce transit-time within the large intestine [49]. The bases act as a vehicle for delivering bisacodyl, the active ingredient. Prior to insertion of a bisacodyl suppository, the rectum should be digitally checked for feces. If present, the feces should be manually evacuated. In addition, the anal canal should be lubricated with a water-based jelly. Within the SCI population, a 10 mg bisacodyl suppository is commonly prescribed as it facilitates independent care [27]. Typically, one bisacodyl suppository is used every 1–2 days for immediate effect, with a bowel movement following 15–60 min after use.

Contraindications for bisacodyl suppository use in the general population are ileus, intestinal obstruction, acute abdominal conditions, including appendicitis, acute inflammatory bowel diseases, severe abdominal pain associated with nausea and vomiting, severe dehydration, and anal fissures or ulcerative proctitis with mucosal damage [50]. Two studies in SCI found that the insertion of rectal medications significantly increased systolic blood pressure [51,52]. This agrees with a retrospective chart review that indicated that rectal medication users had a four-fold increase in the likelihood of reporting autonomic dysreflexia than individuals with SCI, who spontaneously defecated [44]. Care may be necessary when using rectal medications on individuals who are susceptible to autonomic dysreflexia.

An alternative to a suppository, a mini-enema may be used as a first-line rectal medication given that their smaller size and dose may be less irritating and easier to insert. A small tube is inserted, and the liquid contents are squeezed into the rectum. The use of a suppository or mini-enemas may be dependent on local medical practices and reimbursement coverage.

If bowel care is taking too long or is ineffective, then the patient may progress to an enema if the patient is able to self-administer or if a caregiver can assist with administration. Alternatively, a suppository in a water-soluble base (polyethylene glycol) could be considered if that were not already being used. Such PGB suppositories (e.g., Magic Bullet) are generally more expensive but can reduce the time to bowel evacuation by allowing the medication to disperse within minutes after insertion. If bowel evacuation is still taking longer than desired, then one may need to adjust other parts of the bowel program (fluids, fiber, positioning, oral laxatives, etc.).

3.8. Narcotics Antagonist

More than 50% of individuals after SCI [53] and MS [54] have chronic pain stemming from neuropathic or musculoskeletal pain. Opioids are still a common choice option for pain management in SCI and MS, especially in refractory cases, although it is increasingly discouraged for non-malignant pain due to its risk for addiction. Opioids, together with immobility, compounds the risk of constipation. No literature was found specific to SCI and opioid-induced constipation or narcotic antagonist. The American Gastroenterological Association (AGA) Guidelines on the Medical Management of Opioid-Induced Constipation [55] recommend laxatives as the first-line agent. In patients with laxative refractory opioid-induced constipation, the AGA recommends using peripherally acting opioid receptor antagonists, which do not enter the central nervous system but block the opioid receptors in the gut (e.g., naloxegol, methylnaltrexone, naldemedine).

4. Discussion

The first observation from this study was the stark discrepancy between the large number of agents currently prescribed (Table 1) and an extremely limited amount of literature. Despite the common prescription of oral laxatives and narcotic antagonists, there were no studies with NBD and the best evidence was extracted from idiopathic constipation guidelines, which have serious limitations. There was evidence (low-quality) that polyethylene glycol-based bisacodyl suppositories produced faster outcomes than vegetable-based bisacodyl suppositories. While there was a small amount of literature in SCI, there was little to no literature available for MS. There are few randomized controlled trials evaluating medications for NBD in SCI. Many medications commonly used for NBD are generic and are unlikely to receive large funding for adequate research trials to take place. Given that many of these medications are considered "gold standard", it is unlikely that there will ever be a study on these medications to compare with placebo given the ethics of withholding gold standard for the sake of research. Only 42% (12/28) of included studies had any control conditions at all (including case–control studies using retrospective data as controls from chart reviews). Thus, it is difficult to make firm assertions based on the research evidence alone, and any results, positive or negative, should be interpreted with caution, taking into consideration any methodological concerns of the study itself.

There are inconsistencies with how NBD is scored between studies. For example, some studies use validated scales, but many rely on self-report (patient bowel journals) to determine bowel dysfunction. Bowel dysfunction in MS is often scored using the Rome criteria [56], but none of the studies we found testing medications on bowel dysfunction used this scale. Standardized and validated measures, such as the International SCI Bowel Function Basic Data Set or the NBD score, used consistently across researchers and clinicians, would produce more detailed descriptions and objective outcomes for comparison [57]. Variations in measurement approaches may be necessary for dysfunction-specific reasons or to meet experimental standards of any particular study, but a key set of bowel measures with a low data collection burden could be used, thus helping researchers and clinicians to embrace collection and reporting of such outcomes [58].

The time period during which bowel dysfunction is measured also varies greatly. We found studies asking participants about their bowel dysfunction over the last week, the last month, the last three months, the last year, or with no interval at all (i.e., have you ever had bowel dysfunction?) Without any decision on what is an appropriate time period to study, we are left with no standard interval for comparison between studies.

4.1. Clinical Insights

Because the literature provides little guidance on how and when to prescribe medication for the management of NBD in MS or SCI, we will be providing clinical insight in this section based on our clinical experience and understanding of the literature and guidelines. It is important to remember that pharmacologic treatment is only part of a bowel program for NBD in MS or SCI. As noted in the other manuscripts in this special edition and highlighted in recently published clinical practice guidelines, [22,23] modifications to optimize bowel regulation should not be solely focused on medication changes.

4.2. Case 1

History: A 55-year-old female with MS has a power wheelchair and is dependent on transfers and toileting. She has infrequent defecation about 3–5 times per week and abdominal discomfort/bloating. When she has bowel movements, she is able to sense the need to defecate, but she is not able to control the BM (incontinence), and she cannot get to a toilet; thus, the BM occurs in her briefs. She lives with a 65-year-old husband, who is unable to help care for her due to his own health problems. Thus, she has homecare assistance three times per day. When she has a BM into her briefs, she must wait until homecare comes next to get cleaned up. On examination, she has irritation/erythema of the skin of the buttocks with some breakdown and some soiling with stool in the briefs she is wearing. She requires a mechanical lift for transfers and has the weakness of upper limbs, no functional movement in lower limbs, and she needs partial assistance to turn in bed for the exam. She cannot assist at all in lowering pants for examination. She has a relatively preserved sensation of the perineal area and weak anal contraction. There is hard stool present on the rectal exam. She also has significant spasticity in the lower limbs.

Proposed treatment: The main issue here is lack of mobility and independence, thus not being able to toilet when a bowel movement is about to occur. Defecation occurs at times when no assistance is available, leading to being left for up to several hours in soiled briefs with resulting skin breakdown. The second issue is that the infrequency of bowel movements is causing hard stools and discomfort, which may be triggering her spasticity. The goals of treatment would be to have regular, predictable bowel movements, either daily or every second day, in a timely fashion, assisted by her home care workers. If starting with an every-other-day routine, give oral laxative (such as polyethylene glycol 17 mg) every 2 nights, then the next morning administer a rectal bisacodyl suppository, with digital stimulation as needed until the bowel routine is finished. This will allow for a regularly scheduled routine so that bowel incontinence does not occur later when no supports are available and will allow for less discomfort with bloating from infrequent bowel movements. If this approach is not successful, then she may switch the laxative to a more stimulating product, such as sennosides and may switch to a daily schedule if she still has unplanned bowel movements on off days.

4.3. Case 2

History: A 35-year-old male who had a traumatic SCI 15 years ago has a C7 AIS A injury. Since the injury, bowel care has consisted of digital anorectal stimulation performed every other day by a caregiver. However, for the last couple of years, the time for bowel care has increased to more than one hour. The patient has episodes of fecal incontinence approximately two times per month. He has vague abdominal discomfort and bloating that makes breathing difficult. Stools are usually hard (type 2 on the Bristol stool chart). For the last year, the patient has taken opioid analgesics because of neuropathic pain and abdominal discomfort.

Proposed treatment: In order to target difficult rectal evacuation and frequent fecal incontinence, first-line treatment will be a stimulant rectal laxative, either as suppository or enema.

In the present case, oral laxatives will most likely be added to counteract symptoms of prolonged colonic transit. The first choice would be an osmotic laxative. If this failed, we would suggest adding a stimulant laxative and, finally, a prokinetic agent.

If there is insufficient relief of symptoms, an opioid antagonist should be prescribed to treat opioid-induced bowel dysfunction. Long-term, additional focus should be given to optimizing this patient's analgesic regimen using non-opioid options. If the pharmacological treatment failed, consider transanal irrigation or a stoma.

Comments: The case illustrates that NBD usually includes symptoms of constipation as well as fecal incontinence. Treatment with rectal laxatives or an enema is the rational choice as it targets both poor evacuation and fecal incontinence. Patients with spinal cord lesions above the sacral spinal cord often have prolonged transit throughout the colon, which makes oral laxatives or prokinetics a necessary supplement to rectal laxatives. The case also illustrates that NBD is not a stable condition as constipation tends to become increasingly severe with time since injury. Prokinetics and opioid antagonists are usually not prescribed until standard osmotic and stimulant laxatives have failed to provide symptom relief.

4.4. Case 3

History: A 65-year-old female had a ground-level fall two years ago that resulted in an injury to the cauda equina. She has bowel movements once or twice per day. Defecation is difficult and usually lasts at least 45 min. Afterward, she has a strong feeling that rectal evacuation was incomplete. Stool consistency is normal. She has no bloating or abdominal pain. Her daily activities are restricted by the need to keep near a toilet because she has fecal incontinence several times per week. She has no other significant medical problems. On examination, there is reduced perianal sensation and very weak voluntary contraction of the anal canal.

Proposed treatment: The first choice of treatment would be a stimulant rectal laxative administered daily, preferably in the morning, to keep her continent during the day. If this failed, the patient should be offered transanal irrigation.

Comments: Lesions at the conus medullaris or cauda equina often cause poor evacuation of the rectum as well as fecal incontinence. In most cases, transport through the proximal colon is less severely affected. Rational treatment aims at restoring rectal evacuation by rectal laxatives (suppositories or enema) or by transanal irrigation. Oral laxatives are usually not needed unless stools are hard, and then they would be prescribed.

4.5. Recommendations for Future Research

Researchers have suggested that to increase the data quality and effectiveness of clinical research studies, the use of large data sets (like SCI model systems) can facilitate comparisons among treatments, patients, centers, and countries [59]. As SCI and MS are technically "lower frequency" conditions compared to stroke, cancer, or heart disease, it can be difficult to get sample sizes that are large enough to have any statistical power.

The SCI model systems database network has helped contribute to research with greater statistical power, and thus we can have more confidence in results that are generalizable. Some additional suggestions for areas in which SCI and MS research can improve include:

- Matched control research would increase the number of studies with a control group and would also help to establish sorely needed norms in SCI and MS research. Both neurological diseases affect many-body systems and understanding what norms are for individuals with NBD for colon transit time, bowel evacuation time and frequency after nutritional additions, an exercise intervention, or medication changes would be extremely useful;
- Standardizing a bowel treatment training program and evaluating learning and behavioral changes. Education research is rare, and the components of what constitutes a quality bowel training program have not yet appeared in the published literature;
- Research on the long-term effects of bowel medications or medications to reduce side-effects in NBD is much needed. Individuals with NBD can experience more severe bowel-related symptoms over time, although it is not known whether this is due to aging, medications becoming less effective, or the development of conditions, such as megacolon (colonic dilatation) [60];
- Research on biomarkers that precede constipation, incontinence, or more serious bowel problems, such as fecal impaction.

Supplementary Materials: The following are available online at https://www.mdpi.com/2077-0383/10/4/882/s1, S1. Search Terms, S2. Results of the Literature Search and S3. Results by Medication, Quality Ratings and Risk of Bias Assessment.

Author Contributions: Conceptualization: J.S.J., K.E., K.K., M.Q., J.J.E.; methodology: J.J.E., M.Q. Analysis: K.K., J.S.J., K.E., J.J.E., M.Q., J.C.; writing: J.S.J., K.K., K.E., J.C., M.Q., J.J.E. All authors have read and agreed to the published version of the manuscript.

Funding: This research received funding from Praxis Spinal Cord Research, International Collaboration on Repair Discoveries and Ontario Neurotrauma Foundation. The study was supported by an educational grant from Coloplast, Denmark.

Conflicts of Interest: The authors declare no conflict of interest. The funders had no role in the design of the study, in the collection, analyses, or interpretation of data, in the writing of the manuscript, or in the decision to publish the results.

References

1. Tate, D.G.; Forchheimer, M.; Rodriguez, G.; Chiodo, A.; Cameron, A.P.; Meade, M.; Krassioukov, A. Risk Factors Associated With Neurogenic Bowel Complications and Dysfunction in Spinal Cord Injury. *Arch. Phys. Med. Rehabil.* **2016**, *97*, 1679–1686. [CrossRef]
2. Krogh, K.; Nielsen, J.; Djurhuus, J.C.; Mosdal, C.; Sabroe, S.; Laurberg, S. Colorectal function in patients with spinal cord lesions. *Dis. Colon Rectum* **1997**, *40*, 1233–1239. [CrossRef]
3. Nusrat, S.; Gulick, E.; Levinthal, D.; Bielefeldt, K. Anorectal Dysfunction in Multiple Sclerosis: A Systematic Review. *ISRN Neurol.* **2012**, *2012*, 1–9. [CrossRef]
4. Menees, S.B.; Almario, C.V.; Spiegel, B.M.; Chey, W.D. Prevalence of and Factors Associated With Fecal Incontinence: Results From a Population-Based Survey. *Gastroenterology* **2018**, *154*, 1672–1681. [CrossRef]
5. Emmanuel, A. Review of the efficacy and safety of transanal irrigation for neurogenic bowel dysfunction. *Spinal Cord* **2010**, *48*, 664–673. [CrossRef]
6. Coggrave, M.; Norton, C.; Wilson-Barnett, J. Management of neurogenic bowel dysfunction in the community after spinal cord injury: A postal survey in the United Kingdom. *Spinal Cord* **2008**, *47*, 323–333. [CrossRef]
7. Coggrave, M.J.; Norton, C. The need for manual evacuation and oral laxatives in the management of neurogenic bowel dysfunction after spinal cord injury: A randomized controlled trial of a stepwise protocol. *Spinal Cord* **2009**, *48*, 504–510. [CrossRef]
8. Anderson, K.D. Targeting Recovery: Priorities of the Spinal Cord-Injured Population. *J. Neurotrauma* **2004**, *21*, 1371–1383. [CrossRef]
9. Dibley, L.; Coggrave, M.; Mcclurg, D.; Woodward, S.; Norton, C. "It's just horrible": A qualitative study of patients' and carers' experiences of bowel dysfunction in multiple sclerosis. *J Neurol.* **2017**, *264*, 1354–1361. [CrossRef]

10. Simpson, L.A.; Eng, J.J.; Hsieh, J.T.; Wolfe, D.L.; The Spinal Cord Injury Rehabilitation Evidence (SCIRE) Research Team. The Health and Life Priorities of Individuals with Spinal Cord Injury: A Systematic Review. *J. Neurotrauma* **2012**, *29*, 1548–1555. [CrossRef]
11. Bharucha, A.E. Fecal Incontinence: American College of Gastroenterology. Available online: https://gi.org/topics/fecal-incontinence/ (accessed on 11 January 2021).
12. Wald, A. Constipation and Defecation Problems: American College of Gastroenterology. Available online: https://gi.org/topics/constipation-and-defection-problems/ (accessed on 11 January 2021).
13. Vallès, M.; Vidal, J.; Clavé, P.; Mearin, F. Bowel Dysfunction in Patients with Motor Complete Spinal Cord Injury: Clinical, Neurological, and Pathophysiological Associations. *Am. J. Gastroenterol.* **2006**, *101*, 2290–2299. [CrossRef]
14. Liu, C.; Huang, C.; Yang, Y.; Chen, S.; Weng, M.; Huang, M. Relationship between neurogenic bowel dysfunction and health-related quality of life in persons with spinal cord injury. *J. Rehabil. Med.* **2009**, *41*, 35–40. [CrossRef]
15. Liu, C.-W.; Huang, C.-C.; Chen, C.-H.; Yang, Y.-H.; Chen, T.-W.; Huang, M.-H. Prediction of severe neurogenic bowel dysfunction in persons with spinal cord injury. *Spinal Cord* **2010**, *48*, 554–559. [CrossRef]
16. Singal, A.K.; Rosman, A.S.; A Bauman, W.; A Korsten, M. Recent concepts in the management of bowel problems after spinal cord injury. *Adv. Med. Sci.* **2006**, *51*, 15–22.
17. Kurtzke, J.F. Rating neurologic impairment in multiple sclerosis: An expanded disability status scale (EDSS). *Neurology* **1983**, *33*, 1444. [CrossRef]
18. Losseff, N.A.; Webb, S.L.; O'Riordan, J.I.; Page, R.; Wang, L.; Barker, G.J.; Tofts, P.S.; McDonald, W.I.; Miller, D.H.; Thompson, A.J. Spinal cord atrophy and disability in multiple sclerosis. A new reproducible and sensitive MRI method with potential to monitor disease progression. *Brain* **1996**, *119*, 701–708. [CrossRef]
19. Bakke, A.; Myhr, K.M.; Grønning, M.; Nyland, H. Bladder, bowel and sexual dysfunction in patients with multiple sclerosis—A cohort study. *Scand. J. Urol. Nephrol. Suppl.* **1996**, *179*, 61–66.
20. Nakayama, H.; Jørgensen, H.; Pedersen, P.; Raaschou, H.; Olsen, T. Prevalence and Risk Factors of Incontinence After Stroke. *Stroke* **1997**, *28*, 58–62. [CrossRef]
21. Lawthom, C.; Durdey, P.; Hughes, T. Constipation as a presenting symptom. *Lancet* **2003**, *362*, 958. [CrossRef]
22. Johns, J.S. Paralyzed Veterans of America. Management of Neurogenic Bowel Dysfunction in Adults after Spinal Cord Injury. Clinical Practice Guidelines: Spinal Cord Medicine. Available online: https://info.pva.org/receive-your-pdf-of-pvas-neurogenic-bowel-cpg (accessed on 25 October 2020).
23. Coggrave, M. Multidisciplinary Association of Spinal Cord Injured Professionals. Guidelines for Management of Neurogenic Bowel Dysfunction. Available online: https://www.mascip.co.uk/wp-content/uploads/2015/02/CV653N-Neurogenic-Guidelines-Sept-2012.pdf (accessed on 19 February 2021).
24. Musco, S.; Bazzocchi, G.; Martellucci, J.; Amato, M.P.; Manassero, A.; Putignano, D.; Lopatriello, S.; Cafiero, D.; Paoloni, F.; Del Popolo, G. Treatments in neurogenic bowel dysfunctions: Evidence reviews and clinical recommendations in adults. *Eur. J. Phys. Rehabil. Med.* **2021**, *56*, 741–755. [CrossRef]
25. GRADE Working Group. Grading quality of evidence and strength of recommendations. *BMJ* **2004**, *328*, 1490–1494. [CrossRef]
26. House, J.G.; Stiens, S.A. Pharmacologically initiated defecation for persons with spinal cord injury: Effectiveness of three agents. *Arch. Phys. Med. Rehabil.* **1997**, *78*, 1062–1065. [CrossRef]
27. A Stiens, S.; Luttrel, W.; E Binard, J. Polyethylene glycol versus vegetable oil based bisacodyl suppositories to initiate side-lying bowel care: A clinical trial in persons with spinal cord injury. *Spinal Cord* **1998**, *36*, 777–781. [CrossRef]
28. Luthra, P.; Camilleri, M.; E Burr, N.; Quigley, E.M.M.; Black, C.J.; Ford, A.C. Efficacy of drugs in chronic idiopathic constipation: A systematic review and network meta-analysis. *Lancet Gastroenterol. Hepatol.* **2019**, *4*, 831–844. [CrossRef]
29. Alsalimy, N.; Madi, L.; Awaisu, A. Efficacy and safety of laxatives for chronic constipation in long-term care settings: A systematic review. *J. Clin. Pharm. Ther.* **2018**, *43*, 595–605. [CrossRef]
30. Paré, P.; Fedorak, R.N. Systematic Review of Stimulant and Nonstimulant Laxatives for the Treatment of Functional constipation. *Can. J. Gastroenterol. Hepatol.* **2014**, *28*, 549–557. [CrossRef]
31. Nelson, A.D.; Camilleri, M.; Chirapongsathorn, S.; Vijayvargiya, P.; Valentin, N.; Shin, A.; Erwin, P.J.; Wang, Z.; Murad, M.H. Comparison of efficacy of pharmacological treatments for chronic idiopathic constipation: A systematic review and network meta-analysis. *Gut* **2016**, *66*, 1611–1622. [CrossRef]
32. Omar, M.I.; Alexander, C.E. Drug treatment for faecal incontinence in adults. *Cochrane Database Syst. Rev.* **2013**, *6*. [CrossRef]
33. Segal, J.L.; Milne, N.; Brunnemann, S.R.; Lyons, K.P. Metoclopramide-induced normalization of impaired gastric emptying in spinal cord injury. *Am. J. Gastroenterol.* **1987**, *82*, 1143–1148.
34. Korsten, M.A.; Lyons, B.L.; Radulovic, M.; Cummings, T.M.; Sikka, G.; Singh, K.; Hobson, J.C.; Sabiev, A.; Spungen, A.M.; Bauman, W.A. Delivery of neostigmine and glycopyrrolate by iontophoresis: A nonrandomized study in individuals with spinal cord injury. *Spinal Cord* **2017**, *56*, 212–217. [CrossRef]
35. Rosman, A.S.; Chaparala, G.; Monga, A.; Spungen, A.M.; Bauman, W.A.; Korsten, M.A. Intramuscular Neostigmine and Glycopyrrolate Safely Accelerated Bowel Evacuation in Patients with Spinal Cord Injury and Defecatory Disorders. *Dig. Dis. Sci.* **2008**, *53*, 2710–2713. [CrossRef]
36. Srikumar, V.; Chhabra, H.S. Management of neurogenic bowel. In *ISCoS Textbook on Comprehensive Management of Spinal Cord Injuries*; Lippincott Williams and Wilkins: Philadelphia, PA, USA, 2015; pp. 423–432. ISBN 978-93-5129-440-5.

37. Daniali, M.; Nikfar, S.; Abdollahi, M. An overview of the efficacy and safety of prucalopride for the treatment of chronic idiopathic constipation. *Expert Opin Pharmacother.* **2019**, *20*, 2073–2080. [CrossRef]
38. Krogh, K.; Jensen, M.B.; Gandrup, P.; Laurberg, S.; Nilsson, J.; Kerstens, R.; De Pauw, M. Efficacy and tolerability of prucalopride in patients with constipation due to spinal cord injury. *Scand. J. Gastroenterol.* **2002**, *37*, 431–436. [CrossRef]
39. Janssen Inc. Consumer Information Resotran. Available online: https://www.janssen.com/canada/sites/www_janssen_com_canada/files/prod_files/live/resotran_ci.pdf (accessed on 19 February 2021).
40. Polman, C.H.; Bertelsmann, F.W.; van Loenen, A.C.; Koetsier, J.C. 4-Aminopyridine in the treatment of patients with multiple sclerosis: Long-term efficacy and safety. *Arch Neurol.* **1994**, *51*, 292–296. [CrossRef]
41. Cardenas, D.D.; Ditunno, J.; Graziani, V.; Jackson, A.B.; Lammertse, D.; Potter, P.; Sipski, M.; Cohen, R.; Blight, A.R. Phase 2 trial of sustained-release fampridine in chronic spinal cord injury. *Spinal Cord* **2006**, *45*, 158–168. [CrossRef]
42. Cardenas, D.D.; Ditunno, J.F.; Graziani, V.; McLain, A.B.; Lammertse, D.P.; Potter, P.J.; Alexander, M.S.; Cohen, R.; Blight, A.R. Two phase 3, multicenter, randomized, placebo-controlled clinical trials of fampridine-SR for treatment of spasticity in chronic spinal cord injury. *Spinal Cord* **2013**, *52*, 70–76. [CrossRef]
43. Inskip, J.A.; Lucci, V.-E.M.; McGrath, M.S.; Willms, R.; Claydon, V.E. A Community Perspective on Bowel Management and Quality of Life after Spinal Cord Injury: The Influence of Autonomic Dysreflexia. *J. Neurotrauma* **2018**, *35*, 1091–1105. [CrossRef]
44. Furusawa, K.; Tokuhiro, A.; Sugiyama, H.; Ikeda, A.; Tajima, F.; Genda, E.; Uchida, R.; Tominaga, T.; Tanaka, H.; Magara, A.; et al. Incidence of symptomatic autonomic dysreflexia varies according to the bowel and bladder management techniques in patients with spinal cord injury. *Spinal Cord* **2010**, *49*, 49–54. [CrossRef]
45. Adriaansen, J.J.; Van Asbeck, F.W.; Van Kuppevelt, D.; Snoek, G.J.; Post, M.W. Outcomes of Neurogenic Bowel Management in Individuals Living With a Spinal Cord Injury for at Least 10 Years. *Arch. Phys. Med. Rehabil.* **2015**, *96*, 905–912. [CrossRef]
46. Frisbie, J. Improved Bowel Care With a Polyethylene Glycol Based Bisacadyl Suppository. *J. Spinal Cord Med.* **1997**, *20*, 227–229. [CrossRef]
47. Amir, I.; Sharma, R.; Bauman, W.A.; Korsten, M.A. Bowel Care for Individuals with Spinal Cord Injury: Comparison of Four Approaches. *J. Spinal Cord Med.* **1998**, *21*, 21–24. [CrossRef]
48. Dunn, K.L.; Galka, M.L. A Comparison of the Effectiveness of Therevac SB™ and Bisacodyl Suppositories in SCI Patients' Bowel Programs. *Rehabil. Nurs.* **1994**, *19*, 334–338. [CrossRef]
49. Kienzle-Horn, S.; Vix, J.-M.; Schuijt, C.; Peil, H.; Jordan, C.C.; Kamm, M.A. Efficacy and safety of bisacodyl in the acute treatment of constipation: A double-blind, randomized, placebo-controlled study. *Aliment. Pharmacol. Ther.* **2006**, *23*, 1479–1488. [CrossRef]
50. Martindale Pharmaceutical. Bisacodyl 10 mg Suppositories. Available online: https://www.medicines.org.uk/emc/product/8462/smpc#gref. (accessed on 19 February 2021).
51. Furusawa, K.; Sugiyama, H.; Tokuhiro, A.; Takahashi, M.; Nakamura, T.; Tajima, F. Topical anesthesia blunts the pressor response induced by bowel manipulation in subjects with cervical spinal cord injury. *Spinal Cord* **2008**, *47*, 144–148. [CrossRef]
52. Furusawa, K.; Sugiyama, H.; Ikeda, A.; Tokuhiro, A.; Koyoshi, H.; Takahashi, M.; Tajima, F. Autonomic dysreflexia during a bowel program in patients with cervical spinal cord injury. *Acta Med. Okayama* **2007**, *61*, 211–227.
53. Hunt, C.; Moman, R.; Peterson, A.; Wilson, R.; Covington, S.; Mustafa, R.; Murad, M.H.; Hooten, W.M. Prevalence of chronic pain after spinal cord injury: A systematic review and meta-analysis. *Reg. Anesthesia Pain Med.* **2021**. [CrossRef]
54. Hirsh, A.T.; Turner, A.P.; Ehde, D.M.; Haselkorn, J.K. Prevalence and Impact of Pain in Multiple Sclerosis: Physical and Psychologic Contributors. *Arch. Phys. Med. Rehabil.* **2009**, *90*, 646–651. [CrossRef]
55. Crockett, S.D.; Greer, K.B.; Heidelbaugh, J.J.; Falck-Ytter, Y.; Hanson, B.J.; Sultan, S. American Gastroenterological Association Institute Guideline on the Medical Management of Opioid-Induced Constipation. *Gastroenterology* **2019**, *156*, 218–226. [CrossRef]
56. Drossman, D.A. Functional Gastrointestinal Disorders: History, Pathophysiology, Clinical Features, and Rome IV. *Gastroenterology* **2016**, *150*, 1262–1279. [CrossRef]
57. Hwang, M.; Zebracki, K.; Vogel, L.C. Long-Term Outcomes and Longitudinal Changes of Neurogenic Bowel Management in Adults With Pediatric-Onset Spinal Cord Injury. *Arch. Phys. Med. Rehabil.* **2017**, *98*, 241–248. [CrossRef]
58. Wheeler, T.L.; de Groat, W.; Eisner, K.; Emmanuel, A.; French, J.; Grill, W.; Kennelly, M.J.; Krassioukov, A.; Santacruz, B.G.; Biering-Sørensen, F.; et al. Translating promising strategies for bowel and bladder management in spinal cord injury. *Exp. Neurol.* **2018**, *306*, 169–176. [CrossRef]
59. Biering-Sørensen, F.; Charlifue, S.; DeVivo, M.J.; Grinnon, S.T.; Kleitman, N.; Lu, Y.; Odenkirchen, J. Using the Spinal Cord Injury Common Data Elements. *Top. Spinal Cord Inj. Rehabil.* **2012**, *18*, 23–27. [CrossRef]
60. Harai, D.; Minaker, K.L. Megacolon in patients with chronic spinal cord injury. *Spinal Cord.* **2000**, *38*, 331–339. [CrossRef]

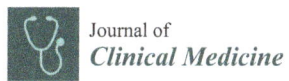

Review

Transanal Irrigation for Neurogenic Bowel Disease, Low Anterior Resection Syndrome, Faecal Incontinence and Chronic Constipation: A Systematic Review

Mira Mekhael [1,2,3,*], Helle Ø Kristensen [1,2], Helene Mathilde Larsen [1,2,3], Therese Juul [1,2,3], Anton Emmanuel [4], Klaus Krogh [2,5] and Peter Christensen [1,2,3]

[1] Department of Surgery, Aarhus University Hospital, DK8200 Aarhus, Denmark; hellkren@rm.dk (H.Ø.K.); hemala@rm.dk (H.M.L.); therjuul@rm.dk (T.J.); petchris@rm.dk (P.C.)
[2] Danish Cancer Society Centre for Research on Survivorship and Late Adverse Effects after Cancer in the Pelvic Organs, DK8200 Aarhus, Denmark; klaukrog@rm.dk
[3] Department of Clinical Medicine, Aarhus University, DK8200 Aarhus, Denmark
[4] GI Physiology Unit, University College London Hospital, London NW1 2BU, UK; anton.emmanuel@nhs.net
[5] Department of Hepatology and Gastroenterology, Aarhus University Hospital, DK8200 Aarhus, Denmark
* Correspondence: mirmek@rm.dk

Citation: Mekhael, M.; Kristensen, H.Ø.; Larsen, H.M.; Juul, T.; Emmanuel, A.; Krogh, K.; Christensen, P. Transanal Irrigation for Neurogenic Bowel Disease, Low Anterior Resection Syndrome, Faecal Incontinence and Chronic Constipation: A Systematic Review. *J. Clin. Med.* **2021**, *10*, 753. https://doi.org/10.3390/jcm10040753

Academic Editor: Bruno Annibale
Received: 30 December 2020
Accepted: 8 February 2021
Published: 13 February 2021

Publisher's Note: MDPI stays neutral with regard to jurisdictional claims in published maps and institutional affiliations.

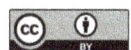

Copyright: © 2021 by the authors. Licensee MDPI, Basel, Switzerland. This article is an open access article distributed under the terms and conditions of the Creative Commons Attribution (CC BY) license (https://creativecommons.org/licenses/by/4.0/).

Abstract: Transanal irrigation (TAI) has received increasing attention as a treatment option in patients with bowel dysfunction. This systematic review was conducted according to the PRISMA guidelines and evaluates the effect of TAI in neurogenic bowel dysfunction (NBD), low anterior resection syndrome (LARS), faecal incontinence (FI) and chronic constipation (CC). The primary outcome was the effect of TAI on bowel function. Secondary outcomes included details on TAI, quality of life (QoL), the discontinuation rate, adverse events, predictive factors for a successful outcome, and health economics. A systematic search for articles reporting original data on the effect of TAI on bowel function was performed, and 27 eligible studies including 1435 individuals were included. Three randomised controlled trials, one non-randomised trial, and 23 observational studies were included; 70% of the studies were assessed to be of excellent or good methodological quality. Results showed an improvement in bowel function among patients with NBD, LARS, FI, and CC with some studies showing improvement in QoL. However, discontinuation rates were high. Side effects were common, but equally prevalent among comparative treatments. No consistent predictive factors for a successful outcome were identified. Results from this review show that TAI improves bowel function and potentially QoL; however, evidence remains limited.

Keywords: transanal irrigation; neurogenic bowel dysfunction; low anterior resection syndrome; faecal incontinence; chronic constipation; bowel dysfunction; quality of life

1. Introduction

Transanal irrigation (TAI) has received increasing attention as a treatment option in patients with bowel dysfunction as it has shown to improve faecal incontinence (FI) and chronic constipation (CC) [1,2]. With TAI, water is introduced into the bowel through the anus, facilitating emptying of the rectosigmoid and the left colon [3]. By performing regular irrigations, control of bowel function including time and place of bowel movements can be re-gained [4]. In patients with FI, efficient and controlled emptying of the bowel can be achieved with TAI. This can prevent episodes of incontinence in between irrigations for an average of two days. In patients with CC, regular evacuation of the rectosigmoid with TAI can prevent constipation [3].

TAI is introduced when conservative treatment fails. At present, TAI is the only minimally invasive treatment option for bowel dysfunction. This has positioned TAI as an important treatment modality before introducing more invasive methods such as sacral nerve stimulation, antegrade colonic irrigation or stoma formation [5].

Neurogenic bowel dysfunction (NBD) affects quality of life (QoL) negatively and is highly prevalent in patients with neurological disorders [1,4]. NBD is caused by neurological disorders such as spinal cord injury (SCI), multiple sclerosis (MS), spina bifida (SB) and Parkinson's disease. FI and CC are very common symptoms in patients suffering from NBD with a prevalence between 23 and 80% depending on the underlying neurological disorder [1]. Patients with SCI report that bowel dysfunction is the most important problem among a wide variety of other sequelae [6]. TAI was introduced into the treatment algorithm of NBD after a randomised controlled trial (RCT) among adult patients with SCI found it to be superior to conservative treatment [7].

TAI has also shown to improve symptoms of low anterior resection syndrome (LARS) [8]. LARS is a defaecation disturbance experienced by up to 80% of patients following low anterior resection for rectal cancer [9]. The syndrome comprises a cluster of FI, emptying difficulties, urgency, increased stool frequency, variable and painful stools, altered stool consistency and soiling [5]. Fifty percent of patients undergoing low anterior resection are affected by severe LARS in the long term, which has a major impact on QoL [10,11].

FI and CC of other origin may also be improved by TAI [12]. This includes among others FI and CC caused by anorectal, gynaecological or urological surgery; prolapse disease; medication; diabetes mellitus or idiopathic FI or CC. Among patients with these diseases, bowel dysfunction also has a significant negative impact on QoL [13].

Even though TAI has been proposed for the managing of bowel dysfunction for decades, the treatment is still not well known or well established. Within the past ten years [12,14], no systematic review has been conducted across NBD, LARS, and FI and CC of heterogeneous origin. We believe that such a review would help disseminate current knowledge on the effect of TAI and be beneficial to patients suffering from NBD, LARS, and FI and CC of other origin.

The aim of this systematic review was to evaluate the effect of TAI in the management of bowel dysfunction in adults with NBD, LARS, and FI and CC of other origin.

2. Materials and Methods

This review was conducted according to the PRISMA guidelines [15], and the protocol was registered with the International Prospective Register of Systematic Reviews (PROSPERO) (CRD42020206262).

2.1. Inclusion and Exclusion Criteria

The review included all study designs reporting original data on the effect of TAI on bowel function for individuals with (1) neurogenic bowel disorders (SCI, cauda equina syndrome, MS, Parkinson's disease, cerebrovascular events, cerebral palsy and SB), (2) low anterior resection syndrome, and (3) FI and CC of heterogeneous origin. The study population included adults ($\geq$18 years), and only articles in English published in peer-reviewed journals were reviewed. Articles were excluded if patients were treated with any other interventions than TAI, if TAI patients were pooled with other treatment modalities, or if enemas were not clearly defined as an irrigation volume $\geq$150 mL.

2.2. Outcomes

The primary outcome for this review was the effect of TAI on bowel function measured by patient-reported outcome measures (PROMs), objective measures of bowel symptoms or compliance as a surrogate measure of clinical benefit on bowel function. Secondary outcomes included details on TAI, QoL, discontinuation rate, adverse events, predictive factors and health economics. Articles with other outcomes were excluded. Studies were defined as having short-term follow-up (FU) if FU was <12 months, as long-term if FU $\geq$ 12 months, and mixed if patients with both short-term and long-term FU were included.

2.3. Search Strategy and Data Extraction

On October 15, 2020, the electronic databases PubMed, Embase, and Cochrane Library were systematically searched for relevant studies. The search strategy was developed by all authors in collaboration with a librarian with expertise in systematic reviews. The search was performed using relevant MeSH- or Emtree terms and text words. The search strategy is presented in Figure 1. Covidence was used for the removal of duplicate publications, article screening and data extraction [16], and Web of Science was used to screen references and citing articles of all included studies.

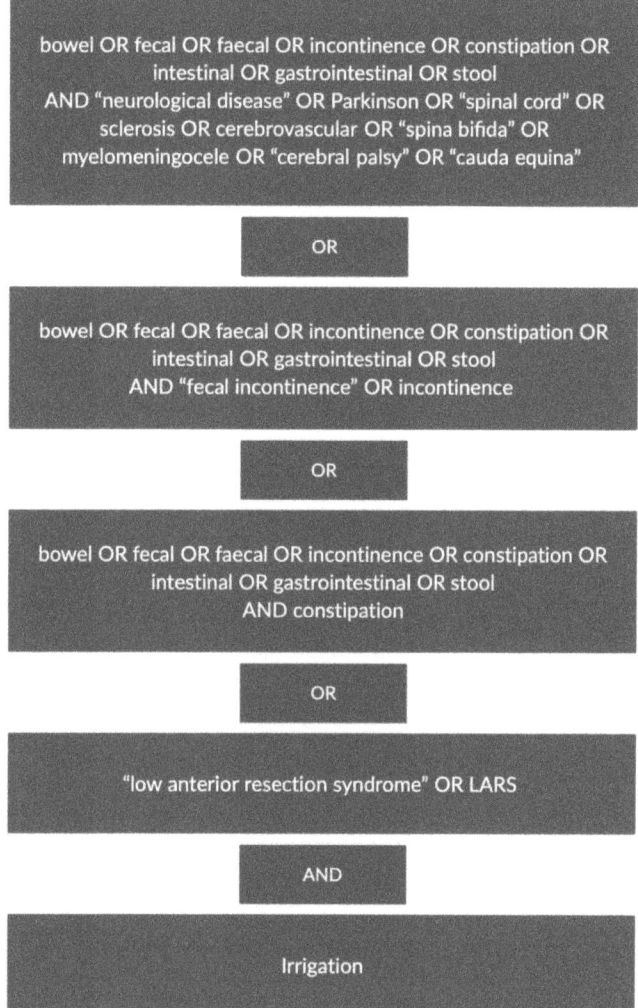

Figure 1. Search strategy.

Two authors (H.Ø.K. and M.M.) independently extracted information on author, study design, study population and outcomes of interest using an electronic spreadsheet in Covidence. Any disagreements during the screening or data extraction process were solved by consensus discussions between H.Ø.K. and M.M. or by a third party (T.J., K.K. or P.C.).

2.4. Risk of Bias and Quality Assessment

The risk of bias was assessed using a modified version of the Downs and Black checklist [17]. The checklist is validated for both RCTs and non-randomised studies [17]. It comprises 27 items covering reporting, external and internal validity, and statistical power. In the present version, item 27 addressing statistical power was modified so that a study was given one point if a power calculation was conducted and zero if it was not. For each question, one point was awarded if the study fulfilled the question (item 5 ranges from 0–2 points). Hence, the maximum score for randomised trials was 28 and non-randomised studies 25. Studies were classified as being excellent (26–28), good (20–25), fair (15–19) or poor (≤14) [18]. The assessment was independently performed by two reviewers (H.Ø.K. and M.M.). Disagreements were solved by consensus discussion between the two authors or by a third party (T.J.).

2.5. Data Synthesis

Results are presented separately for NBD, LARS, and FI and CC of heterogeneous origin. If data regarding NBD or LARS were separately presented in articles reporting data on FI and CC of heterogeneous origin, results were presented along with NBD or LARS results. Study and patient characteristics, details on TAI, primary and secondary outcomes, and quality assessment of each study are presented in tables and summarised descriptively. Due to the heterogeneity of outcomes and study designs, a meta-analysis was not conducted.

3. Results

In total, 1698 studies were identified through the database search. Another two studies were identified through the screening of references from the included studies. After the removal of 383 duplicates, the remaining 1317 studies were screened by title and abstract independently by two authors (H.M.L. and M.M.). As a result, 1151 studies were excluded, leaving 166 studies for full-text screening. Full-text screening was completed independently by two authors (H.M.L. and M.M.). Twenty-seven studies met the inclusion criteria. A flowchart of the screening process is presented in Figure 2.

3.1. Neurogenic Bowel Dysfunction

In total, eleven studies were identified reporting data on the effect of TAI in NBD patients [7,19–28]. The results are presented in Table 1. The articles were published between 2004 and 2019, and included one RCT [7], eight prospective cohort studies [19–23,26–28], one cross-sectional study [25] and one retrospective study [24]. Six studies included patients with various neurological disorders, primarily SCI [7,19–22,24]; two studies included patients with SCI [23,25]; two studies included patients with MS [26,27]; and one study included patients with SB [28]. Eight studies only included patients using TAI [19–24,26,27], one study randomised to TAI or conservative treatment [7], and two studies included patients using conservative treatment, TAI or had surgical treatment [25,28]. In total, 308 patients using TAI were included with between 4 and 62 patients included in each study. Six studies had short-term FU ([7,19–21,23,26], one had long-term FU (≥12 months) [27], two had mixed FU [22,24] and two studies did not report FU [25,28].

One study was assessed to be of excellent methodological quality [7], six of good quality [20,21,23,26–28], two of fair quality [24,25] and two of poor quality [19,22].

The predominant symptoms were FI (13–33%) and CC (55–84%) [7,20,21,23,24,27]. Irrigation volume ranged between 200 mL and 1500 mL [7,20,21,23,24,26]. Irrigation every second day was most common, and 21 to 100% of patients self-administered TAI [7,20,21,23, 24,26,27]. One study reported the mean (standard deviation, SD) daily time spent on bowel management to be 47.0 (25.0) min [7]. Another study reported a mean irrigation time of 20.3 min and a mean defaecation time of 18.3 min with 60% of patients using <30 min [24]. Eight studies reported that patients received TAI training [7,20–24,26,27].

Table 1. Neurogenic bowel dysfunction.

Reference	Study Design	TAI Cohort (Total Cohort)	Follow-Up Time	Inclusion Criteria	Patient Characteristics	Details on TAI	Bowel Function Outcome	Quality of Life Outcome	Discontinuation	Adverse Events	Quality Assessment ° [17]
Gardiner 2004 [19]	Prospective cohort	4	6 weeks	N/A	2 with MS, 1 with epilepsy, 1 with transverse myelitis	N/A	Successful outcome in all patients	N/A	No one discontinued	N/A	Reporting: 2 External: 1 Internal: 4 Power: 0 Total score: 7
Christensen 2006 [7]	Multicentre randomised controlled trial TAI or conservative treatment (CT)	42 (87)	10 weeks	At least 3 months after SCI Presence of one of four predefined bowel symptoms	SCI and SB Age (years), mean (SD): 47.5 (12.8) Male/female: 29/13 Predominant symptoms: CC: 76% FI: 21% Other: 3% Duration of bowel symptoms (months), median (range): 54 (4–780) American Spine Injury Association score (complete/incomplete): T9 and above: 21/10 T10-L2: 3/5 L3-S1: 1/1 S2 and below: 0/1	Peristeen® (Coloplast A/S, Denmark) Volume (mL), median (range): 700 (200–1500) Frequency: 16% every day, 49% every second day, 35% 1–3 times/week 62% self-administered Trained by a specialist nurse	Termination scores: CCCS * [29], mean (SD): TAI: 10.3 (4.4) CT: 13.2 (3.4) ($p = 0.0016$) FICS score * [30], mean (SD): TAI: 5.0 (4.6) CT: 7.3 (4.0) ($p = 0.015$) NBD score * [31], mean (SD): TAI: 10.4 (6.8) CT: 13.3 (6.4) ($p = 0.48$) Total time spent on bowel management daily (min), mean (SD): TAI: 47.0 (25.0) CT: 74.4 (59.8) ($p = 0.040$)	Termination scores, modified FIQLS * [32], mean (SD): Lifestyle: TAI: 3.0 (0.7) CT: 2.8 (0.8) ($p = 0.13$) Coping/behaviour: TAI: 2.8 (0.8) CT: 2.4 (0.7) ($p = 0.013$) Depression/self-perception: TAI: 3.0 (0.8) CT: 2.7 (0.8) ($p = 0.055$) Embarrassment: TAI: 3.2 (0.8) CT: 2.8 (0.9) ($p = 0.024$)	12 (29%) patients discontinued: 25% repeated expulsions of catheter, 17% prior to training, 17% lost to follow-up, 8% lack of compliance, 8% dislike of TAI, 8% burst of rectal balloons, 8% inefficacy; 8% adverse events	14 (36%) patients experienced side effects: 15.7% abdominal pain, 10.5% sweating, 7.0% chills, 5.9% pronounced general discomfort, 5.4% dizziness, 3.0% pounding headache, 2.7% flushing, 1.4% anorectal pain No significant difference in the proportion of patients experiencing side effects between the groups ($p = 0.052$) 4 adverse events in TAI group. 3 serious adverse events	Reporting: 11 External: 3 Internal: 11 Power: 1 Total score: 26

Table 1. Cont.

Reference	Study Design	TAI Cohort (Total Cohort)	Follow-Up Time	Inclusion Criteria	Patient Characteristics	Details on TAI	Bowel Function Outcome	Quality of Life Outcome	Discontinuation	Adverse Events	Quality Assessment [17]
Christensen 2008 [20]	Multicentre prospective cohort	62 42 overlapping with Christensen 2006 [7]	10 weeks	At least 3 months after SCI Presence of one of four predefined bowel symptoms	SCI and SB Age (years), mean (range): 47.5 (25–76) Male/female: 45/17 Predominant symptoms: CC: 76% FI: 18% Other: 6% Duration of bowel symptoms (months), median (range): 60 (4–776) Complete/incomplete: 37/25 Level of injury: Supraconal: 61 Conal/cauda equina (S2–S4): 1	Peristeen® (Coloplast A/S, Denmark) Volume (mL), median (range): 650 (0–1500) Frequency: 20% every day, 48% every second day, 30% 1–3 times/week, 2% never In patients irrigating daily, 40% need assistance; 60% of those who irrigated every second day needed assistance Trained by a specialist nurse	Post-treatment–pre-treatment score, mean (95% CI): CCCS: -3.4 (-4.6; -2.2) ($p < 0.0001$) FICS score: -4.1 (-5.2; -2.9) ($p < 0.0001$) NBD score: -4.5 (-6.6; -2.4) ($p < 0.0001$)	N/A	17 (27%) patients discontinued: 29% repeated expulsions, 24% lost to follow-up, 12% prior to training, 12% inefficacy, 6% leakage of water around catheter, 6% dislike of treatment, 6% bursts of rectal balloons, 6% adverse events,	N/A	Reporting: 11 External: 3 Internal: 8 Power: 0 Total score: 22

Table 1. Cont.

Reference	Study Design	TAI Cohort (Total Cohort)	Follow-Up Time	Inclusion Criteria	Patient Characteristics	Details on TAI	Bowel Function Outcome	Quality of Life Outcome	Discontinuation	Adverse Events	Quality Assessment θ [17]
Del Popolo 2008 [21]	Multicentre prospective cohort	33	3 weeks	Congenital SCI or acquired SCI at least 6 months previously Severe NBD with unsatisfactory bowel management	SCI, MS and SB Age (years), median (SD): 31.6 (13.3) Male/female: 18/15 Predominant symptoms: FI: 13% CC: 84% Not recorded: 3% Complete/incomplete: 13/14	Peristeen® (Coloplast A/S, Denmark) Volume (mL), mean (SD): 789 (222) Frequency: 15% ≥1 time a day, 55% every second day, 30% 1–3 times a week 100% self-administered Trained by a specialist nurse	Pre/post-treatment: Likert like scale: Abdominal discomfort ($p < 0.001$) Incomplete evacuation ($p < 0.001$) Leakage of faeces ($p = 0.002$) Gas incontinence ($p = 0.002$) 11-point Likert scale: Increase in opinion of bowel function $p = 0.001$ Defaecation time: Decrease in time spent on evacuation $p = 0.004$	11-point Likert scale: Increase in QoL score $p = 0.001$	1 (3%) patient discontinued: 3% lost to follow-up	No adverse events recorded	Reporting: 10 External: 3 Internal: 7 Power: 0 Total score: 20
Loftus 2012 [22]	Prospective cohort	11	3–28 months	NBD Unsatisfactorily treated with conservative management	SCI and SB Age (years), mean (range): 44 (27–72) Male/female: 7/4 Complete/incomplete: 4/5 Level of injury: 1 C4, 2 C7, 1 T4, 1 T5, 2 T6, 2 L1	Peristeen® (Coloplast A/S, Denmark) Trained by a specialist nurse	Post-treatment–pre-treatment score, mean: CCCS: −7.55 ($p < 0.001$) FICS score: −5.36 ($p < 0.001$) NBD score: −10.32 ($p < 0.005$)	N/A	N/A	No major adverse events	Reporting: 7 External: 3 Internal: 4 Power: 0 Total score: 14

Table 1. *Cont.*

Reference	Study Design	TAI Cohort (Total Cohort)	Follow-Up Time	Inclusion Criteria	Patient Characteristics	Details on TAI	Bowel Function Outcome	Quality of Life Outcome	Discontinuation	Adverse Events	Quality Assessment [17]
Kim 2013 [23]	Multicentre prospective cohort	52	6 months	SCI at least 6 months previously Unsatisfactorily treated with conservative management	SCI Age (years), median (range): 45.5 (18–65) Male/female: 41/10 Predominant symptoms, multiple choice: FI: 29% CC: 54% Pain/discomfort during defaecation:38% Haemorrhoid or anal bleeding: 35% Autonomic dysreflexia: 17% Injury type: Tetraplegia: 28 Paraplegia: 24	Peristeen® (Coloplast A/S, Denmark) Volume (mL), mean (SD): 789 (153) Frequency: 11% every day, 17% every second day, 72% twice every week 33% self-administered Trained by an investigator	Pre/post-treatment: Self-reported impact of bowel function on QoL increased measured with a ICF qualifier scale * [33] (p = 0.003) Decreased defaecation time (p = 0.003) At 6 months FU: Satisfaction of TAI (10-point Likert scale (10 = perfect satisfaction), mean (SD): 8.33 (1.37)	At 6 months FU: Impact of TAI on QoL (10-point Likert scale (10 = perfect satisfaction), mean (SD): 8.44 (1.34)	34 (66%) patients discontinued (reasons, multiple choice): 26% time-consuming, 25% personal reasons, 24% inefficacy, 15% adverse events, 12% expulsion of catheter, 6% difficulties cleaning up after TAI, 6% dislike of treatment, 3% leakage of irrigation fluid	15 (29%) patients experienced side effects: 17% abdominal pain or discomfort, 6% minor anal bleeding, 2% hot flash, 2% headache, 2% perianal discomfort, 2% perspiration, 2% general discomfort, 2% fatigue	Reporting: 11 External: 3 Internal: 9 Power: 0 Total score: 22
Hamonet-Torny 2013 [24]	Retrospective	16	Mean (range): 31 (7.5–66) months	Patients benefitting from TAI	SCI, MS, SB, multiple system atrophy Age (years), mean: 49 Predominant symptoms: CC: 75% CC + FI: 19% CC + perianal pain: 6% Injury type: Tetraplegia: 3 Paraplegia: 2	Peristeen® (Coloplast A/S, Denmark) Volume (mL), mean: 922 Mean irrigation frequency: twice a week 38% self-administered Irrigation time (min), mean: 20.3 Time to obtain defaecation after irrigation (min), mean: 18.33 Formal education, except one	NBD score, mean: 6.25 CCIS * [34,35]: 0.50 62.5% irrigated after a mean of 31 months Time spent on bowel management < 30 min for 60% of patients Difference in consumption of laxatives, mean: Before: 1.66 After: 1.4 (p = 0.6783)	N/A	6 (38%) patients discontinued: 50% inefficacy, 13% heavy administration, 13% vomiting following administration	1 (6%) patients experienced anal bleeding 1 adverse event	Reporting: 9 External: 1 Internal: 6 Power: 0 Total score: 16

Table 1. *Cont.*

Reference	Study Design	TAI Cohort (Total Cohort)	Follow-Up Time	Inclusion Criteria	Patient Characteristics	Details on TAI	Bowel Function Outcome	Quality of Life Outcome	Discontinuation	Adverse Events	Quality Assessment θ [17]
Adriaansen 2015 [25]	Multicentre cross-sectional	29 (258)	N/A	SCI with time since injury of ≥10 years Age at injury 18–35 years Current age 28–65 years Using a wheelchair ≥500 m	SCI Age (years), mean (range): 45 (29–64) Male: 77% Time since injury (years), mean (range): 22 (10–46) Injury type: Tetraplegia: 12 Paraplegia: 17	N/A	Severe NBD: 41.4% Dissatisfied/very dissatisfied with TAI, 5-point Likert scale: 17.2% Perianal problems: 41.4% CC: 27.6% FI at least once a month: 34.5% Average > 60 min required for defaecation: 24.1%	N/A	N/A	N/A	Reporting: 7 External: 2 Internal: 6 Power: 0 Total score: 15
Preziosi 2012 [26]	Prospective cohort	37	6 weeks	Failure of biofeed-back Not eligible for biofeed-back No response to conservative treatment MS and NBD	MS Age (years), median (range): 49 (42–56) Male/female: 3/27	Peristeen® (Coloplast A/S, Denmark) Recommended volume between 500–1500 mL Recommended irrigation frequency every third day adjusted according to response 93% self-administered Trained by a specialist nurse	Pre/post-treatment: CCCS, median (IQR): Pre: 12 (8.75–16) Post: 8 (4–12.5) ($p = 0.001$) CCIS, median (IQR): Pre: 12 (4.75–16) Post: 4 (2–8) ($p < 0.001$)	Pre/post-treatment: SF-36 * [36], mean (SD): Pre: 51.3 (7.8) Post: 50.4 (7.8) ($p = 0.051$)	7 (19%) patients discontinued prior to irrigation training 14 (47%) patients discontinued during trial At 6 months of follow-up, all responders continued using the irrigation, with the exception of 2 patients	N/A	Reporting: 10 External: 3 Internal: 9 Power: 0 Total score: 22

Table 1. Cont.

Reference	Study Design	TAI Cohort (Total Cohort)	Follow-Up Time	Inclusion Criteria	Patient Characteristics	Details on TAI	Bowel Function Outcome	Quality of Life Outcome	Discontinuation	Adverse Events	Quality Assessment θ [17]
Passananti 2016 [27]	Multicentre prospective cohort	49	Minimum 1 year with a mean of 40 months	MS and NBD for ≥6 months Bowel symptoms for ≥6 months not responding to conservative management	MS Age (years), mean (range): 51 (26–80) Male/female: 12/37 Predominant symptoms: FI: 33% CC: 67%	Peristeen® (Coloplast A/S, Denmark) Frequency: 48% irrigating daily, 48% every second day, 4% every third day 98% self-administered Trained by a specialist nurse	Pre/post-treatment: FI (weekly episodes), mean (range): Pre: 4.8 (1–21) Post: 0.9 (0–7) (p < 0.005) Severe NBD: Pre: 47% Post: 18%	Pre/post-treatment: EQ-5D * [37] utility score, mean (95% CI): Pre: 0.57 (0.5;0.65) Post: 0.52 (0.4;0.63) EQ-VAS score, mean (95% CI): Pre: 44.5 (41.26;47.73) Post: 63.4 (58.41;68.49)	22 (45%) patients discontinued: 55% dislike of treatment, 14% inefficacy, 9% adverse events, 9% other pathology, 9% lost to follow-up, 5% burst of rectal balloons	N/A	Reporting: 10 External: 3 Internal: 8 Power: 0 Total score: 21
Brochard 2019 [28]	Prospective cohort	15 (57)	Not specified for TAI group. FU for entire cohort: 46 (±36) months	Spinal dysraphism Evaluation by gastroenterologist	SB Not specified for the TAI cohort	N/A	Pre/post-treatment: Improvement of CCIS * ≥ 50%: 46.7% Variation of CCIS <50%: 19.5% (p = 0.016)	N/A	N/A	N/A	Reporting: 10 External: 3 Internal: 8 Power: 0 Total score: 21

θ Quality assessment using a modified version of the Downs and Black checklist was performed by authors of this review. * CCCS = Cleveland Clinic Constipation score (Wexner Constipation score), FIGS = St. Mark's Faecal Incontinence Grading System (Vaizey score), NBD = Neurogenic Bowel Dysfunction score, FIQLS = American Society of Colon and Rectal Surgeons Faecal Incontinence Score, ICF = International Classification of Function, Disability and Health scale, CCIS = Cleveland Clinic Incontinence score (Wexner Incontinence score), SF-36 = Short Form (36) Health Survey, EQ-5D = European Quality of Life—5 Dimension, EQ-VAS = European Quality of Life Visual Analogue Scale.

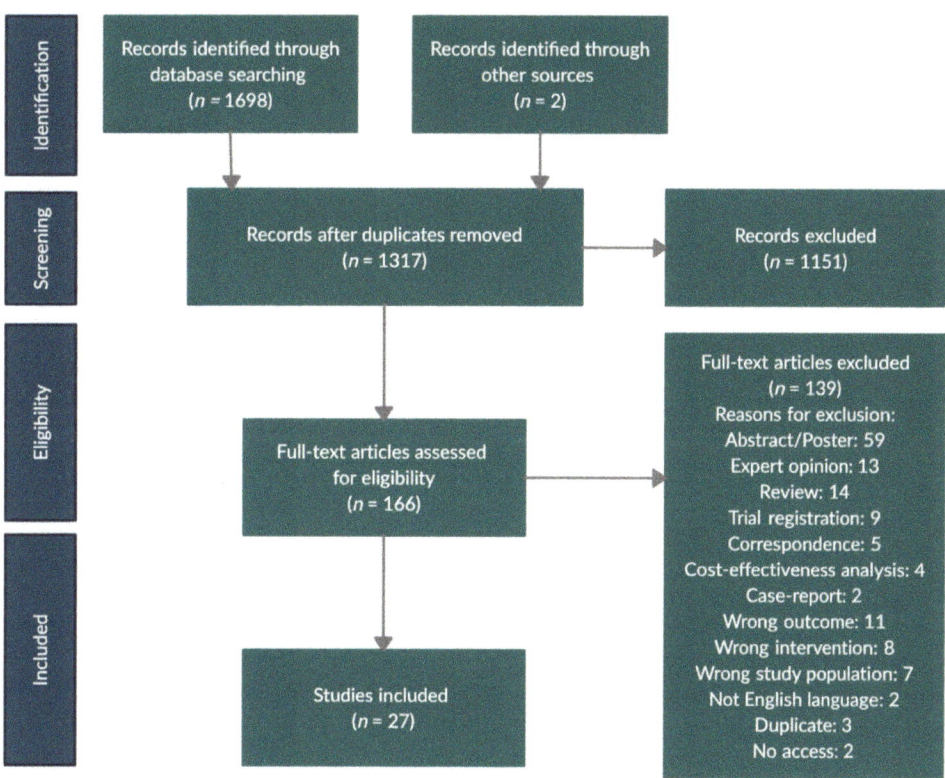

Figure 2. Flow diagram adapted from PRISMA [15].

Bowel function was assessed by validated PROMs in eight studies [7,20,22–28] and by non-validated PROMs in three [21,23]. One study did not report outcome measure [19]. Six studies used the Neurogenic Bowel Dysfunction (NBD) score [7,20,22,24,25,27,31] [34], four the Cleveland Clinic Constipation Score (CCCS) [7,20,22,26,29], three the Cleveland Clinic Incontinence Score (CCIS) [24,26,28,34,35] and three the St. Mark's Faecal Incontinence Grading System (FIGS) score [7,20,22,30].

Eight studies measuring pre- and posttreatment scores including patients with SCI, MS or SB showed a significant improvement in bowel function [7,20–23,26–28]. One cross-sectional study reported a prevalence of severe NBD among TAI users of 41% and a proportion of 17% as being dissatisfied or very dissatisfied with TAI [25]. A retrospective study found a mean NBD score of 6.25 and a mean CCIS of 0.50 among current TAI users [24]. One study showed a successful outcome in all patients [19].

Five studies reported QoL data. Three studies used validated PROMs [7,26,27] and two studies non-validated PROMs [21,23]. Two studies measuring pre- and posttreatment scores including patients with MS measured generic QoL [26,27]. One study showed no significant difference in the Short Form (36) Health Survey (SF-36) scale scores [26,36] and the other no difference in the European Quality of Life–5 Dimension (EQ-5D) score [37], but a significant improvement in the European Quality of Life Visual Analogue Scale (EQ-VAS) score [27]. One study including patients with SCI measured disease-specific QoL using the American Society of Colon and Rectal Surgeons Faecal Incontinence Score (FIQLS) [7,32]. The study showed a significant difference in the coping/ehavior and embarrassment scales, but not in the lifestyle or depression/self-perception scales between patients treated with TAI and conservative treatment [7].

The discontinuation rate ranged between 3 and 66% [7,20,21,23,24,26,27]. Reported reasons for discontinuation were expulsions of the catheter, bursting of rectal balloons, time consumption, heavy administration, dislike of treatment, adverse events and inefficacy. Two studies systematically reported the frequency of side effects with a range between 29 and 36% of patients experiencing side effects [7,23], the most frequent of which were abdominal pain, sweating/hot flushes, general discomfort, headache and perianal/anorectal pain. No studies reported health-economic results; however, two studies showed a reduction in urinary tract infections requiring treatment and reduction in contacts with health care professionals [7,27].

Using a multivariable analysis, one study identified several factors associated with a positive outcome of individual bowel scores; however, no consistent factors were identified [20]. To identify predictive factors for a positive outcome, four studies compared the compliant group with the non-compliant group; one study showed a higher proportion of patients with tetraplegia and patients depending on help in the non-compliant group [23]; one showed a higher baseline CCIS, SF-36 score and maximum tolerated volume to rectal balloon distension in the compliant group; one showed that impaired anal electrosensitivity was predictive for a successful outcome [27]; and one found no significant difference between the groups [24].

3.2. Low Anterior Resection Syndrome

In total, seven studies were identified reporting data on the effect of TAI in patients with LARS [38–44]. Results are presented in Table 2. The articles were published between 1989 and 2020. Five studies investigated TAI as a treatment for LARS [38–42], and two studies investigated TAI as a prophylactic treatment for LARS immediately after ileostomy closure [43,44].

3.2.1. Transanal Irrigation as Treatment for LARS

One RCT and four prospective cohort studies investigated TAI as a treatment for patients diagnosed with LARS [38–42]. Two studies hadshort FU [41,42], one had long FU [40], one had mixed FU [39] and one did not report any FU [38]. In total, 96 patients using TAI were included, with between 10 and 33 patients in each study. Four studies reported reasons for LARS, and the primary reason for LARS was resection for rectal cancer (89%) [39–42]. One study reported the operation type. In this study, 78% of patients had a total mesorectal excision [41]. Three studies were assessed to be of good methodological quality [40–42], one to be of fair methodological quality [39] and one to be of poor methodological quality [38].

One study reported a mean (SD) irrigation volume of 1500 (600) mL [39] and two studies a median (range) of 900 (500–1500) mL and 450 (300–1000) mL, respectively [40,41]. Irrigation every day or every second day was most common, and all patients self-administered TAI [40,42]. One study reported a mean (SD) irrigation time of 43.9 (27.3) min [39]. In three studies, patients received TAI training [40–44].

Bowel function was assessed by validated PROMs in five studies [40–44] and by a non-validated PROM in one study [39]. One study used the William's Incontinence score [39,45], one the CCIS [36,37,40], one used the LARS score [46–48] and the Memorial Sloan Kettering Cancer Centre Bowel Function Instrument (MSKCC BFI) [41,49], and one the LARS score, the FIGS score and the obstructed defaecation syndrome (ODS) score [29,42,50]. QoL was assessed using the SF-36 in two studies [32,40,41] and in one study using the European Organisation for Research and Treatment of Cancer (EORTC-QLQ-C30) questionnaire [42,51].

Table 2. Low anterior resection syndrome.

Reference	Study Design	TAI Cohort (Total Cohort)	Follow-Up Time	Inclusion Criteria	Patient Characteristics	Details on TAI	Bowel Function Outcome	Quality of Life Outcome	Discontinuation	Adverse Events	Quality Assessment
Iwama 1989 [38]	Prospective cohort	10	N/A	N/A	LARS 2 Turnbull-Cutait, 2 extra anal staple sutures, 1 pull-through operation, 5 anterior resections Age (years), mean (range): 61.4 (38–75) Male/female: 7/3 Predominant symptom: Frequent urge to defecate	Colostomy wash-out set (Hollister Incorporated, USA or Eisai Company, Japan) Irrigation volume (mL), range: 200–1000 Irrigation time (min), range: 20–50 Frequency of irrigation: 10% twice a day, 60% every day, 10% every second day, 20% once a week	In all cases, the frequent urge to defecate disappeared	N/A	Two patients continued using irrigation for more than 5 years, approximately once a week without any complications.	N/A	Reporting: 6 External: 1 Internal: 3 Power: 0 Total score: 10
Koch 2009 [39]	Prospective cohort	26	Mean (SD): 1.6 (1.1) years	FI after LAR for rectal cancer	LARS 30 rectal cancer Age (years), mean (SD): 67.6 (7.4) Male/female: 21/5 FU (years) after LAR, mean (SD): 4.7 (3.5)	Biotrol® Irrimatic pump (B. Braun Medical A/S, Germany) Irrigation volume (mL), mean (SD): 1500 (600) Irrigation time + defecation time (min), mean (SD): 43.9 (27.3) Frequency (day), mean (SD): 1.8 (0.7)	Pre-/post-treatment: William's Incontinence Score * [45], mean (SD): Pre: 4.5 (0.6) Post: 1.7 (0.9) ($p < 0.0001$) 57% pseudo continent, 14% incontinent for flatus, 29% incontinent for liquid stools	N/A	5 (19%) discontinued: 10% improved and stopped TAI, 80% were not satisfied	16 (62%) patients experienced side effects: 27% abdominal cramps, 23% leakage after irrigation, 7% time-consuming, 30% other (nausea, pain inserting cone etc.)	Reporting: 10 External: 1 Internal: 8 Power: 0 Total score: 19

Table 2. *Cont.*

Reference	Study Sesign	TAI Cohort (Total Cohort)	Follow-Up Time	Inclusion Criteria	Patient Characteristics	Details on TAI	Bowel Cunction Outcome	Quality of Life Outcome	Discontinuation	Adverse Events	Quality Assessment
Rosen 2011 [40]	Multicentre Prospective cohort	14	Median (range): 29 (15–46) months	LARS Minimum 9 months after stoma reversal Insufficient conservative treatment	LARS 12 rectal cancer, 2 large villous adenomas Age (years), median (range): 68 (45–80) Male/Female: 11/3 Time (months) from LAR or stoma reversal to assessment, median (range): 19 (9–48) Neoadjuvant radiotherapy (n): 10	Peristeen® (Coloplast A/S, Denmark) (2 used a Foley catheter) Volume (mL), median (range): 900 (500–1500) Irrigation frequency: 64% every day, 28% every second day, 7% every third day 100% self-administered Trained by a specialist nurse	Pre-/post-treatment: Defaecation episodes (n)/day, median (range): 8 (4–12) to 1 (1–2) (p < 0.001) Defaecation episodes (n)/night, median (range): 3 (2–5) to 0 (0–0) (p < 0.0001) CCIS, median (range): 17 (15–20) to 5 (4–9) (p < 0.01)	Pre-/post-treatment: MCS SF-36 *: 46 (35–55) to 55 (45–60) (p < 0.01) PCS SF-36 *: 55 (41–60) to 56 (49–62) (p = 0.3061) All domains of FIQLS were improved (p < 0.001)	No patients discontinued	3 (21%) patients experienced transient abdominal pain, 4 (29%) patients experienced minor rectal bleeding	Reporting: 11 External: 2 Internal: 7 Power: 0 Total score: 20
Martellucci 2018 [41]	Prospective cohort	33	6 months TAI follow-ing 3 months enema treat-ment	Short-term or long-term LARS with a LARS score ≥ 30 Failed conservative treatment	LARS 25 rectal cancer, 1 ulcerative colitis, 1 diverticular disease Age (years), median (range): 61 (29–83) Male/Female: 17/10 Neoadjuvant RT (n): 18 21 total mesorectal excision, 3 partial mesorectal excision, sigmoid resection 2, 1 total colectomy	Peristeen® (Coloplast A/S, Denmark) Volume (mL), median (range): 450 (300–1000) Frequency: 3–4 times per week Trained by a specialist nurse	Pre-/post-treatment: Daily number of bowel movements, median (range): Pre: 7 (0–14) Post: 1 (0–4) Post enema: 4 (0–13) LARS score * [46–48], median (range): Pre: 35.1 (30–42) Post: 12.2 (0–21) (p < 0.0001) Post enema: 27 (5–39) (p < 0.0001) MSKCC BFI * [49]: Significant improvement in frequency items, urgency items, incomplete emptying, and clustering of the No difference in effect between short-term and long-term LARS	Four scales of SF-36 significantly improved (mental health, social functioning, role emotional and bodily pain).	6 (18%) patients discontinued: 17% refused participation, 50% cancer recurrence, 17% proctitis, 17% dissatisfaction with protocol 85% continued TAI after the study	N/A	Reporting: 10 External: 3 Internal: 9 Power: 0 Total score: 22

Table 2. Cont.

Reference	Study Design	TAI Cohort (Total Cohort)	Follow-Up Time	Inclusion Criteria	Patient Characteristics	Details on TAI	Bowel Function Outcome	Quality of Life Outcome	Discontinuation	Adverse Events	Quality Assessment
Enriquez-Navascues 2019 [42]	Randomised controlled trial TAI or percutaneous tibial nerve stimulation	13 (27)	6 months	LARS score > 29 Total mesorectal excision for rectal cancer LARS or stoma reversal	LARS 13 rectal cancer Age (years), mean (range): 68 (48–71) Male/female: 9/4 Duration (months) of LARS, median (range): 30 (13–84) Neoadjuvant chemoradiotherapy: 6	Peristeen® (Coloplast A/S, Denmark) Volume: Adjusted for each patient Frequency of irrigation: Initially once a day then adjusted to 3–4 times a week 100% self-administered Trained by a specialist nurse	Intention-to-treat: Reduction in LARS grade in at least 50% of patients: 8 out of 13 patients fell from major to minor LARS Per-protocol: LARS score, median (IQR): 35 (32–39) to 12 (12–26) ($p = 0.021$) 80% of patients treated with TAI reported a reduction of at least 50% in the FIGS score No significant improvement in the ODS * [50] score	For EORTC-QLQ-C30 * [51] VAS scores of Global health status improved ($p = 0.020$)	3 (23%) discontinued: 23% no acceptability of TAI	No significant adverse events	Reporting: 11 External: 3 Internal: 9 Power: 0 Total score: 23
Rosen 2019 [43]	Multicentre randomised controlled trial TAI or best supportive care (BS) as prophylaxis for LARS immediately after ileostomy closure	18 (37) Rectal resection for rectal cancer	One week, 1 month, 3 months	Rectal resection for rectal cancer Anastomotic height < 5 cm above dentate line Complete healing of anastomosis Informed consent and physical and mental capability to perform TAI	LARS 18 rectal cancer Age (years), median (range): 58.5 (52–70) Male/female: 12/6 Neoadjuvant radiotherapy: 15	Peristeen® (Coloplast A/S, Denmark) or Foley catheter (28 French) Irrigation volume: 1000 mL Irrigation frequency: Every 24 h Irrigation time (min), median (range): 45 (30–60) 100% self-administered Trained by a specialist	Maximum number of defaecation episodes during daytime at 1 month, median (range): TAI: 3 (1–10) vs BS: 7 (3–30) ($p = 0.003$) Maximum number of defaecation episodes during night at 3 months, median (range): TAI: 0 (0–2) vs. BS: 1 (1–5) ($p = 0.002$) LARS score at 3 months, median (range): TAI: 9 (0–34) vs. BS: 31 (3–42) ($p = 0.001$) CCIS at 3 months, median (range): TAI: 2 (0–11) vs. BS: 6 (0–17) ($p = 0.046$)	MCS SF-36 at 3 months, median (range): TAI: 55 (31–60) vs. BS: 57 (26–63) ($p = 0.436$) PCS SF-36 at 3 months, median (range): TAI: 50 (39–64) vs. BS: 51 (37–61) ($p = 0.741$)	1 (6%) patients discontinued	No complications related to TAI	Reporting: 11 External: 2 Internal: 11 Power: 1 Total score: 25

Table 2. Cont.

Reference	Study Design	TAI Cohort (Total Cohort)	Follow-Up Time	Inclusion Criteria	Patient Characteristics	Details on TAI	Bowel Function Outcome	Quality of Life Outcome	Discontinuation	Adverse Events	Quality Assessment
Rosen 2020 [44]	Multicentre prospective cohort	19 (37)	12 months FU from Rosen 2019 [43]	See Rosen 2019 [43]	See Rosen 2019 [43]	Peristeen® (Coloplast A/S, Denmark) or Foley catheter Volume (mL), median (range): 600 (range 200–1000) Irrigation frequency: 50% every day, 30% every second day, 20% not on a regular schedule but at least 2/week. 100% self-administered	Maximum number of defaecation episodes during, median (range): Day: TAI: 3 (1–6) ($p = 0.018$) BS: 5 (2–10) Night: TAI: 0 (0–1) vs. BS 1 (0–5) ($p = 0.004$) LARS score, median (range): TAI: 18 (9–32) vs. 30 (3–39) ($p = 0.063$) CCIS: TAI: 4 (0–12) vs. BS: 7 (0–16) ($p = 0.151$)	MCS SF-36, median (range): TAI: 52 (34–59) vs. BS: 56 (28–62) ($p = 0.325$) PCS SF-36, median (range): TAI: 55 (50–67) vs. 5 (31–59) ($p = 0.460$)	9 (47%) patients discontinued: 89% time-consuming, 11% pain during TAI	N/A	Reporting: 10 External: 3 Internal: 9 Power: 0 Total score: 23

* MCS = Mental Component Summary, PCS = Psychical Component Summary, LARS score = Low Anterior Resection Syndrome score, MSKCC BFI = Memorial Sloan Kettering Cancer Centre Bowel Function Instrument ODS score = the obstructed defaecation syndrome score, EORTC-QLQ-C30 = European Organisation for Research and Treatment of Cancer questionnaire.

Comparing pre- and post-treatment scores, all studies showed a significant improvement of bowel function. One study showed a significant improvement of the mental component of the SF-36 and a non-significant improvement in the physical component [32,40]. Another study showed an improvement in four (mental health, social functioning, role emotional, and bodily pain) of eight SF-36 scales [41]. One study using EORTC-QLQ-C30 showed an improvement in VAS scores of the Global health status domain [42].

The discontinuation rate ranged between 0 and 23% [39–41]. Reported reasons for discontinuation were time consumption, dislike of treatment, cancer recurrence, proctitis and pain during TAI. Two studies reported side effects with a range between 29 and 62% experiencing side effects [39,41] including abdominal cramps, minor rectal bleeding, leakage after irrigation, nausea and pain at insertion.

One study investigated predictive factors for a decrease in LARS score, but found none [41].

3.2.2. Transanal Irrigation as a Prophylactic Treatment for LARS

TAI compared to best supportive care as a prophylactic treatment for LARS immediately after ileostomy closure was investigated in an RCT with three months of FU [43]. Eighteen patients were randomised to TAI. One-year FU results were published later [44]. Patients were included if a low anterior resection for rectal cancer was performed. The studies were assessed to be of good methodological quality.

The irrigation volume during the trial was 1000 mL, and at 1-year FU the median (range) volume was 600 (200–1000) mL. During the trial, the median (range) irrigation time was 45 (30–60) min and all patients irrigated daily. At 1-year FU, irrigation was performed daily by 50% of patients. All patients self-administered TAI and were trained in TAI.

Bowel function was assessed by the number of defaecation episodes during the day and night and by the LARS score and the CCIS. QoL was assessed by the mental and physical components of the SF-36.

At 3 months of FU, the studies showed a significant difference between the groups in LARS score and CCIS, and in the number of defaecation episodes during the day and night. At 12 months of FU, a significant difference in the number of defaecation episodes during the day and night was observed, but no significant difference in the LARS score or CCIS was seen. At 3- and 12-months of FU, no significant difference in QoL measured by the SF-36 in patients using TAI compared with patients using best supportive treatment was observed.

After 3 months, 6% of patients had discontinued TAI; at the 1-year FU, 47% had discontinued. Among patients discontinuing at one year, 89% had discontinued because TAI was too time-consuming, and 11% had discontinued due to pain during irrigation.

3.3. Faecal Incontinence and Constipation

In total, ten studies were identified reporting data on the effect of TAI in patients suffering from FI or constipation of heterogeneous origin [52–60]. The results are presented in Table 3. The articles were published between 1996 and 2017, and included one non-randomised trial [59], seven prospective studies [19,52,53,55–57,60], one cross-sectional study [54] and one retrospective study [58]. Eight studies included patients with FI or CC of heterogeneous origin and seven of these studies included both patients with FI and CC or a combination [53–58], and one study included only patients with FI [52]. One study included patients with chronic idiopathic constipation [60], and one study included women with FI because of sphincter damage after birth trauma [59]. In total, 1012 patients using TAI were included with between 16–507 patients in each study. Two studies had short FU [19,60], three studies long FU [54,55,58] and five studies mixed FU [52,53,56,57,59].

Table 3. Faecal incontinence and constipation.

Reference	Study Design	TAI Cohort (Total Cohort)	Follow-Up Time	Inclusion Criteria	Patient Characteristics	Details on TAI	Bowel Function Outcome	Quality of Life Outcome	Discontinuation	Adverse Events	Quality Assessment
Briel 1996 [52]	Prospective cohort	16	Median of 18 months	Impaired continence	Heterogeneous aetiology Age (years), median (range): 52 (25–72) Male/female: 5/11 FI: 16	System unspecified Irrigation time (min), median (range): 30 (10–90) Irrigation frequency: 87% ≥ 1 time a day Trained by enterostomal therapist	38% reported a successful outcome	N/A	6 (38%) patients discontinued	N/A	Reporting: 4 External: 1 Internal: 4 Power: 0 Total score: 9
Crawshaw 2003 [53]	Prospective cohort	48	Median (range): 11 (4–27) months	Absence of correctable pathology or the failure of medical and surgical treatment	Heterogeneous aetiology Age (years), median (IQR): 54 (41–61) Male/female: 13/35 Symptoms: FI: 33 CC: 15	Equipment adapted from a Coloplast Stoma Irrigation set (Coloplast A/S, Denmark) Irrigation volume: 1500 mL Irrigation frequency: 5% twice a day, 38% daily, 17% on alternate days, 15% every 3–7 days, 19% as required Trained by specialist nurse	Bowel control, visual analogue scale: Successful response to TAI in 24 (50%) patients. Bowel rating among these 24 patients, VAS 100 maximum (100 = full control), median (IQR): Pre: 15 (3–24) Post: 50 (34–65)	QoL among 24 patients with successful outcome, median (IQR): 59.16 (46.55–67.43) No difference compared to the 24 patients without successful response	4 (8%) patients discontinued: 50% unacceptable, 50% relief of symptoms with rectopexy	N/A	Reporting: 8 External: 2 Internal: 8 Power: 0 Total score: 18
Gardiner 2004 [19]	Prospective cohort	57	6 weeks		Symptoms: FI: 16 CC: 41	N/A	Proportion of patients with successful outcome: FI: 75% CC: 51% Slow transit CC (n = 15): 57% Obstructed defaecation (n = 26): 42%	N/A	FI: 2 (12.5%) patients discontinued: 6.25% not severe enough symptoms to continue TAI, 6.25% still under review	N/A	Reporting: 2 External: 1 Internal: 4 Power: 0 Total score: 7

Table 3. Cont.

Reference	Study Design	TAI Cohort (Total Cohort)	Follow-Up Time	Inclusion Criteria	Patient Characteristics	Details on TAI	Bowel Function Outcome	Quality of Life Outcome	Discontinuation	Adverse Events	Quality Assessment
Cazemier 2007 [54]	Cross-sectional	40	Time (y) using irrigation, mean (range): 8.5 (2.5–18)	FI or CC TAI No response to medical treatment or biofeedback	Heterogeneous aetiology Includes NBD FI: 28 Age (years): 42 Male/Female: 5/23 CC: 12 Age (years): 45 Male/Female: 3/9	Iryflex® (B. Braun Medical A/S, Germany) Irrigation volume: 500–1000 mL Frequency: 32% daily, 36% 3 times/week, 32% twice or less/week	25 (63%) patients still used TAI Overall satisfaction ($n = 40$): 29 (73%) Actual users ($n = 25$): satisfaction: 22 (88%)	N/A	Overall, 15 (38%) discontinued: FI: 5 (29%) CC: 7 (58%)	Side effects: 37.5% abdominal cramps	Reporting: 9 External: 3 Internal: 10 Power: 0 Total score: 22
Koch 2008 [55]	Prospective cohort	39	3, 6 and 12 months	FI or CC or both after failed conservative treatment or after (partially) unsuccessful surgical treatment for defaecation disorder	Heterogeneous aetiology Age (years), mean (SD): 58 (13.5) Male/Female: 13/26 Symptoms: FI: 18 CC: 11 FI + CC: 10	Biotrol® Irrimatic pump (B. Braun Medical A/S, Germany) or irrigation bag Braun (B. Braun Medical A/S, Germany) 1-year FU: Irrigation volume (L), mean (SD): 1.75 (0.79) Irrigation time (min), mean (SD): 36.39 (16.02) Frequency (time/day), mean (SD): 1.1 (0.49) Trained by physician	3 months FU, number (%) pseudo continent: FI: 11 (61%) ($p < 0.001$) FI + CC: 6 (60%) ($p = 0.009$) Baseline compared with 1-year FU: FI: Park's score [61]: 3.61 (0.5) to 1.6 (0.92) ($p < 0.005$) CCCS: Feeling of incomplete evacuation: 1.60 (2.47) to 2.75 (1.36) ($p = 0.036$)	Improvement in overall QoL measured with SF-36 and the FIQLS ($p = 0.012$)	9 (23%) patients discontinued: 78% unsatisfactory results, 22% appendicostomy	23 (59%) experienced side effects: 7% leakage after irrigation, 16% abdominal cramps, 22% abdominal bloating, 13% combination of the above side effects, 2% other	Reporting: 11 External: 2 Internal: 8 Power: 0 Total score: 21

Table 3. *Cont.*

Reference	Study Design	TAI Cohort (Total Cohort)	Follow-Up Time	Inclusion Criteria	Patient Characteristics	Details on TAI	Bowel Function Outcome	Quality of Life Outcome	Discontinuation	Adverse Events	Quality Assessment
Vollebregt 2016 [56]	Prospective cohort	60	Median FU: 12 months	Chronic defaecatory disorders not responding to conservative treatment	Heterogeneous aetiology Includes NBD and colorectal surgery Age (years), median (range): 49 (21–74) Male/female: 15/45 Symptoms: FI: 8 CC: 44 FI + CC: 8	Peristeen® (Coloplast A/S, Denmark) or Biotrol® Irrimatic pump (B. Braun Medical A/S, Germany) Irrigation volume (mL), median (range): 875 (250–2200) Frequency: 6% twice/day, 52% daily, 33% every second day, 6% when needed Trained by enterostomal therapist	First FU: FIQLS score did not differ between patients continuing or discontinuing TAI	First FU: Using SF-36 patients continuing TAI had more energy and were less fatigued compared with patients discontinuing TAI ($p = 0.01$) Patients continuing TAI had a tendency to have a higher SF-36 social functioning and a higher total SF-36 score, but this was non-significant	33 (55%) of patients had discontinued at the first FU, 37 (62%) at second FU and 38 (63%) at last FU	N/A	Reporting: 10 External: 3 Internal: 8 Power: 0 Total score: 21

Table 3. *Cont.*

Reference	Study Design	TAI Cohort (Total Cohort)	Follow-Up Time	Inclusion Criteria	Patient Characteristics	Details on TAI	Bowel Function Outcome	Quality of Life Outcome	Discontinuation	Adverse Events	Quality Assessment
Juul 2017 [57]	Prospective cohort	507	Mean (range): 1.06 (0.52–1.46) years	Intractable FI and/or CC with unsatisfactory results after conservative treatment	Heterogeneous aetiology Includes NBD and anorectal surgery Age (years), median (range): 56 (19–86) Male/female: 84/423 Symptoms: FI: 238 CC: 171 FI + CC: 98	Coloplast irrigation bag®/Colotip® (Coloplast A/S, Denmark) (majority), Coloplast irrigation bag® (Coloplast A/S, Denmark)/Qufora cone® (MBH International A/S), Aqua colon enema tip with silicone balloon ch 24® (Runfold Plastics Ltd., UK) or Peristeen® (Coloplast A/S, Denmark) Irrigation volume (mL), median (IQR): 1000 (750–1000) Irrigation time (min), median (IQR): 20 (15–30) Frequency: 35% daily, 16% every second day, 20% 2–3 times/week, 21% < once a week Self-administered 99%, assistance 1% Trained by specialist nurse	Patients with FI, pre-/post-treatment, mean change (95% CI): 11-point Likert, FI: 2.7 (2.2–3.2) ($p < 0.001$) CCIS: 2.2 (1.6–2.8) ($p < 0.001$) FIGS score: 2.2 (1.5–2.9) ($p < 0.001$) 65% improvement of FI, 29% stability, and 6% deterioration. Patients with CC, pre-/post-treatment, mean change (95% CI): 11-point Likert, CC: 1.6 (0.9–2.4) ($p < 0.001$) CCCS: 1.9 (1.1–2.7) ($p < 0.001$) ODS score: 3.3 (2.0–4.5) ($p < 0.001$). 48% improvement of CC, 40% stability and 12% deterioration.	Patients with FI and CC, pre-/post-treatment, mean change (95% CI): 11-point Likert, QoL: 1.8 (1.4–2.2) ($p < 0.001$)	174 (34%) discontinued: 49% inefficacy, 18% dislike treatment, 16% symptoms resolved, 13% time consumption, 12% side effects, 8% practical problems, 21% other, 8% undetermined	120 (58%) patients experienced side effects: 23% abdominal pain, 15% anorectal pain, 6% shivering/chills/11% nausea, 8% dizziness, 13% sweating	Reporting: 11 External: 2 Internal: 8 Power: 0 Total score: 21

Table 3. Cont.

Reference	Study Design	TAI Cohort (Total Cohort)	Follow-Up Time	Inclusion Criteria	Patient Characteristics	Details on TAI	Bowel Function Outcome	Quality of Life Outcome	Discontinuation	Adverse Events	Quality Assessment
Bildstein 2017 [58]	Retrospective	108	1-year FU	FI or CC Refractory to conservative treatment	Heterogeneous aetiology Includes NBD Age (years), mean (range): 55 (18–83) Male/female: 21/87 Symptoms CC: 51 FI + CC: 47 FI: 10	Peristeen® (Coloplast A/S, Denmark) Trained by specialist nurse	1-year FU: 46 (42.6%) patients still irrigated 62 (57%) discontinued: 44 had discontinued, 5 failed during first training, 12 lost to follow-up and 1 died	N/A	Reasons for discontinuation: 36.4% technical problems, 40.9% inefficacy, and 22.7% constraints (primary time-consuming) Median (range) time before discontinuation: 3 (0.2–11) months	25 (54.3%) reported minor 47 minor and self-limiting adverse events: 34% leakage of fluid around catheter, 29.9% pain when inserting catheter or water, 19.1% catheter expulsion, 10.6% rectal balloon burst, 6.4% water retention	Reporting: 11 External: 3 Internal: 9 Power: 0 Total score: 23
van der Hagen 2012 [59]	Multicentre non-randomised trial	35 (70)	6 months	History of birth trauma Passive faecal incontinence CCIS ≤ 8 after anal sphincter exercise and biofeedback Defect of the internal anal sphincter	Sphincter damage after birth trauma Age (years), mean (range): 53 (38–74)	REPROP® Clyster Trained by specialist nurse	In 3 (9%) patients faecal incontinence resolved completely Baseline 6-month FU: CCIS, average number of days per week with incontinence for solid or liquid stools, and average number of pads used did not change significantly	N/A	3 (9%) patients discontinued	No severe adverse effects	Reporting: 11 External: 2 Internal: 7 Power: 0 Total score: 20

Table 3. *Cont.*

Reference	Study Design	TAI Cohort (Total Cohort)	Follow-Up Time	Inclusion Criteria	Patient Characteristics	Details on TAI	Bowel Function Outcome	Quality of Life Outcome	Discontinuation	Adverse Events	Quality Assessment
Etherson 2017 [60]	Prospective cohort	102	Length of therapy use, median (range): 30.15 (1–460) weeks	Fulfilled Rome II criteria Past or present TAI treatment Received TAI for chronic idiopathic constipation (CIC) Failed all medical and behavioural therapies	Chronic idiopathic constipation (CIC) Age (years), median (range): 45 (25–84) Male/female: 7/95 Duration (years) of CIC, mean (SD): 21.8 (16.9)	Peristeen® (Coloplast A/S, Denmark) (majority), Qufora® (MBH International A/S) Biotrol® Irrimatic pump (B. Braun Medical A/S, Germany) Frequency: on average every second day	Overall symptom improvement: 42% Bowel frequency: Clearance of rectum: 63% Abdominal pain: 48% Bloating: 49% General well-being: 65% Awareness of urge: 25% Overall satisfaction with TAI was reported by 67% as either moderately better or very much better	N/A	48 (47%) patients discontinued	22 (22%) patients experienced side effects: 6% rectal bleeding, 3% painful irrigations, 2% painful haemorrhoids, 2% new anal fissure, 10% bursting balloons, 3% splitting of catheter	Reporting: 10 External: 2 Internal: 8 Power: 0 Total score: 20

Seven studies were assessed to be of good methodological quality [54–60], one of fair methodological quality [53] and two of poor methodological quality [19,52].

In four studies, irrigation volume ranged between 500 and 2200 mL [53,54,56,57] and one study reported a mean (SD) of 1750 (790) mL [55]. Irrigation every day or every second day was most common [52–56,60], and one study reported 99% of patients to self-administer [57]. One study reported a mean (SD) irrigation time of 36.39 (16.02) min [55] and two studies a median (range) time of 30 (10–90) min and 20 (15–30) min [52,57], respectively. In seven studies, patients received TAI training [52,53,55–59].

In four studies, validated bowel-specific PROMs were used as an outcome measure [55–57,59]; in five studies, non-validated PROMs were used [19,52–54,60]. One study used compliance as an outcome measure [58]. Two studies used the CCIS [57,59], one the CCCS [55], one the FIGS score [57], one the Park's score [55], one the obstructed defaecation syndrome (ODS) score [50,57] and one the FIQL score [56]. QoL was measured in four studies. One measured generic QoL with the SF-36 [32,55], one used the disease-specific FIQLS and two used non-validated PROMs [53,57].

Three prospective studies including patients with FI and CC of heterogeneous origin showed a significant improvement in bowel function with validated PROMs [55–57]. One of the studies showed significant improvement in QoL using the SF-36 [55] and the other an improvement in QoL on a non-validated 11-point Likert scale [57]. The last study showed no significant improvement in the FIQLS [56].

In the studies using non-validated PROMs to measure bowel dysfunction, one study reported an overall satisfaction with TAI of 73% [54], and one study showed a successful response to TAI in 50% of patients [53]. Using compliance as a success criterion, one retrospective study showed that 43% still irrigated at the 1-year FU. The study reporting data on only patients with FI used a non-validated measure and reported a successful outcome in 38% of patients [52].

In patients with chronic idiopathic constipation, overall satisfaction was reported in 67% of patients [60]. In patients with FI following sphincter damage after birth, no difference was seen when comparing the baseline and termination score [59].

The discontinuation rate ranged between 8 and 57% [52–60]. Reasons for discontinuation were inefficacy, pain during TAI, time consumption, side effects, practical problems and disliking the treatment. Side effects were reported to range from 22 to 59% [54,55,57,58,60]. Reported side effects included abdominal cramps, leakage of irrigation fluid, bloating, anorectal pain, chills/shivering, nausea, dizziness and sweating.

Using a multivariate analysis, one study showed a significant association between satisfactory progress of the first training and TAI compliance [58]. A cross-sectional study showed higher satisfaction among younger adults <40 years [54]. One study found no association between incontinence score and anorectal physiology and a successful effect of TAI [53]. Another study found no correlation between baseline measures and duration of TAI treatment [60].

4. Discussion

Results from this review show that TAI is a beneficial treatment for both NBD, LARS, and FI and CC of heterogeneous origin with some studies reporting improvement in disease-specific and generic QoL. With few exceptions, the studies in this review have used TAI as second-line treatment when conservative treatment has failed. Therefore, results from this review mainly evaluate effects on bowel function among patients not responding to conservative treatment, i.e., patients with potentially more severe bowel dysfunction.

Overall, three studies were RCTs [7,42,43] and 16 prospective cohort studies reporting pre- and post-treatment analysis of bowel function [20–23,26–28,39–41,44,53,55,57,59,60]. One study was assessed to be of excellent methodological quality [7] and 18 to be of good methodological quality [20,21,23,26–28,40–44,54–60]. Except from two studies [56,59], all prospective studies comparing pre- and post-treatment scores found a significant improvement in bowel function. Two RCTs supporting the superiority of TAI compared with conservative treatment have been published [7,44]; one in patients with SCI and one as a prophylactic treatment against LARS immediately after ileostomy closure. Another RCT including patients with LARS found a significant improvement in the TAI group, but not in the tibial nerve stimulation group [42].

Change in bowel function and QoL was primarily measured with PROMs. PROMs allow for the evaluation of patients' perspectives on functionality and QoL [62] and have gained acceptance within this research field. The use of validated instruments has previously been identified as a limitation in TAI research [12]. Overall, 67% of the included studies used at least one validated bowel-specific PROM. However, 82% of studies published within the last ten years used validated measures, showing that this limitation is no longer prominent. Nine different PROMs were used to evaluate bowel function, and this inconsistency of outcome measures compromises comparability. Numerous bowel function measures exist, which have been developed and validated differently. The NBD score and the LARS score have been developed and validated to evaluate bowel function based on a correlation with QoL, whereas the CCCS and FIGS are correlated to physiological or clinical assessment. Consensus regarding core outcome measures would ensure comparability in future research.

Half of the studies measured QoL by generic and/or disease-specific QoL measures. Three studies used a disease-specific QoL measure [7,40,56] and two of these showed improvement [7,40]. Although the NBD and LARS scores are not QoL measures, their items correlate with an impact on QoL. The reported improvement of these scores in many of the included studies could therefore suggest an improvement in disease-specific QoL. Some studies showed improvement in generic QoL measured with SF36, EQ-5D, or EORTC-QLQ-C30 [27,40–42,55], while other studies showed no significant change [26,43,44,56]. Two of the studies showing no improvement in generic QoL used TAI as a prophylactic rather than a symptomatic treatment [43,44]. Four studies used non-validated questions to measure QoL; three studies showed significant improvement in QoL [21,23,57]. The wording or themes explored by generic QoL instruments might be insensitive to changes in QoL resulting from an improvement in bowel function. We encourage research into generic QoL instruments sensitive to changes in bowel function that allow for a subjective valuation of the aspects of QoL that are most important to the individual patient.

Results show a high discontinuation rate at the 1-year FU of 19 to 57%, and several studies have based effect analyses solely on patients still performing irrigation at FU. Irrigation is known to be time-consuming and may involve practical difficulties. In order to overcome these challenges, patients have to experience a beneficial effect to continue the use of TAI [12]. Therefore, many studies consider the continuation of TAI as a successful outcome, and the high discontinuation rates in the studies included in this review suggest that TAI is beneficial only for a selected group of patients.

To predict a successful outcome and target the introduction of TAI to patients most likely to benefit from treatment, predictors of discontinuation have been studied. The studies included in this review reported no consistent predictive factors for a successful outcome. Using a multivariate analysis, Bildstein et al. found the progress of the first training to be a predictive factor for a successful outcome [58]. Almost all included studies in the present review reported that patients received TAI training prior to initiation, stressing that training is considered as an important part of the process. However, it is not evident which parameters the training comprises. In our clinic, all patients are taught irrigation by a specialised nurse, and the first irrigation performed by the patient or a caregiver is carried out under supervision at the clinic. In our experience, adequate training and patient support are important factors for patient compliance. Findings in this review partially support this; however, this must be further explored in future studies. Typically, clinical factors or basic demographic variables have been studied, such as age and sex, level of injury in SCI, mobility, tumour characteristics, stoma details, anorectal physiology, baseline bowel function and QoL scores. However, a successful outcome of TAI may also depend on personal characteristics such as the psychological profile and compliance with other treatment and hospital FU [5]. Future research should be directed towards better phenotyping TAI candidates. Among possible predicting factors for a successful outcome, socio-economic factors or personality traits should also be included.

Three of the major reasons for discontinuation identified through this review were technical problems, inefficacy and TAI being too timeconsuming. The primary technical problems reported were expulsion of the catheter, bursting of rectal balloons, and leakage around the catheter. Interestingly, technical problems were not reported as a reason for discontinuation amongst patients with LARS. Possible explanations might be the absence of a hyperreflective rectum in patients with LARS, which is seen in patients with NBD and can complicate rectal installation [63], or that data on technical problems was not reported.

Side effects were systematically reported in eight studies [7,23,39,40,55,57,58,60]. For NBD, side effects were reported to be experienced by 29 to 36% of patients, while this ranged between 29 and 62% for LARS and 22 and 59% for FI and CC of heterogeneous origin. There was no difference in the type of side effects reported among the different conditions. The most frequent side effects were abdominal cramps/pain, anorectal pain, nausea, sweating/hot flushes, minor bleeding and leakage of irrigation fluid. Christensen et al. reported no significant difference in the proportion of patients experiencing side effects during or immediately after TAI when comparing patients treated with TAI and those treated with conservative treatment [7]. This suggests that the side effects are not related to TAI, but to NBD itself. In SCI, autonomic dysreflexia during and after defaecation is even less pronounced when using TAI than with the usual digital manoeuvres to facilitate bowel emptying [64]. However, this finding has not been investigated for the LARS, FI or CC of heterogeneous origin. Only one study reported three serious adverse events, with no serious outcome [7], implying that such events are rare with the use of TAI. Bowel perforation is a potential risk related to TAI, and the risk has been reported to be 1 per 50,000 irrigations [65]. None of the included studies reported bowel perforations.

There are limitations to the included studies. So far, no RCTs have been conducted supporting the treatment of TAI compared with optimal conservative treatment in patients suffering from LARS, MS, FI or CC of other origin, and the risk of confounding as well as publication bias is known to be higher in non-randomised studies. FU varied between the studies, with the majority of studies having short FU time. Furthermore, conclusions may be limited by the fact that only a few studies have made power calculations, and the sample sizes of the included studies are generally modest, which may introduce type 2 errors. Generally, external validation was assessed to be of good quality in most studies; however, the modest sample size might indicate selection bias in the recruitment of patients. Systematic inclusion methods in prospective studies in the future could strengthen the evidence.

Another limitation is that many of the studies only included patients in their analysis who were still irrigating at FU. Therefore, the results primarily reflect improvements in a selected cohort. Future studies should include both intention-to-treat and per-protocol analysis. This is not necessarily a limitation; however, it should be taking into consideration when introducing TAI to patients. Since no consistent predictors supporting which patients could benefit from TAI have been identified until now, this selection process is difficult for the clinician. Therefore, a trial-and-error strategy for the introduction of TAI with focus on an individualised course of treatment has been suggested [5]. TAI is often combined with conservative modalities to optimize treatment; however, the majority of studies do not report concomitant treatment. Reporting of concomitant conservative modalities could help clinicians to optimize treatment. Another limitation to the studies is the missing reporting of clinical significance, and future studies should report results in a manner allowing for this to be assessed.

Limitations to this systematic review include a potential risk of publication bias if studies investigating TAI that found no significant results were not published. Inclusion criteria were restricted to the English language, which could have excluded relevant articles. In some early studies, different terms have been used for TAI — for example, wash-out—

which were not included in the search. This may be a limitation to our search. However, we consider our search using irrigation sufficient as recent literature has used the terms TAI and rectal irrigation, which would have been included in our search. Furthermore, the literature search was limited to three databases, and additional eligible studies might have been identified through other databases.

5. Conclusions

Results from this review show that TAI improves bowel function and potentially improves QoL among patients with NBD, LARS, and FI and CC of heterogeneous origin; however, the evidence remains limited. Until now, the highest evidence of TAI improving bowel function and QoL is from three RCTs showing superiority of TAI over best supportive care [7,43] and TAI as more efficient than tibial nerve stimulation [42] In NBD, the majority of the evidence is for patients with SCI, MS or SB. A high discontinuation rate calls for improved patient selection to TAI. However, no consistent predictive factors for a successful outcome have been identified. In order to identify patients benefiting from TAI, a trial-and-error approach may be used to assess if patients benefit from treatment. To optimize the possibility of a successful outcome of TAI treatment, it is important to conduct a personalised treatment course with supervision from specialised health-care personnel and to monitor outcomes of TAI.

Author Contributions: Conceptualisation, M.M., H.Ø.K., H.M.L., T.J., A.E., K.K., P.C.; methodology, M.M., H.Ø.K., H.M.L., T.J., A.E., K.K., P.C.; data curation, M.M., H.Ø.K., H.M.L.; writing-original draft preparation, M.M.; writing–review and editing, M.M., H.Ø.K., H.M.L., T.J., A.E., K.K., P.C.; supervision, T.J., A.E., K.K., P.C. All authors have read and agreed to the published version of the manuscript.

Funding: This research received no external funding.

Data Availability Statement: Not applicable.

Conflicts of Interest: Mira Mekhael has received grant support from MBH International A/S, Denmark. Professor Klaus Krogh has served as an advisory board member for Coloplast A/S and Wellspect HealthCare, Sweden. Professor Anton Emmanuel has served as an advisory board member for Coloplast A/S, Wellspect HealthCare, Sweden and MBH International. Professor Peter Christensen has served as an advisory board member for Coloplast A/S and Wellspect HealthCare, Sweden and has received grant support from MBH International A/S, Denmark.

References

1. Coggrave, M.; Norton, C.; Cody, J.D. Management of faecal incontinence and constipation in adults with central neurological diseases. *Cochrane Database Syst. Rev.* **2014**, *13*, CD002115. [CrossRef]
2. Dale, M.; Morgan, H.; Carter, K.; White, J.; Carolan-Rees, G. Peristeen Transanal Irrigation System to Manage Bowel Dysfunction: A NICE Medical Technology Guidance. *Appl. Health Econ. Health Policy* **2019**, *17*, 25–34. [CrossRef]
3. Christensen, P.; Olsen, N.; Krogh, K.; Bacher, T.; Laurberg, S. Scintigraphic assessment of retrograde colonic washout in fecal incontinence and constipation. *Dis. Colon Rectum* **2003**, *46*, 68–76. [CrossRef]
4. Emmanuel, A. Neurogenic bowel dysfunction. *F1000Research* **2019**, *8*. [CrossRef]
5. Emmanuel, A.V.; Krogh, K.; Bazzocchi, G.; Leroi, A.M.; Bremers, A.; Leder, D.; van Kuppevelt, D.; Mosiello, G.; Vogel, M.; Perrouin-Verbe, B.; et al. Consensus review of best practice of transanal irrigation in adults. *Spinal Cord* **2013**, *51*, 732–738. [CrossRef] [PubMed]
6. Glickman, S.; Kamm, M.A. Bowel dysfunction in spinal-cord-injury patients. *Lancet* **1996**, *347*, 1651–1653. [CrossRef]
7. Christensen, P.; Bazzocchi, G.; Coggrave, M.; Abel, R.; Hultling, C.; Krogh, K.; Media, S.; Laurberg, S. A randomized, controlled trial of transanal irrigation versus conservative bowel management in spinal cord-injured patients. *Gastroenterology* **2006**, *131*, 738–747. [CrossRef] [PubMed]
8. Christensen, P.; Fearnhead, N.S.; Martellucci, J. Transanal irrigation: Another hope for patients with LARS. *Tech. Coloproctol.* **2020**, *24*, 1231–1232. [CrossRef]
9. Dulskas, A.; Smolskas, E.; Kildusiene, I.; Samalavicius, N.E. Treatment possibilities for low anterior resection syndrome: A review of the literature. *Int. J. Colorectal Dis.* **2018**, *33*, 251–260. [CrossRef]
10. Pieniowski, E.H.A.; Palmer, G.J.; Juul, T.; Lagergren, P.; Johar, A.; Emmertsen, K.J.; Nordenvall, C.; Abraham-Nordling, M. Low Anterior Resection Syndrome and Quality of Life After Sphincter-Sparing Rectal Cancer Surgery: A Long-term Longitudinal Follow-up. *Dis. Colon Rectum* **2019**, *62*, 14–20. [CrossRef] [PubMed]

11. Chen, T.Y.; Wiltink, L.M.; Nout, R.A.; Meershoek-Klein Kranenbarg, E.; Laurberg, S.; Marijnen, C.A.; van de Velde, C.J. Bowel function 14 years after preoperative short-course radiotherapy and total mesorectal excision for rectal cancer: Report of a multicenter randomized trial. *Clin. Colorectal Cancer* **2015**, *14*, 106–114. [CrossRef]
12. Christensen, P.; Krogh, K. Transanal irrigation for disordered defecation: A systematic review. *Scand. J. Gastroenterol.* **2010**, *45*, 517–527. [CrossRef] [PubMed]
13. Christensen, P.; Krogh, K.; Buntzen, S.; Payandeh, F.; Laurberg, S. Long-term outcome and safety of transanal irrigation for constipation and fecal incontinence. *Dis. Colon Rectum* **2009**, *52*, 286–292. [CrossRef]
14. Emmanuel, A. Managing neurogenic bowel dysfunction. *Clin. Rehabil.* **2010**, *24*, 483–488. [CrossRef]
15. Moher, D.; Liberati, A.; Tetzlaff, J.; Altman, D.G. Preferred reporting items for systematic reviews and meta-analyses: The PRISMA statement. *BMJ* **2009**, *339*, b2535. [CrossRef]
16. Covidence Systematic Review Software, Veritas Health Innovation, Melbourne, Australia. Available online: www.covidence.org (accessed on 1 December 2020).
17. Downs, S.H.; Black, N. The feasibility of creating a checklist for the assessment of the methodological quality both of randomised and non-randomised studies of health care interventions. *J. Epidemiol. Community Health* **1998**, *52*, 377–384. [CrossRef]
18. Hooper, P.; Jutai, J.W.; Strong, G.; Russell-Minda, E. Age-related macular degeneration and low-vision rehabilitation: A systematic review. *Can. J. Ophthalmol.* **2008**, *43*, 180–187. [CrossRef] [PubMed]
19. Gardiner, A.; Marshall, J.; Duthie, G. Rectal irrigation for relief of functional bowel disorders. *Nurs. Stand.* **2004**, *19*, 39–42. [CrossRef] [PubMed]
20. Christensen, P.; Bazzocchi, G.; Coggrave, M.; Abel, R.; Hulting, C.; Krogh, K.; Media, S.; Laurberg, S. Outcome of transanal irrigation for bowel dysfunction in patients with spinal cord injury. *J. Spinal Cord Med.* **2008**, *31*, 560–567. [CrossRef]
21. Del Popolo, G.; Mosiello, G.; Pilati, C.; Lamartina, M.; Battaglino, F.; Buffa, P.; Redaelli, T.; Lamberti, G.; Menarini, M.; Di Benedetto, P.; et al. Treatment of neurogenic bowel dysfunction using transanal irrigation: A multicenter Italian study. *Spinal Cord* **2008**, *46*, 517–522. [CrossRef]
22. Loftus, C.; Wallace, E.; McCaughey, M.; Smith, E. Transanal irrigation in the management of neurogenic bowel dysfunction. *Ir. Med. J.* **2012**, *105*, 241–243.
23. Kim, H.R.; Lee, B.S.; Lee, J.E.; Shin, H.I. Application of transanal irrigation for patients with spinal cord injury in South Korea: A 6-month follow-up study. *Spinal Cord* **2013**, *51*, 389–394. [CrossRef] [PubMed]
24. Hamonet-Torny, J.; Bordes, J.; Daviet, J.C.; Dalmay, F.; Joslin, F.; Salle, J.Y. Long-term transanal irrigation's continuation at home. Preliminary study. *Ann. Phys. Rehabil. Med.* **2013**, *56*, 134–142. [CrossRef]
25. Adriaansen, J.J.; van Asbeck, F.W.; van Kuppevelt, D.; Snoek, G.J.; Post, M.W. Outcomes of neurogenic bowel management in individuals living with a spinal cord injury for at least 10 years. *Arch. Phys. Med. Rehabil.* **2015**, *96*, 905–912. [CrossRef] [PubMed]
26. Preziosi, G.; Gosling, J.; Raeburn, A.; Storrie, J.; Panicker, J.; Emmanuel, A. Transanal irrigation for bowel symptoms in patients with multiple sclerosis. *Dis. Colon Rectum* **2012**, *55*, 1066–1073. [CrossRef] [PubMed]
27. Passananti, V.; Wilton, A.; Preziosi, G.; Storrie, J.B.; Emmanuel, A. Long-term efficacy and safety of transanal irrigation in multiple sclerosis. *Neurogastroenterol. Motil.* **2016**, *28*, 1349–1355. [CrossRef] [PubMed]
28. Brochard, C.; Peyronnet, B.; Hascoet, J.; Olivier, R.; Manunta, A.; Jezequel, M.; Alimi, Q.; Ropert, A.; Neunlist, M.; Bouguen, G.; et al. Defecation disorders in Spina Bifida: Realistic goals and best therapeutic approaches. *Neurourol. Urodyn.* **2019**, *38*, 719–725. [CrossRef] [PubMed]
29. Agachan, F.; Chen, T.; Pfeifer, J.; Reissman, P.; Wexner, S.D. A constipation scoring system to simplify evaluation and management of constipated patients. *Dis. Colon Rectum* **1996**, *39*, 681–685. [CrossRef]
30. Vaizey, C.J.; Carapeti, E.; Cahill, J.A.; Kamm, M.A. Prospective comparison of faecal incontinence grading systems. *Gut* **1999**, *44*, 77–80. [CrossRef]
31. Krogh, K.; Christensen, P.; Sabroe, S.; Laurberg, S. Neurogenic bowel dysfunction score. *Spinal Cord* **2006**, *44*, 625–631. [CrossRef]
32. Rockwood, T.H.; Church, J.M.; Fleshman, J.W.; Kane, R.L.; Mavrantonis, C.; Thorson, A.G.; Wexner, S.D.; Bliss, D.; Lowry, A.C. Fecal Incontinence Quality of Life Scale: Quality of life instrument for patients with fecal incontinence. *Dis. Colon Rectum* **2000**, *43*, 9–16, discussion 16–17. [CrossRef]
33. *International Classification of Functioning, Disability, and Health*; ICF World Health Organization: Geneva, Switzerland, 2001.
34. Jorge, J.M.; Wexner, S.D. Etiology and management of fecal incontinence. *Dis. Colon Rectum* **1993**, *36*, 77–97. [CrossRef] [PubMed]
35. Fallon, A.; Westaway, J.; Moloney, C. A systematic review of psychometric evidence and expert opinion regarding the assessment of faecal incontinence in older community-dwelling adults. *Int. J. Evid. Based Healthc.* **2008**, *6*, 225–259. [CrossRef]
36. Ware, J.E., Jr.; Sherbourne, C.D. The MOS 36-item short-form health survey (SF-36). I. Conceptual framework and item selection. *Med. Care* **1992**, *30*, 473–483. [CrossRef] [PubMed]
37. EQ-5D-5L User Guide. EuroQol Research Foundation. 2019. Available online: https://euroqol.org/publications/user-guides (accessed on 1 December 2020).
38. Iwama, T.; Imajo, M.; Yaegashi, K.; Mishima, Y. Self washout method for defecational complaints following low anterior rectal resection. *Jpn. J. Surg.* **1989**, *19*, 251–253. [CrossRef]
39. Koch, S.M.; Rietveld, M.P.; Govaert, B.; van Gemert, W.G.; Baeten, C.G. Retrograde colonic irrigation for faecal incontinence after low anterior resection. *Int. J. Colorectal Dis.* **2009**, *24*, 1019–1022. [CrossRef]

40. Rosen, H.; Robert-Yap, J.; Tentschert, G.; Lechner, M.; Roche, B. Transanal irrigation improves quality of life in patients with low anterior resection syndrome. *Colorectal Dis.* **2011**, *13*, e335–e338. [CrossRef]

41. Martellucci, J.; Sturiale, A.; Bergamini, C.; Boni, L.; Cianchi, F.; Coratti, A.; Valeri, A. Role of transanal irrigation in the treatment of anterior resection syndrome. *Tech. Coloproctol.* **2018**, *22*, 519–527. [CrossRef] [PubMed]

42. Enriquez-Navascues, J.M.; Labaka-Arteaga, I.; Aguirre-Allende, I.; Artola-Etxeberria, M.; Saralegui-Ansorena, Y.; Elorza-Echaniz, G.; Borda-Arrizabalaga, N.; Placer-Galan, C. A randomized trial comparing transanal irrigation and percutaneous tibial nerve stimulation in the management of low anterior resection syndrome. *Colorectal Dis.* **2020**, *22*, 303–309. [CrossRef]

43. Rosen, H.R.; Kneist, W.; Fürst, A.; Krämer, G.; Hebenstreit, J.; Schiemer, J.F. Randomized clinical trial of prophylactic transanal irrigation versus supportive therapy to prevent symptoms of low anterior resection syndrome after rectal resection. *BJS Open* **2019**, *3*, 461–465. [CrossRef]

44. Rosen, H.R.; Boedecker, C.; Fürst, A.; Krämer, G.; Hebenstreit, J.; Kneist, W. "Prophylactic" transanal irrigation (TAI) to prevent symptoms of low anterior resection syndrome (LARS) after rectal resection: Results at 12-month follow-up of a controlled randomized multicenter trial. *Tech. Coloproctol.* **2020**, *24*, 1247–1253. [CrossRef]

45. Williams, N.S.; Patel, J.; George, B.D.; Hallan, R.I.; Watkins, E.S. Development of an electrically stimulated neoanal sphincter. *Lancet* **1991**, *338*, 1166–1169. [CrossRef]

46. Emmertsen, K.J.; Laurberg, S. Low anterior resection syndrome score: Development and validation of a symptom-based scoring system for bowel dysfunction after low anterior resection for rectal cancer. *Ann. Surg.* **2012**, *255*, 922–928. [CrossRef]

47. Juul, T.; Battersby, N.J.; Christensen, P.; Janjua, A.Z.; Branagan, G.; Laurberg, S.; Emmertsen, K.J.; Moran, B. Validation of the English translation of the low anterior resection syndrome score. *Colorectal Dis.* **2015**, *17*, 908–916. [CrossRef]

48. Juul, T.; Ahlberg, M.; Biondo, S.; Emmertsen, K.J.; Espin, E.; Jimenez, L.M.; Matzel, K.E.; Palmer, G.; Sauermann, A.; Trenti, L.; et al. International validation of the low anterior resection syndrome score. *Ann. Surg.* **2014**, *259*, 728–734. [CrossRef] [PubMed]

49. Temple, L.K.; Bacik, J.; Savatta, S.G.; Gottesman, L.; Paty, P.B.; Weiser, M.R.; Guillem, J.G.; Minsky, B.D.; Kalman, M.; Thaler, H.T.; et al. The development of a validated instrument to evaluate bowel function after sphincter-preserving surgery for rectal cancer. *Dis. Colon Rectum* **2005**, *48*, 1353–1365. [CrossRef]

50. Altomare, D.F.; Spazzafumo, L.; Rinaldi, M.; Dodi, G.; Ghiselli, R.; Piloni, V. Set-up and statistical validation of a new scoring system for obstructed defaecation syndrome. *Colorectal Dis.* **2008**, *10*, 84–88. [CrossRef] [PubMed]

51. Aaronson, N.K.; Ahmedzai, S.; Bergman, B.; Bullinger, M.; Cull, A.; Duez, N.J.; Filiberti, A.; Flechtner, H.; Fleishman, S.B.; de Haes, J.C.; et al. The European Organization for Research and Treatment of Cancer QLQ-C30: A quality-of-life instrument for use in international clinical trials in oncology. *J. Natl. Cancer Inst.* **1993**, *85*, 365–376. [CrossRef] [PubMed]

52. Briel, J.W.; Schouten, W.R.; Vlot, E.A.; Smits, S.; van Kessel, I. Clinical value of colonic irrigation in patients with continence disturbances. *Dis. Colon Rectum* **1997**, *40*, 802–805. [CrossRef]

53. Crawshaw, A.P.; Pigott, L.; Potter, M.A.; Bartolo, D.C. A retrospective evaluation of rectal irrigation in the treatment of disorders of faecal continence. *Colorectal Dis.* **2004**, *6*, 185–190. [CrossRef]

54. Cazemier, M.; Felt-Bersma, R.J.; Mulder, C.J. Anal plugs and retrograde colonic irrigation are helpful in fecal incontinence or constipation. *World J. Gastroenterol.* **2007**, *13*, 3101–3105. [CrossRef]

55. Koch, S.M.; Melenhorst, J.; van Gemert, W.G.; Baeten, C.G. Prospective study of colonic irrigation for the treatment of defaecation disorders. *Br. J. Surg.* **2008**, *95*, 1273–1279. [CrossRef]

56. Vollebregt, P.F.; Elfrink, A.K.; Meijerink, W.J.; Felt-Bersma, R.J. Results of long-term retrograde rectal cleansing in patients with constipation or fecal incontinence. *Tech. Coloproctol.* **2016**, *20*, 633–639. [CrossRef]

57. Juul, T.; Christensen, P. Prospective evaluation of transanal irrigation for fecal incontinence and constipation. *Tech. Coloproctol.* **2017**, *21*, 363–371. [CrossRef]

58. Bildstein, C.; Melchior, C.; Gourcerol, G.; Boueyre, E.; Bridoux, V.; Vérin, E.; Leroi, A.M. Predictive factors for compliance with transanal irrigation for the treatment of defecation disorders. *World J. Gastroenterol.* **2017**, *23*, 2029–2036. [CrossRef]

59. van der Hagen, S.J.; van der Meer, W.; Soeters, P.B.; Baeten, C.G.; van Gemert, W.G. A prospective non-randomized two-centre study of patients with passive faecal incontinence after birth trauma and patients with soiling after anal surgery, treated by elastomer implants versus rectal irrigation. *Int. J. Colorectal Dis.* **2012**, *27*, 1191–1198. [CrossRef]

60. Etherson, K.J.; Minty, I.; Bain, I.M.; Cundall, J.; Yiannakou, Y. Transanal Irrigation for Refractory Chronic Idiopathic Constipation: Patients Perceive a Safe and Effective Therapy. *Gastroenterol. Res. Pract.* **2017**, *2017*, 3826087. [CrossRef] [PubMed]

61. Parks, A.G. Royal Society of Medicine, Section of Proctology; Meeting 27 November 1974. President's Address. Anorectal incontinence. *Proc. R. Soc. Med.* **1975**, *68*, 681–690. [PubMed]

62. Habashy, E.; Mahdy, A.E. Patient-Reported Outcome Measures (PROMs) in Pelvic Floor Disorders. *Curr. Urol. Rep.* **2019**, *20*, 22. [CrossRef] [PubMed]

63. Preziosi, G.; Emmanuel, A. Neurogenic bowel dysfunction: Pathophysiology, clinical manifestations and treatment. *Expert Rev. Gastroenterol. Hepatol.* **2009**, *3*, 417–423. [CrossRef] [PubMed]

64. Faaborg, P.M.; Christensen, P.; Krassioukov, A.; Laurberg, S.; Frandsen, E.; Krogh, K. Autonomic dysreflexia during bowel evacuation procedures and bladder filling in subjects with spinal cord injury. *Spinal Cord* **2014**, *52*, 494–498. [CrossRef] [PubMed]

65. Faaborg, P.M.; Christensen, P.; Kvitsau, B.; Buntzen, S.; Laurberg, S.; Krogh, K. Long-term outcome and safety of transanal colonic irrigation for neurogenic bowel dysfunction. *Spinal Cord* **2009**, *47*, 545–549. [CrossRef] [PubMed]

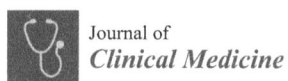

Journal of
Clinical Medicine

MDPI

Article

The Addition of Transdermal Delivery of Neostigmine and Glycopyrrolate by Iontophoresis to Thrice Weekly Bowel Care in Persons with Spinal Cord Injury: A Pilot Study

William A. Bauman [1,2,3,*], Anton Sabiev [1,2], Shahzad Shallwani [2], Ann M. Spungen [1,3], Christopher M. Cirnigliaro [1] and Mark A. Korsten [1,2,3]

[1] Veterans Affairs Rehabilitation Research and Development Service's National Center for the Medical Consequences of Spinal Cord Injury, James J. Peters Veterans Affairs Medical Center, Bronx, NY 10468, USA; anton.sabiev@va.gov (A.S.); ann.spungen@va.gov (A.M.S.); christopher.cirnigliaro@va.gov (C.M.C.); mark.korsten@va.gov (M.A.K.)

[2] Medical Service, James J. Peters Veterans Affairs Medical Center, Bronx, NY 10468, USA; shahzad.shallwani@va.gov

[3] Departments of Medicine and Rehabilitation and Human Performance, The Icahn School of Medicine at Mount Sinai, New York, NY 10029, USA

* Correspondence: william.bauman@va.gov; Tel.: +1-(718)-584-9000 (ext. 5428)

Citation: Bauman, W.A.; Sabiev, A.; Shallwani, S.; Spungen, A.M.; Cirnigliaro, C.M.; Korsten, M.A. The Addition of Transdermal Delivery of Neostigmine and Glycopyrrolate by Iontophoresis to Thrice Weekly Bowel Care in Persons with Spinal Cord Injury: A Pilot Study. *J. Clin. Med.* **2021**, *10*, 1135. https://doi.org/10.3390/jcm10051135

Academic Editor: Alexandra Lucas

Received: 15 January 2021
Accepted: 3 March 2021
Published: 8 March 2021

Publisher's Note: MDPI stays neutral with regard to jurisdictional claims in published maps and institutional affiliations.

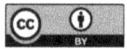

Copyright: © 2021 by the authors. Licensee MDPI, Basel, Switzerland. This article is an open access article distributed under the terms and conditions of the Creative Commons Attribution (CC BY) license (https://creativecommons.org/licenses/by/4.0/).

Abstract: Persons with spinal cord injury (SCI) have neurogenic bowel disorders characterized by difficulty with evacuation (DWE), fecal incontinence, and discoordination of defecation. Six medically stable in-patients with SCI with a mean age of 57 ± 10 years (range: 39–66 years) and time since injury of 18 ± 17 years (range: 3–47 years) were investigated. Standard of care (SOC) for bowel care was followed by two weeks of SOC plus neostigmine (0.07 mg/kg) and glycopyrrolate (0.014 mg/kg) administered transcutaneously by iontophoresis thrice weekly for two weeks while patients continued to receive SOC. The primary endpoint was time to bowel evacuation. Body weights and abdominal radiographs were obtained. Ten questions related to bowel function and the Treatment Satisfaction Questionnaire for Medication were acquired after each arm. Bowel evacuation time decreased after the dual drug intervention arm (106.9 ± 68.4 vs. 40.8 ± 19.6 min; $p < 0.0001$). Body weight decreased (2.78 ± 0.98 kg; $p < 0.0001$), a finding confirmed on abdominal radiograph. Both questionnaires demonstrated improvement after the dual drug intervention arm. No major adverse events occurred. The addition of neostigmine and glycopyrrolate by transcutaneous administration to SOC for bowel care in persons with SCI and DWE resulted in the safe, effective, and predictable bowel evacuation with subjective improvement in bowel care.

Keywords: spinal cord injury; neurogenic bowel; difficulty with evacuation; neostigmine; glycopyrrolate; iontophoresis

1. Introduction

Persons with motor-complete spinal cord injury (SCI), as well as the majority of persons with motor-incomplete spinal cord lesions, have bowel dysfunction, which is a condition that is characterized by difficulty with evacuation (DWE), fecal incontinence, and discoordination of defecation due to dyssynergia between colonic motility and the external anal tone [1]. The clinician prescribing a bowel care regimen for the patient with SCI strives to lessen morbidity by maintaining continence and, if possible, providing the ability to defecate at will. This is frequently accomplished by identifying an individualized bowel regimen by empiric trial and error that may include diet, stool softeners, enemas, and scheduling of bowel care. Despite these approaches, bowel care is frequently unpredictable, time consuming, and often unsatisfactory for those with SCI, adversely affecting quality of life [2–4].

Our group has demonstrated the safety and efficacy of the intravenous and intramuscular administration of neostigmine and glycopyrrolate to induce a safe and predictable bowel evacuation [5,6]. However, the practical utility of the parenteral administration of medication for bowel care is limited due to personal, practical, and medical reasons. As such, to be of any clinical value for routine bowel care in patients with SCI, an alternative mode of administration for this dual drug combination needed to be identified.

To date, the transcutaneous administration of drugs by iontophoresis has been used somewhat sparingly in clinical medicine, and its application has been predominantly to target the delivery of agents to local tissues [7]. Iontophoresis is pain-free, does not require adherence to aseptic technique, allows for low-risk self-administration and, obviously, obviates the role for needles and injection. In addition, a potential therapeutic advantage of transdermal administration of some drugs is their direct delivery into the systemic circulation, avoiding first-pass hepatic metabolism. The application of this methodology may have practical utility in the treatment of certain conditions that require repetitive systemic administration in the home setting, such as that for bowel care in those with SCI or other conditions associated with neurogenic bowel disorders, as well as for those in the general population without a diagnosis of neurogenic bowel but associated with DWE. Our group has reported that a single transcutaneous administration of neostigmine and glycopyrrolate stimulates a predictable bowel movement without adverse local or systemic events [8]. The question remains, and is the subject of the work presented herein, as to whether the addition of this dual drug approach by transcutaneous route to standard of care (SOC) for the bowel management confers any clinical or patient-reported benefits over that of SOC alone.

2. Subjects and Methods

Six medically stable male patients with chronic SCI (>1 year) and DWE (bowel evacuation time > 60 min) with varying degrees of completeness of lesion who were hospitalized on the Spinal Cord Injury Service of the James J. Peters Veterans Affairs Medical Center (JJP VAMC) were recruited for study participation. A history of cardiac or pulmonary disease, uncontrolled hypertension, current infection, and/or pregnancy excluded patients from study participation. Each patient who was recruited for study participation continued to receive his individualized bowel care regimen thrice weekly during the course of the study. The study was performed in agreement with good Clinical Practice guidelines and according to the guidelines of the Declaration of Helsinki. The protocol was approved by the Institutional Review Board of the JJP VAMC. Written informed consent was obtained from each participant. The clinical trial was registered with ClinicalTrials.gov (NCT04671030).

The study consisted of two arms: (1) SOC for bowel three times a week for one week or (2) SOC plus the dual drug combination of neostigmine 0.07 mg/kg and glycopyrrolate 0.014 mg/kg administered transcutaneously by iontophoresis three times a week for two weeks. Bowel care was provided on alternate days, either Monday-Wednesday-Friday or Tuesday-Thursday-Saturday. Baseline and follow-up evaluations were performed before and after each arm of the study and included body weight and an anteroposterior abdominal radiograph. The abdominal radiograph was performed prior to treatment and on the last day of the 2-week treatment period. The images were read for the level of fecal impaction by the radiologists who were blinded as to the phase of the protocol. Using a list of questions from Lynch et al. [9], ten questions were selected and assigned a response score on a five-point scale with a "1" (best) to "5" (worst) response score; this survey was entitled the Ten Question Bowel Survey (10Q), which is not a validated survey vehicle. Rather than only questions 1 to 3 and question 14 being scored on a 7-point scale, the Treatment Satisfaction Questionnaire for Medications [10] was adapted by having all questions scored on a 7-point scale, except question 4 which had a dichotomous answer ("yes" or "no"); as such, the Treatment Satisfaction Questionnaire for Medications, as adapted for this study, is not a validated survey vehicle. The Treatment Satisfaction Questionnaire for Medications and the 10Q Survey were performed at the end of each study arm. Time to stool evacuation was averaged for the bowel care sessions of each subject for each study arm and then averaged for all subjects for that arm of the study. To capture potential adverse events after administration of the agents, blood pressure, heart rate and pulse oximetry were monitored throughout each bowel care session with assessments performed every five minutes for the initial 60 min and then at 90 min.

The skin was prepared at the sites of placement for the anode and cathode electrodes prior to placing the iontophoresis patches. At the placement site for the anode patch, the skin of the anterior thigh was cleaned with 70% alcohol preparation pads and then sprayed with 20% benzocaine followed by epilation and the application of 0.2% sodium lauryl sulfate in deionized water. At the placement site for the cathode patch, which was approximately 4 to 6 inches distant from the anode patch electrode on the lower extremity, the skin was cleaned with 70% alcohol preparation pads. The anode patch was loaded with neostigmine and glycopyrrolate mixed in distilled water in concentrations previously described [8]. The cathode patch was loaded with 0.5 mL 0.9% normal saline with 1.0% citric acid. The electrodes were connected to Dynatron® iBox™ (Salt Lake City, UT, USA) which delivered an electric current (4.0 mA/min) that was insensible to the subject and applied for 20 min.

Statistical Analyses

The results are expressed as the group mean plus or minus standard deviation (SD). For the time to bowel evacuation and change in body weight, a two-tailed paired *t*-tests was performed. The survey scores are presented for descriptive purposes only for the Ten Question Bowel Survey and Treatment Satisfaction Survey for Medications, which were performed following each arm of the study. An *a priori* level of significance was set at $p \leq 0.05$. Statistical analyses were completed using IBM SPSS Statistics (IBM, version 27 for Windows, Armonk, NY, USA) and graphs were generated by Prism (GraphPad Software, version 9.0 for Windows, San Diego, CA, USA).

3. Results

The mean age of the male subjects was 57 ± 10 years (range: 39–66 years) with a mean duration since SCI of 18 ± 17 years (range: 3–47 years) (Table 1). Three patients had a complete motor lesion with partial sensory sparing (International Standards for Neurological Classification of Spinal Cord Injury (ISNCSCI) grade B) and three patients had motor-incomplete lesions with partial sensory (ISNCSCI grade C and D) (Table 1); five of six subjects had spinal cord lesions above thoracic level-6.

Table 1. Characteristics of the Study Participants.

						SOC and NEO + GLY Treatment		
Subject ID	Age (year)	TSI (year)	ISNCSCI (A/B/C/D)	MI (C/I)	SI (C/I)	Baseline Body Weight (kg)	Week-2 Body Weight (kg)	Body Weight △
001	62	3	B	C	I	96.4	93.8	−2.6
002	39	29	C	I	I	74.6	71.5	−3.1
003	54	8	D	I	I	77.8	73.4	−4.4
004	62	13	C	I	I	132	129.6	−2.4
005	66	47	B	C	I	61.4	60.0	−1.4
006	64	5	B	C	I	71.8	69.0	−2.8
Mean (SD)	57.8 (10.1)	17.5 (17.2)	0/3/2/1	3/3	0/6	85.7 (25.4)	82.9 (25.5) *	−2.8 (0.98)

Values are expressed for individual participants and as a group mean ± standard deviation (SD). Abbreviations: ISNCSCI = International Standards for Neurological Classification of Spinal Cord Injury; TSI = time since injury; kg = kilogram; MI = motor impairment; SI = sensory impairment; C = complete; I = incomplete; SOC = standard of care; NEO = neostigmine, GLY = glycopyrrolate; △ = difference. * Baseline Body Weight vs. Week-2 Body Weight (post dual drug treatment): $p < 0.001$.

One-week SOC in six subjects consisted of 18 bowel care sessions, and the two-week SOC plus neostigmine and glycopyrrolate consisted of 36 bowel care sessions. At the conclusion of the SOC arm, the average length of time to complete a bowel care session was 107 ± 68 min, whereas at the termination of the SOC arm plus neostigmine and glycopyrrolate arm the average length of a bowel care session was markedly shortened to 41 ± 20 min (Figure 1; $p < 0.0001$); the difference in the length of bowel care between the control and drug-treatment arms ranged from 42 to 88 min (CI: 95%). After one-week of SOC, there was no significant change in body weight (0.33 ± 0.21 kg) and, as expected, no change in abdominal radiographic images of stool burden. In contrast, at the end of two weeks of SOC plus the dual drug-treatment, an average 2.8 ± 1.0 kg loss of body weight was observed (86 ± 25 kg vs. 83 ± 26 kg; $p < 0.0001$), with an initial 1.2 ± 1.2 kg loss of weight at the end of the first week. The values for individual weight loss after the dual drug intervention arm are provided (Table 1). The loss of body weight was confirmed on abdominal radiographs to be due to a reduction in retained stool (Figure 2). After two weeks of the dual drug treatment, the 10Q Survey showed an improvement in bowel care (Figure 3), and the Treatment Satisfaction Questionnaire for Medications revealed that the medications were well tolerated and that bowel care appeared to be improved as well (Figure 4).

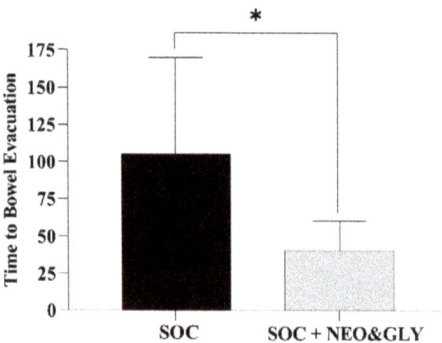

Figure 1. Comparison of the time to bowel evacuation between the standard of bowel care or standard of bowel care plus neostigmine and glypyrrolate arms of the study. SOC = standard of care; NEO = neostigmine; GLY = glycopyrrolate. * $p < 0.0001$.

No severe cardiopulmonary adverse events were observed in the dual drug treatment arm. Heart rate and blood pressure, while affected by the dual drug intervention, were well within acceptable clinical limits for a treatment protocol and were not associated with any reported symptoms attributable to these minor perturbations in vital signs. Heart rate at baseline was reduced to a nadir heart rate at 40 min after the start of the dual drug intervention (72 ± 10 beats per minute (range: 59–83) to 61 ± 9 beats per minute (range: 52–77); $p < 0.05$). Systolic blood pressure increased from 108 ± 15 to 123 ± 16 mg Hg at 40 min after the start of the dual drug intervention, which was not a significant rise in systolic blood pressure and likely represented an autonomic response to stool evacuation. Pulse oximetry values were stable throughout both arms of the study. Abdominal discomfort, or cramping, occurred in all patients, was on average 2/5 in severity and persisted for 24 ± 14 min. As appreciated, abdominal cramping was an expected effect of the dual-drug intervention and represented an increase in bowel motility being sensed by the subject. The sensation of dry mouth occurred in 4 of 36 bowel care sessions at 20 to 35 min after beginning the dual drug-treatment and persisted, on average, for 35 min. Headache of 1/10 severity, which lasted an average of 13 min, was reported twice in one subject. No episodes of autonomic dysreflexia occurred.

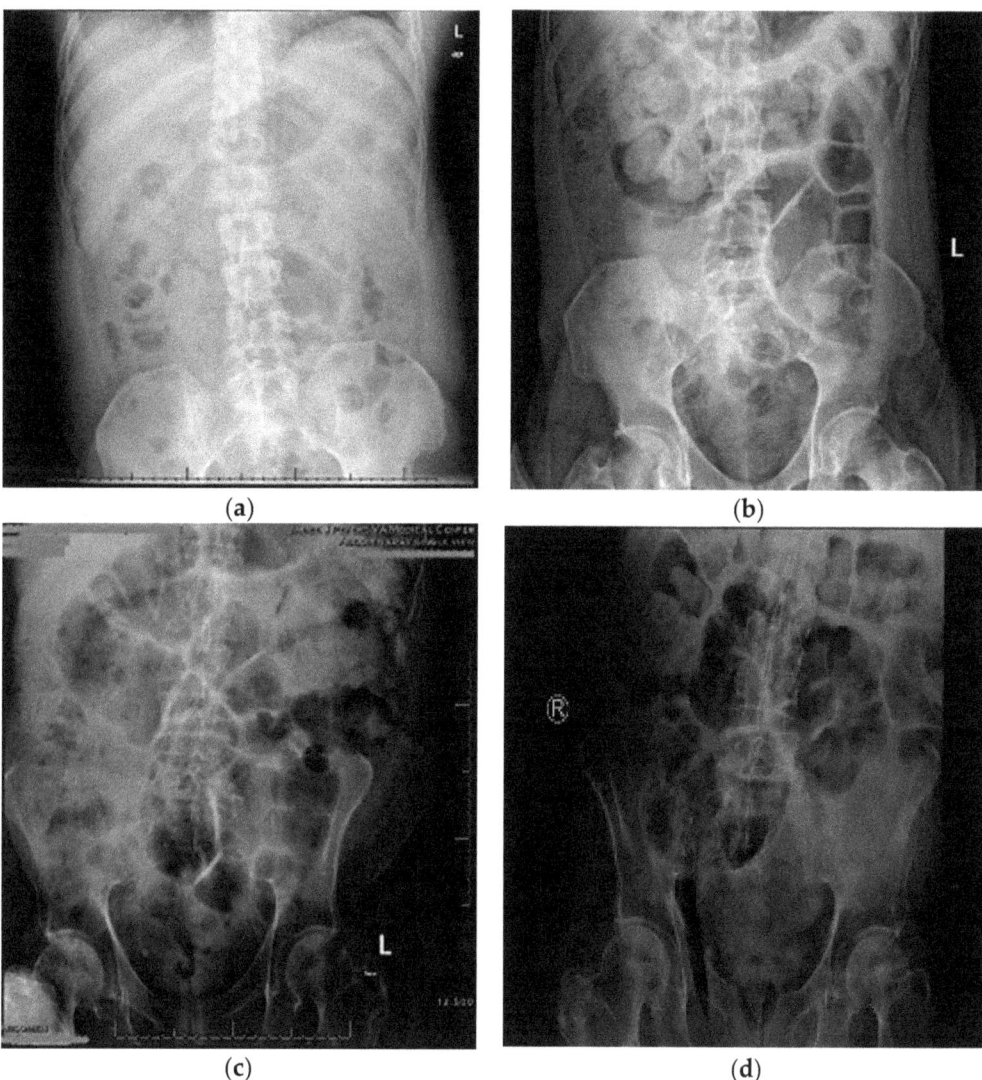

Figure 2. Representative qualitative measure of stool burden on abdominal radiograph after standard of care or standard of care plus neostigmine and glypyrrolate. Fecal burden: (**a**) marked stool throughout the colon, (**b**) moderate stool in the cecum; (**c**) moderate stool in the transverse and left colon, (**d**) moderate stool in the cecum. Loss of body weight after two weeks of standard of bowel care and the dual drug combination: (**a,b**), −4.4 kg; (**c,d**), −2.6 kg.

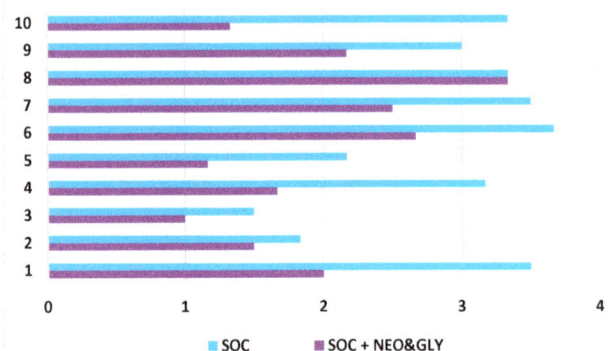

Figure 3. Findings of the ten question bowel survey after standard of care or standard of care plus neostigmine and glypyrrolate. Abscissa axis: A score of "1" represent fully satisfied or the best response; a score of "5" represents fully dissatisfied or the worse response score. Ordinate axis labels: 1. Satisfaction with overall bowel management program during the past month; 2. Bowel control over the past month; Questions 3 to 7, 9, and 10 are asked during the past 7 days: 3. Bowel control over; 4. Use of enemas for bowel control; 5. Use of laxatives; 6. Digital stimulation; 7. Number of bowel movements (1: 7 times or more, 2: 5–6 times, 3: 3–4 times, 4: 1–2 times, 5: none); 8. Average time spent to have a bowel evacuation per bowel care session; 9. Total time in the past week; and 10. Discomfort rating. SOC = standard of care; SOC and NEO + GLY = standard of care plus neostigmine and glycopyrrolate.

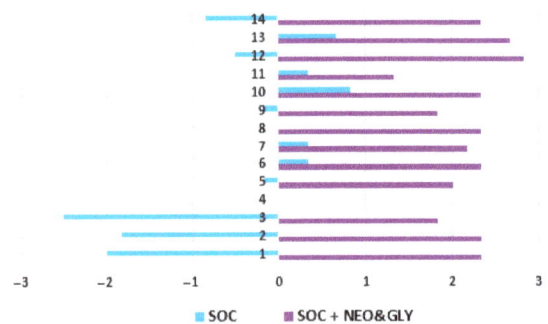

Figure 4. Findings of the Treatment Satisfaction Survey after Standard of Care or after Standard of Care plus Neostigmine and Glypyrrolate. The treatment satisfaction questionnaire for medications [10] was adapted by having all questions scored on a 7-point scale, except question 4 which had a dichotomous answer Abscissa: (−3) Extremely dissatisfied, (−2) Dissatisfied, (−1) Mildly dissatisfied, (0) Ambivalent, (1) Mildly Satisfied, (2) Satisfied, (3) Extremely Satisfied. Ordinate Axis: 1. Ability of medication to treat DWE; 2. Ability of medication to relieve symptoms; 3. Delay in its effect; 4. Side-effects of SOC and NEO + GLY, 5 subjects answered "yes", 1 subjects answered "no"; 5. How bothersome are the side-effects? 6. Side-effects and physical function and health; 7. Side-effects and mental function and health; 8. Side-effects affecting satisfaction with the medication; 9. Difficulty in use; 10. Difficulty in planning; 11. Convenience in following instructions; 12. General satisfaction with the medication; 13. How certain are you that the good things about your medication outweigh the bad things? 14. Taking all things into account, how satisfied or dissatisfied are you with this medication? SOC = standard of care; SOC and NEO + GLY = standard of care plus neostigmine and glycopyrrolate.

4. Discussion

The transdermal delivery of neostigmine and glycopyrrolate by iontophoresis substantially reduced the time to bowel evacuation in patients undergoing routine bowel care and resulted in a more complete stool evacuation, as determined by body weight and abdominal radiographic evidence. Subjectively, the patients showed improvement in all indicators of bowel care and were more satisfied with their bowel treatment regimens.

Individuals with complete SCI have neurogenic bowel, and most of those with incomplete SCI have varying degree of bowel dysfunction. The neurological manifestations of bowel dysfunction in those with SCI may include reduced gastrointestinal motility, loss of external anal sphincter voluntary control, and impaired anal sensation; these neurogenic bowel manifestations may result in abdominal distension, intractable constipation, prolonged defecation, fecal incontinence, and eventually hemorrhoids, rectal prolapses and perianal skin complications, all of which adversely impacts quality of life. Other than bladder problems, gastrointestinal disorders are the most common secondary complication reported in patients with SCI. In a survey of 241 individuals with SCI, only about half were satisfied with their bowel care routine because of the amount of time required, pain or discomfort, and generally unsatisfactory results, which were associated with reduced quality of life in the domains of bowel care, employment, and social function [3]. A safe and effective pharmacological approach to bowel care would be a welcome addition to clinical care for the individual with SCI and DWE.

Persons with SCI require at least one therapeutic intervention to initiate defecation, and most patients report bowel dysfunction as a major life-limiting problem. In one report, constipation (56%, 31/55) and incontinence (42%, 23/55) were the most common gastrointestinal problems. Digital rectal stimulation was the most common method for bowel evacuation, regardless of whether patients participated in a bowel program or not [11]. In a retrospective analysis of a cross-sectional phone survey of 64 patients determined which bowel management methods were evaluated and a Likert-type questionnaire was applied to assess the impact of neurogenic bowel disorders on both the International Classification of Function, Disability and Health (ICF) domains and on quality of life [4]. The most common bowel management methods were laxatives, suppositories and osmotic laxatives; of note, 50.1% of patients scored moderate or severe NBD. For reporting by patient for the ICF domains of Environmental and Personal factors, 46.9% had loss of privacy, 45.3% had a need of assistance for bowel management, 45.3% had feelings of frustration, anxiety or depression, and 39.1% reported neurogenic bowel to be associated with increased economics costs [4]. There was also a significant impact on the ICF category of Body Structures, with 26.6% of patients reporting complaints of pain associated with neurogenic bowel problems; for the ICF Activity domain, 28.1% reported an impact to achieve scheduled activities, 26.6% reported impact on the time spent in defecation, and 23.4% reported the need of diet adaptions [4]. A significant association was found between severity of neurogenic bowel disorder and a negative impact on quality of life ($p < 0.05$) [4]. Inskip et al. reported that management of bowel dysfunction was a problem for 78% of 287 individuals with SCI who were surveyed, and this condition proved to be a problem with personal relationships (60%), prevented from leaving home (62%), and interfered with employment outside the home (41%) [12]. In 24% of respondents with SCI, the routine bowel care regimen lasted longer than 60 min and most persons (59%) and required digital rectal stimulation to complete the bowel care session. Despite the best efforts of patients, bowel incontinence was reported at least monthly in 33% of those queried [12]. Autonomic dysreflexia due to bowel care interfered with activities of daily living in 51% of subjects. Longer durations of bowel care were highly significantly correlated with lower quality of life [12]. There are also economic costs associated with bowel dysfunction. In a survey of 332 patients with fecal incontinence for more than a year with at least monthly leakage of stool, the average annual total cost per person was $4110, with the severity of fecal incontinence correlated to higher annual direct costs [13].

The development of a successful bowel care routine in an individual with SCI is approached empirically. Medications that are employed in the management of bowel dysfunction may be divided by route of administration (e.g., by mouth or per rectum) or by their pharmacological mechanism of action. The categories of agents include bulk-forming agents, stool softeners, and laxatives. Various direct bowel wall stimulants have been used, and include senna preparations by mouth or per rectum, castor oil, magnesium preparations by mouth, and sodium phosphate/biphosphate by mouth. Even after applying these measures to induce a regular bowel evacuation, persons with SCI frequently have incomplete and unpredictable bowel evacuation, which may result in discomfort, autonomic dysreflexia, and/or stool incontinence. The inability to empty the colon predictably and completely results in a high risk of incontinence. Fecal incontinence is a source of hummiliation, lost time, increased caregiver support and additional expense. The possibility of bowel accidents is often provided as a reason that those with SCI remain homebound and have a tendency to avoid activities in the community. Prior to our work, few, if any, evidence-based pharmacologic interventions improve fecal transit time and bowel evacuation in a predictable manner in those with SCI. Trans-anal irrigation has been employed as a treatment to reduce constipation and fecal incontinence when other more conservative modalities prove unsatisfactory. When conservative treatments are not effective, surgical interventions may be considered.

The drug combination of neostigmine, a cholinergic agent, and glycopyrrolate, a selective cardiopulmonary anticholinergic agent, administered by intravenous [5], and intramuscular [6] route was demonstrated by our group to predictably stimulate bowel evacuation without life-threatening cholinergic effects on heart rate or airway [5,14]. The effectiveness and reliability of this dual pharmacological approach to induce bowel evacuation is appreciably greater than that of oral or rectal cathartics. However, the practical utility of prescribing agents by infusion for routine bowel care is limited because certified medical personnel are required to administer medications, as well as the inconvenience and risks of infection with intravenous drug delivery. In addition, the parenteral route of drug delivery often meets resistance from patients. Intramuscular delivery of agents, if administered above the level of lesion, would be painful and may be associated with pain and hematomas that may impair mobility and transfers and, if delivered below the level of lesion, may precipitate autonomic dysreflexia in those with higher cord lesions (e.g., above thoracic level-6). The transdermal administration of these agents by iontophoresis was identified as an alternative route of administration [8]. In three subjects with spinal cord lesions above thoracic level-6, each with a history of autonomic dysreflexia, Faaborg et al. reported that performing digital rectal evacuation or transanal irrigation resulted in substantial blood pressure elevations [15]. Five of the six subjects reported herein had higher spinal cord lesions and each had a history of intermittent autonomic dysreflexia; despite their histories of autonomic dysreflexia, the dual drug combination appeared to be at least as safe as the two bowel interventions reported by Faaborg et al., but additional work should be performed in a larger number of patients with higher cord lesions to confirm this finding. As reported in an earlier report, a 40% success rate was attained to induce bowel evacuation by transcutaneous administration of neostigmine and glycopyrrolate; however, when employing a modified protocol for the transcutaneous administration of these agents, the ability to induce a bowel evacuation was accomplished in each subject for all six of their bowel care sessions in the work reported herein.

The administration of the dual drug combination may result in untoward cholinergic or anti-cholinergic side-effects. Neostigmine may be safely administered by transcutaneous route when the ratio of neostigmine to glycopyrrolate is 5:1, which appears to antagonize the cholinergic effects of neostigmine on the heart and lungs to a clinically sufficient extent but spares the prokinetic effect of neostigmine on the bowel; our group is posed to further define the most clinically beneficial ratio of neostigmine to glycopyrrolate by transcutaneous administration to successfully induce bowel evacuation with the least adverse, albeit relatively minor, side effects. In our prior work with the intravenous

J. Clin. Med. **2021**, *10*, 1135

administration of these agents, which had a greater frequency and intensity of minor adverse events, the major adverse cardiopulmonary manifestations of neostigmine (e.g., severe bradycardia and/or bronchoconstriction) did not occur [8].

This research has high, as well as immediate, translational potential to clinical care for persons with SCI who have difficulty with bowel evacuation. The work presented herein included only hospitalized patients who required greater than an hour for routine bowel care. Thus, it remains to be established if the transdermal delivery of neostigmine and glycopyrrolate has utility for those with shorter durations of bowel care in the home setting. However, the dual drug combination appears to have advantages over other bowel care approaches, including other prokinetic agents such as prucalopride [16], because the approach studied herein induces a prompt, predictable, and a more complete bowel evacuation. The dual drug combination may also be considered as an alternative approach for patients with severe neurogenic bowel following SCI who may otherwise be receiving transanal irrigation as their method for performing routine bowel care [17] or for those considering an intestinal diversion procedure [18]. However, the use of a relatively difficult to use, wired iontophoresis device for a person with SCI remains a major obstacle for this drug delivery approach to be transferred to routine clinical care. However, the development and commercialization of a wireless iontophoresis patch system that is user-friendly and is currently being developed would overcome this obstacle, allowing individuals with SCI to regain far greater control over bowel function than is possible with the bowel care regimens that are currently available. Such an advance in bowel care should markedly reduce the occurrence of complications due to constipation, stool impaction, stool incontinence, and anal pathologies. A far more successful approach to bowel care would permit those with SCI to regain a degree of independence, as well as prove useful as an adjunctive therapy for individuals with other disabilities who suffer from chronic constipation.

In summary, the addition of neostigmine and glycopyrrolate by transcutaneous administration to standard bowel care regimens in persons with SCI and DWE resulted in the safe, effective, and predictable bowel evacuation with subjective improvement in bowel care. The adverse events reported with this approach to bowel care were minor and transient.

Author Contributions: Conceptualization, M.A.K., W.A.B. and A.M.S.; Methodology, A.S., W.A.B. and M.A.K.; Formal Analysis, A.S., C.M.C. and W.A.B.; Investigation, A.S., W.A.B., M.A.K. and S.S.; Resources, W.A.B. and M.A.K.; Data Curation, A.S.; Writing–Original Draft Preparation, W.A.B. and A.S.; Writing—and Review and Editing, M.A.K., A.M.S. and C.M.C.; Supervision, W.A.B., M.A.K. and A.S.; Project Administration, W.A.B. and M.A.K.; Funding Acquisition, W.A.B. and A.M.S. All authors have read and agreed to the published version of the manuscript.

Funding: This research was supported by Veterans Affairs Rehabilitation Research and Development Service's National Center for the Medical Consequences of Spinal Cord Injury (B2020-C).

Institutional Review Board Statement: The study was conducted according to the guidelines of the Declaration of Helsinki and approved by the Institutional Review Board of James J. Peters Veterans Affairs Medical Cener (Protocol IRB ID: 01465; date of original IRB approval: 11 December 2012).

Informed Consent Statement: Informed consent was obtained from all subjects who participated in the study prior to initiating any experimental procedures.

Data Availability Statement: Data presented are contained within the article.

Acknowledgments: The authors also wish to thank the James J. Peters VA Medical Center, Bronx, NY, the Department of Veterans Affairs Rehabilitation Research and Development Service for their support, and the Veterans who participated in making this work possible. The work reported herein does not represent the views of the US Department of Veterans Affairs or the US Government.

Conflicts of Interest: Authors (W.A.B. and M.A.K.) are the inventors of the dual drug combination of neostigmine and glycopyrrolate for the treatment of difficulty with evacuation. The Department of Veterans Affairs holds the patent to this invention.

References

1. Stiens, S.A.; Bergman, S.B.; Goetz, L.L. Neurogenic bowel dysfunction after spinal cord injury: Clinical evaluation and rehabilitative management. *Arch. Phys. Med. Rehabil.* **1997**, *78* (Suppl. 3), S86–S102. [CrossRef]
2. Krassioukov, A.; Eng, J.J.; Claxton, G.; Sakakibara, B.M.; Shum, S. Neurogenic bowel management after spinal cord injury: A systematic review of the evidence. *Spinal Cord* **2010**, *48*, 718–733. [CrossRef] [PubMed]
3. Pardee, C.; Bricker, D.; Rundquist, J.; MacRae, C.; Tebben, C. Characteristics of neurogenic bowel in spinal cord injury and perceived quality of life. *Rehabil. Nurs.* **2012**, *37*, 128–135. [CrossRef] [PubMed]
4. Pires, J.M.; Ferreira, A.M.; Rocha, F.; Andrade, L.G.; Campos, I.; Margalho, P.; Laíns, J. Assessment of neurogenic bowel dysfunction impact after spinal cord injury using the International Classification of Functioning, Disability and Health. *Eur. J. Phys. Rehabil. Med.* **2019**, *54*, 873–879. [CrossRef]
5. Korsten, M.A.; Rosman, A.S.; Ng, A.; Cavusoglu, E.; Spungen, A.M.; Radulovic, M.; Wecht, J.M.; Bauman, W.A. Infusion of neostigmine-glycopyrrolate for bowel evacuation in persons with spinal cord injury. *Am. J. Gastroenterol.* **2005**, *100*, 1560–1565. [CrossRef]
6. Rosman, A.S.; Chaparala, G.; Monga, A.; Spungen, A.M.; Bauman, W.A.; Korsten, M.A. Intramuscular neostigmine and glycopyrrolate safely accelerated bowel evacuation in patients with spinal cord injury and defecatory disorders. *Dig. Dis. Sci.* **2008**, *53*, 2710–2713. [CrossRef]
7. Kumar, M.; Chawla, R.; Goyal, M. Topical anesthesia. *J. Anaesthesiol. Clin. Pharmacol.* **2015**, *31*, 450–456. [CrossRef] [PubMed]
8. Korsten, M.A.; Lyons, B.L.; Radulovic, M.; Cummings, T.M.; Sikka, G.; Singh, K.; Hobson, J.C.; Sabiev, A.; Spungen, A.M.; Bauman, W.A. Delivery of neostigmine and glycopyrrolate by iontophoresis: A nonrandomized study in individuals with spinal cord injury. *Spinal Cord* **2017**, *56*, 212–217. [CrossRef] [PubMed]
9. Lynch, A.C.; Wong, C.; Anthony, A.; Dobbs, B.R.; A Frizelle, F. Bowel dysfunction following spinal cord injury: A description of bowel function in a spinal cord-injured population and comparison with age and gender matched controls. *Spinal Cord* **2000**, *38*, 717–723. [CrossRef] [PubMed]
10. Atkinson, M.J.; Sinha, A.; Hass, S.L.; Colman, S.S.; Kumar, R.N.; Brod, M.; Rowland, C.R. Validation of a general measure of treatment satisfaction, the Treatment Satisfaction Questionnaire for Medication (TSQM), using a national panel study of chronic disease. *Health Qual. Life Outcomes* **2004**, *2*, 12. [CrossRef] [PubMed]
11. Ozisler, Z.; Koklu, K.; Ozel, S.; Unsal-Delialioglu, S. Outcomes of bowel program in spinal cord injury patients with neurogenic bowel dysfunction. *Neural Regen. Res.* **2015**, *10*, 1153. [CrossRef]
12. Inskip, J.A.; Lucci, V.-E.M.; McGrath, M.S.; Willms, R.; Claydon, V.E. A Community Perspective on Bowel Management and Quality of Life after Spinal Cord Injury: The Influence of Autonomic Dysreflexia. *J. Neurotrauma* **2018**, *35*, 1091–1105. [CrossRef]
13. Xu, X.; Menees, S.B.; Zochowski, M.K.; Fenner, D.E. Economic cost of fecal incontinence. *Dis. Colon Rectum* **2012**, *55*, 586–598. [CrossRef] [PubMed]
14. Radulovic, M.; Spungen, A.M.; Wecht, J.M.; Korsten, M.A.; Schilero, G.J.; Bauman, W.A.; Lesser, M. Effects of neostigmine and glycopyrrolate on pulmonary resistance in spinal cord injury. *J. Rehabil. Res. Dev.* **2004**, *41*, 53. [CrossRef] [PubMed]
15. Faaborg, P.M.; Christensen, P.; Krassioukov, A.V.; Laurberg, S.; Frandsen, E.; Krogh, K. Autonomic dysreflexia during bowel evacuation procedures and bladder filling in subjects with spinal cord injury. *Spinal Cord* **2014**, *52*, 494–498. [CrossRef] [PubMed]
16. Krogh, K.; Jensen, M.B.; Gandrup, P.; Laurberg, S.; Nilsson, J.; Kerstens, R.; De Pauw, M. Efficacy and tolerability of prucalopride in patients with constipation due to spinal cord injury. *Scand. J. Gastroenterol.* **2002**, *37*, 431–436. [CrossRef] [PubMed]
17. Christensen, P.; Bazzocchi, G.; Coggrave, M.; Abel, R.; Hultling, C.; Krogh, K.; Media, S.; Laurberg, S. A randomized, controlled trial of transanal irrigation versus management in spinal cord-injured patients. *Gastroenterology* **2006**, *131*, 738–747. [CrossRef] [PubMed]
18. Coggrave, M.; Ingram, R.; Gardner, B.; Norton, C. The impact of stoma for bowel management after spinal cord injury. *Spinal Cord* **2012**, *50*, 848–852. [CrossRef] [PubMed]

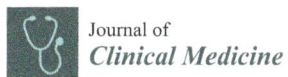

Journal of
Clinical Medicine

MDPI

Article

The Effect of Exoskeletal-Assisted Walking on Spinal Cord Injury Bowel Function: Results from a Randomized Trial and Comparison to Other Physical Interventions

Peter H. Gorman [1,2,*], Gail F. Forrest [3,4], Pierre K. Asselin [5,6], William Scott [7], Stephen Kornfeld [5,6], Eunkyoung Hong [5,6] and Ann M. Spungen [5,6]

[1] Department of Neurology, University of Maryland School of Medicine, Baltimore, MD 21201, USA
[2] Division of Rehabilitation Medicine, University of Maryland Rehabilitation and Orthopaedic Institute, Baltimore, MD 21207, USA
[3] Kessler Foundation, West Orange, NJ 07052, USA; gforrest@kesslerfoundation.org
[4] Department of Physical Medicine and Rehabilitation, Rutgers New Jersey Medical School-Rutgers University, Newark, NJ 07103, USA
[5] Spinal Cord Damage Research Center, James J. Peters VA Medical Center, Bronx, NY 10468, USA; Pierre.Asselin@va.gov (P.K.A.); Stephen.Kornfeld@va.gov (S.K.); Eunkyoung.Hong@va.gov (E.H.); Ann.Spungen@va.gov (A.M.S.)
[6] Department of Rehabilitation and Human Performance, Icahn School of Medicine at Mount Sinai, New York, NY 10029, USA
[7] VA Maryland Healthcare System, Baltimore, MD 21201, USA; William.scott5@va.gov
* Correspondence: pgorman@som.umaryland.edu; Tel.: +1-410-448-6265

Citation: Gorman, P.H.; Forrest, G.F.; Asselin, P.K.; Scott, W.; Kornfeld, S.; Hong, E.; Spungen, A.M. The Effect of Exoskeletal-Assisted Walking on Spinal Cord Injury Bowel Function: Results from a Randomized Trial and Comparison to Other Physical Interventions. *J. Clin. Med.* **2021**, *10*, 964. https://doi.org/10.3390/jcm10050964

Academic Editor: Klaus Krogh

Received: 30 December 2020
Accepted: 17 February 2021
Published: 2 March 2021

Publisher's Note: MDPI stays neutral with regard to jurisdictional claims in published maps and institutional affiliations.

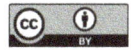

Copyright: © 2021 by the authors. Licensee MDPI, Basel, Switzerland. This article is an open access article distributed under the terms and conditions of the Creative Commons Attribution (CC BY) license (https://creativecommons.org/licenses/by/4.0/).

Abstract: Bowel function after spinal cord injury (SCI) is compromised because of a lack of voluntary control and reduction in bowel motility, often leading to incontinence and constipation not easily managed. Physical activity and upright posture may play a role in dealing with these issues. We performed a three-center, randomized, controlled, crossover clinical trial of exoskeletal-assisted walking (EAW) compared to usual activity (UA) in people with chronic SCI. As a secondary outcome measure, the effect of this intervention on bowel function was assessed using a 10-question bowel function survey, the Bristol Stool Form Scale (BSS) and the Spinal Cord Injury Quality of Life (SCI-QOL) Bowel Management Difficulties instrument. Fifty participants completed the study, with bowel data available for 49. The amount of time needed for the bowel program on average was reduced in 24% of the participants after EAW. A trend toward normalization of stool form was noted. There were no significant effects on patient-reported outcomes for bowel function for the SCI-QOL components, although the time since injury may have played a role. Subset analysis suggested that EAW produces a greater positive effect in men than women and may be more effective in motor-complete individuals with respect to stool consistency. EAW, along with other physical interventions previously investigated, may be able to play a previously underappreciated role in assisting with SCI-related bowel dysfunction.

Keywords: spinal cord injury; bowel function; exoskeletal walking; constipation

1. Introduction

Spinal cord injury (SCI) is well known to adversely affect bowel function [1–3]. Constipation related to slowed colonic transit time is a major issue related to positioning in non-ambulatory individuals and has been specifically demonstrated in SCI [4]. Greater than one third of male participants with SCI reported via a survey that bowel and bladder dysfunction had the most significant effect on life after SCI [5]. Standard bowel management approaches include the manipulation of the diet, oral laxatives and stool softeners, rectal suppositories and enemas, digital rectal stimulation, the use of evacuation equipment, and the timing or scheduling of bowel care [6]. There are some suggestions that a frequent upright posture might help with bowel function. In a Canadian survey study of adults with SCI, 30% of the respondents (38 out of 126) indicated that they participated in prolonged standing (40 min per session, 3 to 4 times per week) in order to improve or maintain health. Of those respondents, 20 out of 38 indicated that bowel and bladder function was one of the main perceived benefits, and 17 indicated that "digestion" was improved [7]. An Australian study [8] explored the specific question as to whether a six-week standing protocol in wheelchair-dependent persons with chronic SCI would improve the time to first stool as well as several other secondary outcomes (the time to complete bowel care, neurogenic bowel dysfunction (NBD) score [9], Cleveland Clinic Constipation Score [10], and St Mark's Incontinence Score [11]). This was a single-blind, randomized, crossover, controlled study with a four-week washout period, and standing was accomplished through the use of a tilt table for 30 min, five times per week for six weeks. The study demonstrated no effect on the time to first stool, nor any treatment effect on any of the other secondary outcome measures. There was, however, a perception on the part of eight out of the 20 participants that standing "improved" bowel function, although what, exactly, this meant was not reported [8].

In the able-bodied population, it is well established that walking as a form of exercise can enhance bowel motility [12,13]. In a study of inactive middle-aged patients with chronic idiopathic constipation, a 12-week physical activity program, which included brisk walking, statistically reduced total colonic transit time when compared to sedentary controls [14]. This phenomenon may be more related to activity than upright posture, as a study comparing treadmill running, bicycle ergometry and rest in a chair demonstrated improvements in bowel transit time in the two active arms but not the sedentary one [15]. It is therefore reasonable to consider the effect of locomotor interventions on bowel function in those with SCI. In a prospective observational cohort study of locomotor training as well as overground standing and stepping activities in those with motor-incomplete chronic SCI, significant improvement was documented in the sensation of bowel movement, and although not statistically significant, improvements in stool continence occurred in 7 out of 16 individuals with reduced or absent continence at baseline [16]. In a prospective cohort study of seven chronic participants with a range of SCI from C4-through-T5 including both complete and incomplete injuries, who underwent 80 sessions of locomotor training alone, there was a significant decrease in the time required for defecation and a decrease in fecal incontinence as well [17]. Exoskeletal-assisted walking may be another intervention that could potentially improve bowel function in this population [18]. In this prospective single-group case series, ten persons with motor-complete SCI who completed 25–63 sessions of exoskeletal-assisted training over 12 to 14 weeks were provided bowel function surveys at baseline and post-training. These included the total bowel evacuation time per bowel day, frequency of bowel evacuations per week, and Bristol Stool Form Scale (BSS) [19] stool consistency assessments. More than 50% of the participants reported some aspect of improvement in bowel management and/or bowel function. Four participants went on to participate in an additional two months of exoskeletal-assisted walking training, and post-measurements were performed at one-month post-training. All four of these participants reported a decrease in total bowel evacuation time during exoskeletal training [20]. Three out of four reported normalization of stool consistency on the BSS, and three out of four reported the elimination of the need for bowel medications during training, although they required them prior to and after training. These pilot data were encouraging. Therefore, we proposed studying bowel management and function as secondary outcome variables in more detail in the context of a randomized clinical trial of the effects of 36 sessions of exoskeletal-assisted walking in individuals with chronic non-ambulatory SCI.

2. Experimental Section

2.1. Recruitment

This study was approved by the Institutional Review Boards (IRBs) of three collaborating clinical sites: (1) The James J. Peters VA Medical Center (JJPVAMC), Bronx, NY; (2) The

University of Maryland, Baltimore, IRB for the University of Maryland Rehabilitation and Orthopaedic Institute (UM Rehab and Ortho), Baltimore, MD; and (3) The Kessler Foundation (KF), West Orange, NJ. In addition, the Department of Defense Congressionally Directed Medical Research Program, Spinal Cord Injury Research Program (SCIRP) Human Research Protection Office (HRPO) approved the overall study. Several recruitment strategies were employed. Study physicians at each site were the primary source for identifying potential participants. Additionally, IRB-approved flyers and brochures were distributed at each site. Third, some participants self-identified through the clinicaltrials.gov website listing (NCT02314221). All the potential participants were informed about the details and eligibility for the study. The targeted study population was those with chronic SCI (≥6 months) who were non-ambulatory and therefore used wheelchairs for mobility.

2.2. Protocol

A three-center, randomized, crossover, controlled clinical trial of exoskeletal-assisted walking (EAW) was designed and implemented in non-ambulatory individuals with chronic SCI (>6 months post-injury). The primary aim of the study was to determine the number of sessions necessary to achieve adequate EAW skills and hypothesized velocity milestones. The mobility component of the study, as well as the detailed eligibility criteria, has been published elsewhere [21]. Briefly, individuals with paraplegia or tetraplegia greater than six months in duration, between 18 and 65 years old, unable to ambulate faster than 0.17 m/s on level ground, wheelchair dependent for mobility, and without any history of concurrent medical or neurologic disease or history of lower extremity fracture within the past two years were eligible for the study. There were no specific inclusion or exclusion criteria that were based specifically on bowel function. As a secondary outcome measure, we investigated whether an EAW intervention would improve bowel function as compared to usual activity (UA).

Individuals were screened using a complete history and physical examination incorporating the following: the International Standards for Neurological Classification of SCI (ISNCSCI) examination to determine the level and completeness of injury (the American Spinal Injury Association Impairment Scale (AIS A to D)) and the ranges of motion at the hips, knees and ankles bilaterally; an Ashworth spasticity examination in the lower extremities; a standing orthostatic tolerance test; and the bone mineral density (BMD) scanning of bilateral knees (proximal tibia and distal femur) and hips (femoral neck and total hip) by dual energy X-ray absorptiometry (DXA).

The eligible participants were randomized within the site to one of two groups for 12 weeks (three months): Group 1 received EAW first, three times per week for 12 weeks, and then crossed over to UA for a second 12 weeks; Group 2 received UA first for 12 weeks and then crossed over to EAW for 12 weeks of training.

Two powered exoskeleton devices were used in this study, namely, the ReWalk™ (ReWalk Robotics, Marlborough, MA) [22,23] and the Ekso GT™ (Ekso Bionics, Richmond, CA) [24]. These powered exoskeletons were chosen because they were the only devices commercially available and Food and Drug Administration (FDA)-approved for use within rehabilitation centers at the time of study development. The ReWalk™ was approved for FDA market clearance in 2014, and the Ekso™, in 2016. The two exoskeletal systems are similar in that the external frame supports the user at the feet, ankles, legs, pelvis and lower trunk. Lofstrand crutches or a walker are required for balance and stability during standing, stepping and walking. Additional information about the exoskeletal training and decision tree for the devices has been published elsewhere [21].

Within the first two sessions, standing balance skills were practiced and achieved prior to progression to walking skills. Walking skills were then initiated utilizing a weight-shifting pattern. Continuous walking resulted from a serial performance of weight shifting. Participants were advanced in their degrees of activity and numbers of steps based on individual progress as determined by the instructing trainer. Missed sessions were added to the end of the 12 weeks to achieve a 36-session total intervention.

The effect of exoskeletal-assisted walking on bowel function was assessed using three instruments: a modified bowel survey modelled after Lynch et al. [25] that we called the 10 Question Bowel Function Survey (10Q), the BSS [19,26], and the short-form item bank for Bowel Management Difficulties from the SCI-Quality of Life instrument (SCI-QOL) [27,28]. These instruments were used three times: at baseline, at crossover, and after the second arm for both the UA and the EAW group. The 10Q consisted of questions felt to be important to the principal investigators in assessing patient-reported bowl management issues, specifically with regard to bowel program satisfaction, the time it took to perform a bowel program, the amount of enema assistance needed, the amounts of oral laxatives and stool softeners used, the frequency of digital stimulation needed, and the frequency of unwanted bowel evacuation episodes. The 10Q has not previously been validated. The BSS provided information about stool consistency. The BSS rates stool consistency from 1 (hard to pass) to 7 (watery liquid), where 4 is the desired medium consistency in persons with upper-motor-neuron bowel dysfunction. It has been validated in the context of other disease entities [26]. The Bowel Management Difficulties item bank from the SCI-QOL instrument consisted of 26 items scored on a five-point Likert scale (possible score range, 26–130). The SCI-QOL scores were standardized on a T-metric, according to a previously published T-score conversion table for SCI-QOL Bowel Management Difficulties [29]. Lower scores indicate greater satisfaction with management. The items included such statements as the following: bowel accidents limited my independence, I worried about performing my bowel program, and I was frustrated by repeated bowel accidents. Validation of the SCI-QOL has been performed [28,29]. The 10Q survey and the BSS scales are available in the Appendix A as is information on how to access the SCI-QOL instrument.

3. Results

A total of 50 participants completed the exoskeletal-assisted walking protocol including crossover. Of these, 49 individuals completed the bowel surveys and the BSS at all the time points. Males represented 76% of the participants ($n = 38$). The percent of paraplegic individuals was 72%. The duration of SCI was greater than two years for 52% of the participants, while 48% of the participants were six months to two years out from their injury. Participants with motor-complete injury (American Spinal Injury Impairment Scale (AIS) A and B) represented 62% of the participants, and those with motor-incomplete injury (AIS C and D) made up the remaining 38%. More complete demographic data have been previously presented [21].

The 10Q Bowel Function survey results specifically related to external assistance needed and bowel evacuation times are presented in Table 1. Results from five out of the 10 questions are presented in this table, with the responses from three similar questions detailing the extent of external help needed combined for the purposes of analysis. The five-point scales used in the 10Q survey (see the Appendix A for specifics) were then coded into a binary categorization to allow for qualitative comparisons pre- and post-EAW. In looking at the whole group (regardless of the randomization order), 12% of the participants reported a reduced need for external help, and 24% of the participants reported a reduced evacuation time during each session and across a full week after the 36 sessions of EAW. Analysis of the other five questions did not demonstrate any effect from the EAW or the UA intervention.

Table 1. Selected patient-reported outcomes from the 10Q Function Survey. Results from three of the 10Q questions were combined in the first category in the table in order to represent the degree of external assistance needed in order to accomplish a bowel evacuation. The other two categories represent results from one individual question from the 10Q. For each category, a new binary response was created by lumping responses in order to qualitatively compare pre -and post-EAW results. For the purpose of the results in the last column, improvement was defined as either reduction in external assistance or reduction in bowel evacuation time.

Category	Frequency Reported	Pre-EAW	Post-EAW	Percent of Participants Improved
Enema, oral medication and/or manual digital stimulation needed for each bowel evacuation in the past week	Never to a few times	57%	63%	12%
	Most to every time	41%	35%	
Average bowel evacuation time needed per bowel day during the past week	5 to 60 min	80%	92%	24%
	>1 to 3 h	18%	6%	
Average bowel evacuation time needed in the past week	1 to 6 h	80%	92%	24%
	>6 to 8 h	16%	6%	

The BSS data suggested a qualitative improvement, as the participants reported an improvement (i.e., trend towards a medium stool consistency of 4) after EAW not seen in the UA group. By chance, the UA group at baseline tended to do better than the baseline EAW group, and further improvement in the UA group was not seen (Figure 1). When the BSS grades 5 and 6, representing loose stools, were grouped together, the percentage of loose stools changed from 19.1% pre-EAW to 9.3% post-EAW, whereas there was less of a change with usual activity (19.0% pre- to 15.2% post-UA). In an analysis based on gender as an independent variable, the percentage of men with loose stools decreased with EAW (22.2% pre- to 9.1% post-EAW), but the percentage did not change in women (9.1% pre- to 10.0% post-EAW), although the baseline percentages were different in men versus women. According to an analysis comparing motor-complete versus motor-incomplete cohorts, the EAW intervention reduced the percentage of loose stools from 23.3% to 6.9% ($n = 31$) in the motor-complete participants, whereas there was a slight worsening in the motor-incomplete subgroup (11.8% pre- to 14.3% post-EAW, $n = 17$).

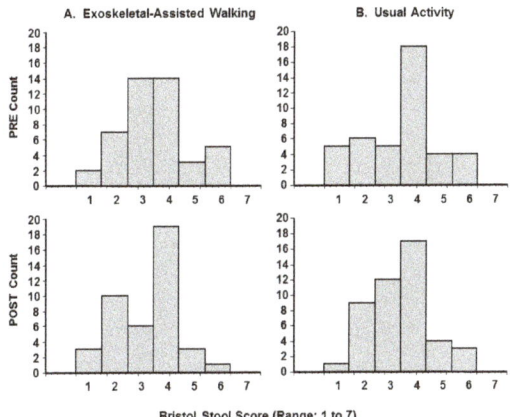

Figure 1. Bristol Stool Form Scale (BSS) results. Frequency distribution of pre- and post-exoskeletal-assisted walking and pre- and post-usual activity. The top row represents preintervention, and the bottom row, postintervention data. Larger values on the 1 to 7 BSS represent looser stools. Details of the BSS can be found in the Appendix A.

The results from the Bowel Management Item Bank components of the SCI-QOL are presented in Table 2. Overall, for the whole group, there were no significant effects found for changes in patient-reported outcomes for the Bowel Management Difficulties SCI-QOL survey after EAW in comparison to UA. The only statistically significant beneficial preintervention–postintervention change was seen during the EAW phase for the participants who started in the UA-first group. An improvement from 49.5 ± 9.2 to 46.5 ± 9.8 (*p* = 0.028) was noted (a lower score indicating better satisfaction).

Table 2. Bowel Management Item Bank from the Spinal Cord Injury Quality of Life (SCI-QOL).

Category	Exoskeletal-Assisted Walking (EAW) Phase (*n* = 50)				Usual Activity (UA) Phase (*n* = 49)				EAW vs. UA Diff (*p* Value)
	Pre	Post	Paired T-Test (*p*)	Pre–Post Diff	Pre	Post	Paired T-Test (*p*)	Pre–Post Diff	
All (*n* = 49) (± SD)	49.7 (8.7)	48.4 (9.2)	0.207	−1.3 (7.1)	50.8 (8.6)	49.3 (9.2)	0.071	−1.5 (5.8)	0.88
(range)	36.1–79.4	36.1–74.4			36.1–75.0	36.1–79.4			
EAW first (*n* = 24)	49.9 (8.4)	50.4 (8.3)	0.292	0.5 (7.4)	50.4 (8.3)	49.1 (9.5)	0.292	−1.3 (5.8)	0.46
UA first (*n* = 25)	49.5 (9.0)	46.5 (9.8)	0.028	−3.0 (6.5)	51.2 (8.9)	49.5 (9.1)	0.145	−1.8 (5.8)	0.54
DOI > 2.0 y (*n* = 26)	51.0 (9.5)	48.8 (10.2)	0.144	−2.2 (7.3)	52.0 (9.4)	50.9 (9.6)	0.299	−1.1 (5.4)	0.60
DOI ≤ 2.0 y (*n* = 23)	47.9. (7.6)	47.5 (8.3)	0.823	−0.4 (6.9)	49.1 (7.5)	47.0 (8.5)	0.143	−2.0 (6.2)	0.51
Male (*n* = 38)	50.1 (9.1)	47.6(9.8)	0.041	−2.5 (7.1)	50.8 (9.0)	49.5 (9.3)	0.109	−1.3 (5.0)	0.49
Female (*n* = 11)	48.5 (6.5)	51.2 (5.3)	0.108	2.8 (4.9)	50.8 (6.3)	48.6 (8.3)	0.398	−2.1 (7.7)	0.23
Complete (*n* = 31)	51.6 (9.3)	49.9 (9.6)	0.243	−1.7 (7.8)	52.1 (9.1)	51.4 (9.7)	0.489	−0.7 (5.7)	0.65
Incomplete (*n* = 18)	46.5 (6.6)	45.9 (8.1)	0.642	−0.6 (5.8)	48.6 (7.4)	45.7 (7.0)	0.047	−2.9 (5.8)	0.32

Note that a lower score represents a better outcome. *n* = 49 for the usual activity (UA) group, as one participant in UA-first group was lost to follow-up after the UA arm for this outcome; values in parentheses are ± standard deviation; EAW = exoskeletal-assisted-walking-first group; UA = usual-activity-first group; DOI = duration of injury; y = years; Diff = the difference from pre- to postintervention; shaded area indicates statistically significant value from pre- to postintervention; bold type font represents statistically significant changes. Thicker lines are placed between sets of rows for easier comparisons.

We performed several *post hoc* subgroup analyses based on (1) the time since injury, (2) gender and (3) motor-complete (AIS A/B) versus motor-incomplete (AIS C/D) injury. The time since injury analysis was considered important since it was noticed that the more newly injured participants (less than two years since injury) were often still learning to maximize their bowel management. Stratification by the duration of injury (DOI) subcategories for the outcomes of bowel function showed that those persons injured for more than two years demonstrated an improvement trend in the Bowel Management SCI-QOL survey after EAW. By contrast, the more newly injured cohort (DOI < 2 y) did not show improvement. A comparison of the effects of EAW on the SCI-QOL bowel management item bank in men vs. women was performed. For men (*n* = 38), the average score decreased from 50.1 to 47.6 with EAW (*p* = 0.041), but in women, there was an average score increase from 48.5 to 51.2, albeit, non-significant (ns). When those with motor-complete injury were compared with those with motor-incomplete injury, the EAW intervention did not produce any beneficial effect in either group. Surprisingly, however, the usual activity intervention produced a statistically significant preintervention–postintervention change in the motor-incomplete cohort. Comparisons between the changes observed with the EAW and the UA interventions, when examined in total and in all the subgroup analyses, demonstrated no statistically significant differences.

4. Discussion

EAW training had a positive effect on about one quarter of the participants for the patient-reported outcomes for bowel function and management. There were also trends towards normalization of stool consistency in the EAW group not seen in the UA group. Men responded better than women to EAW in terms of reductions in loose stools. Those with motor-complete injury responded to EAW in terms of reductions in loose stools, whereas the motor-incomplete group did not. The overall results from the Bowel SCI-QOL batteries did not show a significant improvement in patients' perceptions of their evacuation management with the EAW intervention. The time-since-injury sub-analysis suggested that those with newer SCI may still be adjusting and becoming competent with their bowel program, thus negating any potential positive effect from the EAW intervention. When the bowel SCI-QOL results were examined by gender, it was noted that men responded to EAW significantly, whereas women did not, although the enrolled women started off scoring slightly better (lower) on this scale (48.5 vs. 50.1). When the results were examined by the presence or absence of motor completeness, the usual activity intervention was associated with a significant improvement, whereas the EAW intervention was not. It is to be noted, however, that in both the EAW and UA groups, the baseline bowel SCI-QOL scores were better in the participants with motor-incomplete (AIS C/D) SCI. This makes intuitive sense, as these individuals at baseline had more intact corticospinal tracts in their spinal cords (as demonstrated by preserved motor control) and, therefore, would be expected to have better bowel control. It is difficult to draw direct conclusions as to the clinical significance of the observed effect of usual activity in the participants with motor-incomplete injury.

The effect of exoskeletal-assisted walking on bowel function in spinal cord injury was not as dramatic as was hypothesized. Our 25-to-63-session EAW pilot investigation had suggested a more robust finding. Indeed, in 10 participants, there were a reported reduction in the time spent having a bowel movement (5/10), fewer bowel accidents (6/10), a decreased frequency of laxative and/or stool softener use over the prior week (7/10), and a reported improvement in overall satisfaction with the bowel program (6/10) [18]. This much larger randomized study did not confirm these findings. Rather, more subtle improvements were noted, and only one out of the two preintervention–postintervention comparisons demonstrated a significant improvement with the EAW intervention. When all of the preintervention–postintervention EAW data were evaluated together, irrespective of the order of the EAW intervention, the statistical significance of the effect was lost.

With regard to the self-reported outcomes, the improvement in approximately one quarter of the participants in bowel evacuation time did confirm prior pilot data. This contrasts with the lack of improvement in bowel evacuation time found by Kwok et al. in a study of standing alone discussed previously [8]. One might therefore postulate that the actual activity associated with exoskeletal walking rather than just the upright posture alone was the causative agent leading to improved transit times. This might be related to the trunk exertion needed to shift weight during stepping, although further work would be needed to confirm this.

The Bristol stool form scale perhaps provided the most intriguing results. Normalization of the stool consistency (i.e., towards the middle category 4 on the 1–7 scale) after EAW walking was noted and appeared not to have occurred after UA. The baseline values prior to UA included a number of category 4 reports, which likely made it more difficult to make a comparison statistically significant. Nonetheless, this effect is a relevant one with regard to the risk of incontinence in those with spinal cord injury. The fact that the motor-complete subgroup responded to EAW in terms of a reduction in loose stools is likely due to the fact that they were worse off at baseline, and achieving overground walking through the robotic intervention likely represented a more dramatic change in physiology than in the motor-incomplete group.

The results provided here lend support to the idea that upright overground activity (i.e., walking) and not just standing may have a beneficial effect on bowel function in those with chronic spinal cord injury, but the size of the effect was not as profound as hypothesized. Nonetheless, the collection of these secondary outcome data was not excessively burdensome and likely should be included in the future study of any type of mobility intervention in people with spinal cord injury.

5. Conclusions

A 36-session exoskeletal-assisted walking program implemented over three months in non-ambulatory persons with spinal cord injury provided some, albeit limited, improvement in several measures of bowel function when compared to a usual activity control group. The most notable improvement (i.e., reduction) was seen in average bowel evacuation time and in a trend to the normalization of bowel form consistency. The degree of subjective improvement as determined by quality-of-life bowel survey instruments may be, in part, related to the time since injury, and exoskeletal-assisted walking may have a predilection to benefit men more than women. The bowel survey quality-of-life results at baseline were confirmed to be better in motor-incomplete persons than those with motor-complete injuries, but individuals with motor-complete injury may improve more readily with an EAW intervention in terms of stool consistency.

Author Contributions: Conceptualization, A.M.S. and P.H.G.; methodology, A.M.S., P.H.G. and G.F.F.; validation, P.K.A., W.S. and E.H.; formal analysis, E.H. and A.M.S.; investigation, all authors; resources, P.H.G., G.F.F. and A.M.S.; data curation, E.H.; writing—original draft preparation, P.H.G.; writing—review and editing, G.F.F., P.K.A., S.K. and A.M.S.; project administration, A.M.S.; funding acquisition, A.M.S. and P.H.G. All authors have read and agreed to the published version of the manuscript.

Funding: This research was funded by the Department of Defense/CDMRP SC130234, Award: W81XWH-14-2-0170, and National Center for the Medical Consequences of SCI (B9212-C, B2020-C) at the James J. Peters Veterans Affairs Medical Center. Additional local support was provided by the James Lawrence Kernan Endowment Fund, Baltimore, Maryland; a philanthropic gift from Dr. Bert Glaser at the Baltimore site; and The Bronx Veterans Medical Research Foundation at the Bronx site.

Institutional Review Board Statement: The study was conducted according to the guidelines of the Declaration of Helsinki, and approved by the Institutional Review Boards (IRB) of the three collaborating clinical sites, namely the James J. Peters VA Medical Center (JJPVAMC), Bronx, NY, Kessler Institute for Rehabilitation/Kessler Foundation (KIR/KF), West Orange, NJ, and the University of Maryland, Baltimore IRB for the University of Maryland Rehabilitation and Orthopedic Institute (UM Rehab and Ortho), Baltimore, MD). In addition, the Department of Defense Congressionally Directed Medical Research Program (DOD CDMRP) IRB approved the total study.

Informed Consent Statement: Informed consent was obtained at each site for each participant prior to being enrolled in the study.

Data Availability Statement: The data presented in this study are available on request from the corresponding author. The data are not publicly available due to restrictions based on Department of Veterans Affairs regulations.

Acknowledgments: The authors would like to acknowledge the efforts of therapist Marni Kallins, PT, and research coordinators Michael Elliot, Denis Doyle Green, Rebecca Webb and Leigh Casey. The contents of this paper do not represent the views of the Department of Veterans Affairs or the United States Government.

Conflicts of Interest: The authors declare that the research was conducted in the absence of any commercial or financial relationships that could be construed as a potential conflict of interest. The funders had no role in the design of the study; in the collection, analyses or interpretation of data; in the writing of the manuscript; or in the decision to publish the results.

Appendix A

The Ten Question Bowel Function Survey (10Q) and the Bristol Stool Form Scale (BSS) are provided as appendices to this manuscript. For access to the 9-item SCI-QOL: Bowel Management Difficulties Short Form, readers are encouraged to request access directly from the authors of the original source manuscript by sending an e-mail to Dr. David Tulsky and Pamela Kisala at SCI-QOL@udel.edu or in REDCap for use free of charge.

TEN QUESTION BOWEL SURVEY

Questions 1 and 2 refer to events within the last MONTH

1. How satisfied have you been with your overall bowel management program?
   Fully satisfied _____
   Almost fully satisfied _____
   Somewhat satisfied _____
   Moderately dissatisfied, generally unhappy _____
   Not satisfied at all, fully dissatisfied _____

2. How would you best describe you bowel control?
   No leakage or accidents _____
   Leakage or an accident 1-2 times _____
   Leakage or an accident 3-4 times _____
   Leakage or an accident 5-6 times _____
   Leakage or an accident 7 or more times _____

Questions 3 – 10 refer to events within the last 7 DAYS

3. How would you best describe your bowel control?
   No leakage or accidents _____
   Leakage or an accident 1-2 times _____
   Leakage or an accident 3-4 times _____
   Leakage or an accident 5-6 times _____
   Leakage or an accident 7 or more times _____

4. How often did you require enemas or irrigations to help you with each bowel movement?
   None/never _____
   Only once _____
   A few times _____
   Most times (but not for ALL bowel movements) _____
   Every time _____

5. How often did you require oral medications, such as laxative or stool softener, to help you have each bowel movement?
   None/never _____
   Only once _____
   A few times _____
   Most times (but not for ALL bowel movements) _____
   Every time _____

6. How often did you need manual/digit stimulation for each bowel movement?
   None/never _____
   Only once _____
   A few times _____
   Most times (but not for ALL bowel movements) _____
   Every time _____

7. How often did you have a bowel movement?
   7 times or more _____
   5-6 times _____
   3-4 times _____
   1-2 times _____
   None _____

8. On average, how much <u>time per bowel day</u> did you spend to have a bowel movement?
   5 to 15 minutes _____
   15 to 30 minutes _____
   30 to 60 minutes _____
   1 to 3 hours _____
   More than 3 hours _____

9. How much <u>total time in the week</u> did you spend to move your bowels?
   1 to 2 total hours _____
   2 to 4 total hours _____
   4 to 6 total hours _____
   6 to 8 total hours _____
   More than 8 total hours _____

10. Have you felt bloated, distended or other such bowel related discomfort?
    Not at all. _____
    Once (1 day) _____
    A few times (2 or more days) _____
    Most of the time (but not every day) _____
    Every day; felt discomfort all the time _____

Other signs or symptoms: _____

_____

Figure A1. Ten Question Bowel Function Survey (10Q).

J. Clin. Med. **2021**, *10*, 964

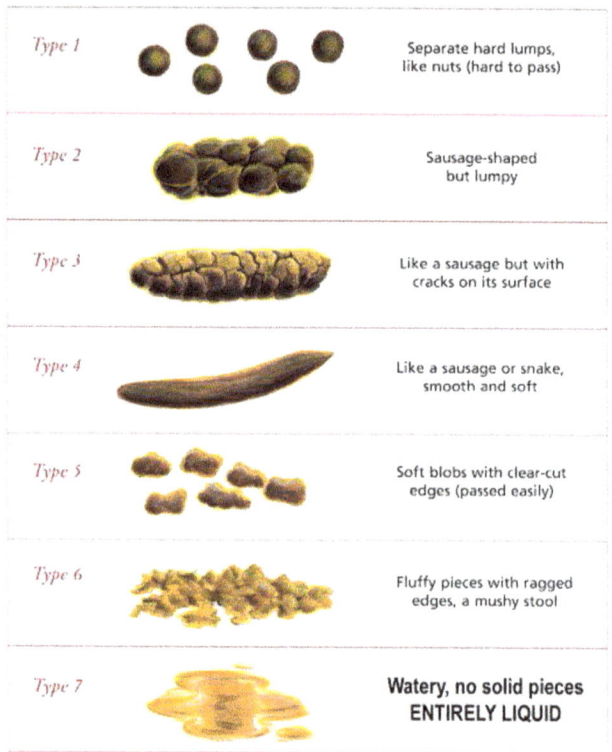

Figure A2. Bristol Stool Form Scale. From: Blake M.R., Raker J.M. and Whelan K. Validity and reliability of the Bristol Stool Form Scale in healthy adults and patients with diarrhoea-predominant irritable bowel syndrome. Aliment Pharmacol Ther. 2016;44(7):693-703 (reference [26] in this manuscript).

References

1. Korsten, M.A.; Fajardo, N.R.; Rosman, A.S.; Creasey, G.H.; Spungen, A.M.; Bauman, W.A. Difficulty with evacuation after spinal cord injury: Colonic motility during sleep and effects of abdominal wall stimulation. *J. Rehabil. Res. Dev.* **2004**, *41*, 95–100. [CrossRef]
2. Adriaansen, J.J.; Van Asbeck, F.W.; Van Kuppevelt, D.; Snoek, G.J.; Post, M.W. Outcomes of Neurogenic Bowel Management in Individuals Living With a Spinal Cord Injury for at Least 10 Years. *Arch. Phys. Med. Rehabil.* **2015**, *96*, 905–912. [CrossRef] [PubMed]
3. Faaborg, P.M.; Christensen, P.; Finnerup, N.; Laurberg, S.; Krogh, K. The pattern of colorectal dysfunction changes with time since spinal cord injury. *Spinal Cord* **2007**, *46*, 234–238. [CrossRef]
4. Rasmussen, M.M.; Krogh, K.; Clemmensen, D.; Bluhme, H.; Rawashdeh, Y.; Christensen, P. Colorectal transport during defecation in participants with supraconal spinal cord injury. *Spinal Cord* **2013**, *51*, 683–687. [CrossRef]
5. Hanson, R.W.; Franklin, M.R. Sexual loss in relation to other functional losses for spinal cord injured males. *Arch. Phys. Med. Rehabil.* **1976**, *57*, 291–293.
6. Steins, S.A.; Bergman, S.B.; Goetz, L.L. Neurogenic bowel dysfunction after spinal cord injury: Clinical evaluation and rehabiliative management. *Arch. Phys. Med. Rehabil.* **1997**, *78*, S86–S100. [CrossRef]

7. Eng, J.J.; Levins, S.M.; Townson, A.F.; Mah-Jones, D.; Bremner, J.; Huston, G. Use of Prolonged Standing for Individuals With Spinal Cord Injuries. *Phys. Ther.* **2001**, *81*, 1392–1399. [CrossRef]
8. Kwok, S.; Harvey, L.A.; Glinsky, J.V.; Bowden, J.L.; Coggrave, M.; Tussler, D. Does regular standing improve bowel function in people with spinal cord injury? A randomised crossover trial. *Spinal Cord* **2015**, *53*, 36–41. [CrossRef] [PubMed]
9. Krogh, K.; Christensen, P.; Sabroe, S.; Laurberg, S. Neurogenic bowel dysfunction score. *Spinal Cord* **2005**, *44*, 625–631. [CrossRef] [PubMed]
10. Agachan, F.; Chen, T.; Pfeifer, J.; Reissman, P.; Wexner, S.D. A constipation scoring system to simplify evaluation and management of constipated patients. *Dis. Colon Rectum* **1996**, *39*, 681–685. [CrossRef] [PubMed]
11. Vaizey, C.J.; Carapeti, E.; Cahill, J.A.; Kamm, M.A. Prospective comparison of faecal incontinence grading systems. *Gut* **1999**, *44*, 77–80. [CrossRef] [PubMed]
12. Bi, L.; Triadafilopoulos, G. Exercise and gastrointestinal function and disease: An evidence-based review of risks and benefits. *Clin. Gastroenterol. Hepatol.* **2003**, *1*, 345–355. [CrossRef]
13. Moses, F.M. The Effect of Exercise on the Gastrointestinal Tract1. *Sports Med.* **1990**, *9*, 159–172. [CrossRef] [PubMed]
14. De Schryver, A.M.; Keulemans, Y.C.; Peters, H.P.; Akkermans, L.M.; Smout, A.J.; De Vries, W.R.; Van Berge-Henegouen, G.P. Effects of regular physical activity on defecation pattern in middle-aged patients complaining of chronic constipation. *Scand. J. Gastroenterol.* **2005**, *40*, 422–429. [CrossRef] [PubMed]
15. Oettle, G.J. Effect of moderate exercise on bowel habit. *Gut* **1991**, *32*, 941–944. [CrossRef] [PubMed]
16. Morrison, S.A.; Lorenz, D.; Eskay, C.P.; Forrest, G.F.; Basso, D.M. Longitudinal Recovery and Reduced Costs After 120 Sessions of Locomotor Training for Motor Incomplete Spinal Cord Injury. *Arch. Phys. Med. Rehabil.* **2018**, *99*, 555–562. [CrossRef] [PubMed]
17. Hubscher, C.H.; Herrity, A.N.; Williams, C.S.; Montgomery, L.R.; Willhite, A.M.; Angeli, C.A.; Harkema, S.J. Improvements in bladder, bowel and sexual outcomes following task-specific locomotor training in human spinal cord injury. *PLoS ONE* **2018**, *13*, e0190998. [CrossRef]
18. Chun, A.; Asselin, P.K.; Knezevic, S.; Kornfeld, S.; Bauman, W.A.; Korsten, M.A.; Harel, N.Y.; Huang, V.; Spungen, A.M. Changes in bowel function following exoskeletal-assisted walking in persons with spinal cord injury: An observational pilot study. *Spinal Cord* **2020**, *58*, 459–466. [CrossRef]
19. Perez, M.M.; Martinez, A.B. The Bristol scale—A useful system to assess stool form? *Rev. Esp. Enferm. Dig.* **2009**, *101*, 305–311.
20. Fineberg, D.B.; Asselin, P.; Harel, N.Y.; Agranova-Breyter, I.; Kornfeld, S.D.; Bauman, W.A.; Spungen, A.M. Vertical ground reaction force-based analysis of powered exoskeleton-assisted walking in persons with motor-complete paraplegia. *J. Spinal Cord Med.* **2013**, *36*, 313–321. [CrossRef]
21. Hong, E.; Gorman, P.H.; Forrest, G.F.; Asselin, P.K.; Knezevic, S.; Scott, W.; Wojciehowski, S.B.; Kornfeld, S.; Spungen, A.M. Mobility Skills With Exoskeletal-Assisted Walking in Persons With SCI: Results From a Three Center Randomized Clinical Trial. *Front. Robot. AI* **2020**, *7*. [CrossRef]
22. Esquenazi, A.; Talaty, M.; Packel, A.; Saulino, M. The ReWalk Powered Exoskeleton to Restore Ambulatory Function to Individuals with Thoracic-Level Motor-Complete Spinal Cord Injury. *Am. J. Phys. Med. Rehabil.* **2012**, *91*, 911–921. [CrossRef]
23. Zeilig, G.; Weingarden, H.; Zwecker, M.; Dudkiewicz, I.; Bloch, A.; Esquenazi, A. Safety and tolerance of the ReWalk exoskeleton suit for ambulation by people with complete spinal cord injury: A pilot study. *J. Spinal Cord Med.* **2012**, *35*, 96–101. [CrossRef] [PubMed]
24. Palermo, A.E.; Maher, J.L.; Baunsgaard, C.B.; Nash, M.S. Clinician-Focused Overview of Bionic Exoskeleton Use After Spinal Cord Injury. *Top. Spinal Cord Inj. Rehabil.* **2017**, *23*, 234–244. [CrossRef] [PubMed]
25. Lynch, A.C.; Wong, C.; Anthony, A.; Dobbs, B.R.; Frizelle, F.A. Bowel dysfunction following spinal cord injury: A description of bowel function in a spinal cord-injured population and comparison with age and gender matched controls. *Spinal Cord* **2000**, *38*, 717–723. [CrossRef] [PubMed]
26. Blake, M.R.; Raker, J.M.; Whelan, K. Validity and reliability of the Bristol Stool Form Scale in healthy adults and patients with diarrhoea-predominant irritable bowel syndrome. *Aliment. Pharmacol. Ther.* **2016**, *44*, 693–703. [CrossRef]
27. Tulsky, D.S.; Kisala, P.A.; Victorson, D.; Tate, D.; Heinemann, A.W.; Amtmann, D.; Cella, D. Developing a Contemporary Patient-Reported Outcomes Measure for Spinal Cord Injury. *Arch. Phys. Med. Rehabil.* **2011**, *92* (Suppl. 10), S44–S51. [CrossRef]
28. Tulsky, D.S.; Kisala, P.A. The Spinal Cord Injury—Quality of Life (SCI-QOL) measurement system: Development, psychometrics, and item bank calibration. *J. Spinal Cord Med.* **2015**, *38*, 251–256. [CrossRef] [PubMed]
29. Tulsky, D.S.; Kisala, P.A.; Tate, D.G.; Spungen, A.M.; Kirshblum, S.C. Development and psychometric characteristics of the SCI-QOL Bladder Management Difficulties and Bowel Management Difficulties item banks and short forms and the SCI-QOL Bladder Complications scale. *J. Spinal Cord Med.* **2015**, *38*, 288–302. [CrossRef]

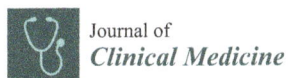

Journal of
Clinical Medicine

MDPI

Review

Gastrointestinal Dysfunction in Parkinson's Disease

Casper Skjærbæk *, Karoline Knudsen, Jacob Horsager and Per Borghammer

Department of Nuclear Medicine & PET, Aarhus University Hospital, Palle Juul-Jensens Boulevard 165, J220, 8200 Aarhus N, Denmark; karoknud@rm.dk (K.K.); jacobnls@rm.dk (J.H.); perborgh@rm.dk (P.B.)
* Correspondence: cas@clin.au.dk

Abstract: Parkinson's disease (PD) is the second most common neurodegenerative disease. Patients show deposits of pathological, aggregated α-synuclein not only in the brain but throughout almost the entire length of the digestive tract. This gives rise to non-motor symptoms particularly within the gastrointestinal tract and patients experience a wide range of frequent and burdensome symptoms such as dysphagia, bloating, and constipation. Recent evidence suggests that progressive accumulation of gastrointestinal pathology is underway several years before a clinical diagnosis of PD. Notably, constipation has been shown to increase the risk of developing PD and in contrast, truncal vagotomy seems to decrease the risk of PD. Animal models have demonstrated gut-to-brain spreading of pathological α-synuclein and it is currently being intensely studied whether PD begins in the gut of some patients. Gastrointestinal symptoms in PD have been investigated by the use of several different questionnaires. However, there is limited correspondence between subjective gastrointestinal symptoms and objective dysfunction along the gastrointestinal tract, and often the magnitude of dysfunction is underestimated by the use of questionnaires. Therefore, objective measures are important tools to clarify the degree of dysfunction in future studies of PD. Here, we summarize the types and prevalence of subjective gastrointestinal symptoms and objective dysfunction in PD. The potential importance of the gastrointestinal tract in the etiopathogenesis of PD is briefly discussed.

Keywords: Parkinson's disease; autonomic; gastrointestinal; constipation; alpha-synuclein; parasympathetic

Citation: Skjærbæk, C.; Knudsen, K.; Horsager, J.; Borghammer, P. Gastrointestinal Dysfunction in Parkinson's Disease. *J. Clin. Med.* **2021**, *10*, 493. https://doi.org/10.3390/jcm10030493

Academic Editor: Klaus Krogh
Received: 4 January 2021
Accepted: 26 January 2021
Published: 31 January 2021

Publisher's Note: MDPI stays neutral with regard to jurisdictional claims in published maps and institutional affiliations.

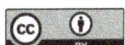

Copyright: © 2021 by the authors. Licensee MDPI, Basel, Switzerland. This article is an open access article distributed under the terms and conditions of the Creative Commons Attribution (CC BY) license (https://creativecommons.org/licenses/by/4.0/).

1. Introduction

Parkinson's disease (PD) is the second most common neurodegenerative disease affecting 2–3% of the population above 65 years of age [1]. Slowness of movements (bradykinesia) in combination with rigidity or tremor constitute the motor symptoms necessary for a clinical diagnosis [2] but non-motor symptoms (NMS) are numerous and often burdensome [3].

NMS attributable to the digestive system are particularly common and dysfunction along the entire length of the digestive tract give rise to symptoms such as dysphagia, bloating, early satiety, and constipation [4]. Interestingly, constipation may precede PD by more than a decade [5], supporting the relatively recent hypothesis that PD may in fact originate in the enteric nervous system and spread to the CNS via the vagus nerve [6]. In support, pathological aggregates of α-synuclein have been detected in gastrointestinal tissues removed several years prior to clinical diagnosis of PD [7], and epidemiological studies have shown that truncal vagotomy decreases the risk of PD by 40–50% [8,9]. In addition, injections of preformed α-synuclein fibrils into the gut wall of rodents leads to initiation and gut-to-brain spreading of α-synuclein aggregates in a pattern highly similar to that seen in human patients—and similar findings were seen after exposing the stomach to the pesticide rotenone [10,11].

Therefore, it is of considerable importance to unravel the etiopathogenic role of the gastrointestinal tract in PD, and to improve our understanding and assessment methods of subjective gastrointestinal symptoms and objective gastrointestinal dysfunction.

This review provides a brief summary of gastrointestinal pathophysiology of PD and highlights specific gastrointestinal symptoms and objective measures of dysfunction relevant for further research. The current approaches to treatment of gastrointestinal symptoms in PD will also be briefly touched upon.

2. Gastrointestinal Pathology in PD

The loss of dopaminergic neurons in the substantia nigra of the brainstem plays a pivotal role in onset and progression of motor symptoms [2]. The distinctive aggregates of α-synuclein, now termed Lewy pathology (LP), were first identified by Friedrich Lewy in 1912 and since then, the distribution of LP in PD has been extensively studied [12].

In most patients, the dorsal motor nucleus of vagus (DMV) in the medulla oblongata is severely affected by LP with a 50% loss of neurons [13–15] and the vagal nerve containing the visceromotor fibers from the DMV also shows involvement [13]. The density of LP in the gastrointestinal tract follows a rostro-caudal gradient corresponding to the density of vagal motor terminals [16] with the lower esophagus and the stomach representing the most affected areas, while the upper esophagus is spared corresponding to its innervation by somatomotor fibers from the relatively unaffected ambiguus nucleus [13,17,18]. Only sparse pathology is found throughout the colon including the distal third of the colon and rectum that are not innervated by the vagal nerve but by fibers from sacral nuclei in which LP is also found [13,17,18]. Notably, this rostro-caudal gradient of pathology is in sharp contrast to the relative magnitude of reported symptoms as constipation and defecatory problems are more prevalent than dysphagia especially in early disease [19,20]. Constipation may present more than a decade prior to clinical diagnosis [5,21].

The link between the gastrointestinal tract and development of PD is also supported by the finding that truncal vagotomy lowers the risk of PD when compared to a super-selective vagotomy in which only a few fibers to the stomach are cut [8,9]. Naturally, these are observational studies, but the idea of retrograde spreading of pathology in PD, as initially postulated Braak et al. [6,22,23], has found additional support in animal models capable of reproducing a formation and spreading of α-synuclein aggregates after injection of either preformed α-synuclein fibrils into the gut wall or by exposing the gut to the pesticide rotenone [10,11].

In vivo studies of human intestinal biopsies have found α-synuclein to be frequent in PD patients compared to controls [24–26]. Interestingly, the appendix vermiformis is a hot spot of α-synuclein aggregation in healthy adults [27], but conflicting epidemiological studies of appendectomized individuals' risk of PD later in life has raised doubts about the importance of appendicular α-synuclein aggregation in the development of PD [28–30]. Importantly, the pathological studies have been cross-sectional and do not clarify whether the pathology is spreading from one gastrointestinal hot spot prior to disease as in the aforementioned animal models. Additionally, the specificity and sensitivity of α-synuclein staining may be suboptimal and further limited by insufficient availability of full-thickness gastrointestinal tissue making such human longitudinal in vivo studies difficult [31,32].

The intestinal mucosa, only millimeters away from the enteric nervous system (ENS), is exposed to not only environmental toxins but also potentially toxic microbial metabolites creating high demands for the epithelial barrier, which could be potential trigger factors for initiating PD [33]. Interestingly, exposure to *Escherichia coli* producing the protein curli enhances the aggregation of α-syn in aged Fischer rats [34]. Furthermore, in a transgenic mouse model of PD with overexpression of α-synuclein it was demonstrated that colonization of germ-free mice with microbiota transplants from PD patients enhance the development of physical impairments compared to microbiota transplants from healthy volunteers [35]. Studies of the human microbiome in PD have recently been reviewed elsewhere [36] and although some studies point to interesting differences suggestive of a pro-inflammatory microbiome in PD patients the findings are heterogenous and mainly from cross-sectional studies of manifest PD. Elevated levels of pro-inflammatory markers such as IL-1α have also been found in stool samples when comparing PD patients with controls [37]. Furthermore, levels of zonulin in stool samples were also found to be elevated in PD indication a degradation of intestinal tight junctions in PD [38]. Signs compatible with increased intestinal permeability *(leaky gut)* in PD was demonstrated in a small sample of 9 PD patients and 7 controls. That study found that the gastrointestinal permeability for sucralose, but not lactulose or mannitol, was increased in the PD group [39]. In support of the role for gastrointestinal inflammation in PD is the finding that inflammatory bowel disease increases the risk of PD later in life [40]

Ideally, these hypotheses about the etiology of PD should be tested in longitudinal human studies, but as it is inherently difficult to study the silent onset of pathology this has so far not been possible. However, a peculiar sleep disorder characterized by disruption of the normal atonia during REM-sleep together with dream enactment has gained interest. Nearly all people with this sleep disorder, called REM-sleep behavior disorder (RBD), progresses to manifest PD or the highly similar condition dementia with Lewy bodies (DLB) within 15 years [41]. The disorder arises as a consequence of damage to certain nuclei in the pons and is the strongest prodromal marker of PD [42]. Remarkably, patients with RBD display a greater density of gastrointestinal LP than patients without [43]. Likewise, loss of cardiac sympathetic innervation and colonic acetylcholinesterase in RBD cases have been shown to be comparable to that of diagnosed PD patients, although the dopaminergic system in the RBD cases was still intact [44]. Consequently, it has been proposed that RBD represents a prodromal biomarker of a gastrointestinal, body-first onset of PD [45].

Overall, widespread pathology of the gastrointestinal tract is indeed present already in prodromal stages of PD at least in a considerable fraction of cases. Yet, there are no longitudinal studies in humans to confirm the idea of a gastrointestinal onset of disease, but the relevance of gastrointestinal symptoms and objectives measures of dysfunction is clearly present.

3. Gastrointestinal Symptoms in PD

A wide range of NMS in PD arise from the gastrointestinal tract and several questionnaires have been developed to quantify the symptoms including the Scales for Outcomes in Parkinson's Disease—Autonomic [19,46] (SCOPA-AUT), the Non-Motor Symptoms Scale [47,48] (NMSS) and the Non-motor Symptoms Questionnaire [49] (NMSQuest). These are validated for use in PD and all include a section on gastrointestinal symptoms.

3.1. Upper Gastrointestinal Symptoms

Dysphagia in PD involves difficulty in the initiation and efficient completion of swallowing leading to decreased pace and comfort of eating and a reduction in quality of life [50,51]. Swallowing impairments might also contribute to malnutrition and weight loss and the occurrence of aspiration pneumonia constitute a major cause of death in PD [50].

Swallowing can be divided into an oral, pharyngeal, and esophageal phase. Generally, complaints of oropharyngeal dysphagia, e.g., difficulties swallowing or choking, are present in 35% of patients with a clear tendency to increase in prevalence and severity with disease progression [52]. Thus, marked dysphagia is often considered a late symptom of PD while severe dysphagia in early disease raises the suspicion of an atypical Parkinsonian disorder [2]. The presence of substantial dysphagia is not always reported by patients, but significant predictors of dysphagia include advanced clinical disease stage, drooling, significant weight loss, or body mass index below 20 [53]. Notably, drooling is a very common and troublesome feature of PD. However, it is not a consequence of hypersecretion of saliva, as the secretion is often decreased, but occurs when swallowing is impaired or infrequent causing accumulation of saliva in the mouth [54].

Oropharyngeal dysfunction includes inadequate mastication, poor formation of the bolus, difficulties in initiating swallowing, and choking as a sign of aspiration. As such, it has been considered as a motor symptom rather than a non-motor symptom. Accordingly, it often improves upon initiating medication [55] and it also improves during the on-state of medication even in the presence of dyskinesias [56,57]. Whether isolated esophageal dysfunction gives rise to distinct symptoms is unclear, although dysfunction of the lower esophageal sphincter might contribute to gastroesophageal reflux [52].

Symptoms attributed to gastroparesis are common in PD. Bloating and abdominal fullness has been reported by up to 50% of patients, while nausea and vomiting are reported by 15% [58,59]. Yet, rapid gastric emptying known as gastric dumping has also been reported [60]. Gastroparesis and gastric dumping are possible etiologies for unpredictable absorption of L-dopa with delayed onset of effect from anti-Parkinson medications as well as rapid effect resulting in dyskinesias.

Small intestinal bacterial overgrowth (SIBO) is a condition with increased bacterial density in the small intestines and has also been associated with disturbances in absorption and effect of anti-Parkinson medications. Furthermore, the condition is suspected to cause bloating, abdominal discomfort, and diarrhea [61]. However, these symptoms can also arise directly because of progressive neurodegeneration of the enteric and autonomic nervous system in PD, and the relative contribution from SIBO to the development of such symptoms is unclear.

3.2. Lower Gastrointestinal Symptoms

Infrequent bowel movements and straining during defecation are key symptoms of constipation [62]. Additionally, the perception of incomplete rectal emptying, abdominal discomfort, and pain that may be relieved by defecation are also attributable to constipation [63]. Studies of constipation are hampered by the lack of standardization and more than 10 different definitions of constipation have been applied in the PD literature alone [62].

The most frequently used definition of constipation is "less than 3 bowel movements per week," which is used by the SCOPA-AUT and NMSS questionnaires, while "straining" alone is sufficient to fulfill the definition of constipation in the NMSQuest. A common feature of these widely used questionnaires is the aim of measuring the full burden of NMS in PD and not constipation in detail. Better suited for the latter is the Rome Functional Constipation questionnaires [63,64]. Although it has not been validated for use in PD, it provides a more detailed and quantifiable measure of constipation symptoms as is also the case with the Cleveland Constipation Scoring System [65].

A recent meta-analysis found that 40–50% of PD patients report less than 3 bowel movements per week compared to ~15% of matched controls [62]. However, the prevalence estimates in individual studies ranged from 8% to 70% in patients and from 0% to 34% in healthy controls underlining the questionable reliability associated with symptom-based investigations of constipation. This substantial variance is not only a consequence of different settings and questionnaires but possibly also aggravated by individuals slowly getting accustomed to symptoms as they develop over time. A significant recollection bias when reporting bowel movement frequencies as found by Ashraf et al. [66] may also contribute to the variance. Notably, a definition based purely on bowel movement frequency will also tend to overlook the presence of constipation if the patient suffers from co-existing diarrhea as seen when watery stools leak around a blockage of hard stool in cases of fecal impaction [67].

Interestingly, a meta-analysis has found that constipation in otherwise healthy adults increases the risk of subsequent PD diagnosis [5]. This association was present with an OR of 2.13 even in those patients whose constipation preceded the diagnosis of PD by more than 10 years [5]. The finding is supported by a more recent study of a large Danish cohort [21]. Similarly, constipation is frequent in RBD cases [68] and the prevalence is higher in PD patients with RBD than those without [69]. The causal mechanisms behind this association are unclear but might be related to pathological processes affecting the ENS and the DMV prior to recognizable loss of motor function.

Anorectal symptoms are very common in PD with straining being one of the most commonly reported gastrointestinal symptoms in PD. The prevalence of straining is ~70% in PD compared to around 40% in controls while incomplete emptying is reported by ~55%

of patients and 28–42% of controls [19,20]. The considerable burden of anorectal symptoms in PD is further substantiated by the finding that 66% of early PD patients report defecatory symptoms, whereas only 29% reported a weekly bowel movement frequency of fewer than 3 times [70].

In summary, PD patients frequently suffer from a variety of gastrointestinal symptoms, although these symptoms remain difficult to define and measure using questionnaires. Consequently, objective measures are needed to assess functional disturbances of the gastrointestinal tract in order to advance our understanding of the underlying pathologies.

4. Objective Measures of Gastrointestinal Dysfunction

Gastrointestinal dysfunction can sometimes be subclinical, so measurable dysfunction is often more frequent than the corresponding subjective symptoms assessed by questionnaires. The following section covers the principles behind the most useful objective measures and summarizes key findings.

4.1. Swallowing Dysfunction

Successful swallowing involves complex voluntarily initiated movements followed by reflexes involving motor as well as sensory neurons of somatic and visceral origin [50,71]. As such, the basal ganglia are involved primarily in the oral and pharyngeal phase of swallowing during which the bolus is formed and by coordinated effort of striated muscles transported to the top of the esophagus [50,71]. The visceral fibers of the vagal nerve innervate the lower third of the esophagus [72]. The DMV and the vagal nerve are among the earliest and most severely affected structures in PD and show marked involvement in most patients [13]. LP has also been found in the peripheral pharyngeal nerve fibers [73,74] although the ambiguus nucleus innervating the pharyngeal muscles and the upper esophagus is relatively unaffected by LP [13,72]. Consequently, oropharyngeal and lower esophageal dysfunction are inherently different from a functional as well as a neuropathological perspective in the context of PD.

Oropharyngeal dysfunction can be visualized using fiberoptic endoscopic evaluation of swallowing (FEES) and by videofluoroscopic swallowing studies (VFSS). These methods are suitable for evaluating risk of aspiration in relation to different food consistencies and liquids being swallowed during visualization [50]. In PD, abnormalities during FEES are reported in as many as 95% of patients with residues being the most common finding (93%) but also with a significant finding of aspiration in 16% of asymptomatic PD patients [75].

These methods do not sufficiently evaluate esophageal dysfunction and thus, high-resolution manometry (HRM) compliments the use FEES and VFSS. HRM is performed by passing a thin pressure-sensitive tube through the nose to the stomach. Using HRM and FEES Suttrup et al. examined 65 PD patients of different disease stages and reported that 95% of cases had measurable impairments of esophageal motility [76]. These changes were seen almost evenly across all stages of disease and was without clear association to the FEES scores of oropharyngeal dysphagia [76]. Esophageal motility can also be evaluated by esophageal scintigraphy where a radioactively labeled bolus is swallowed during the dynamic recording of gamma emission. Using this principle Potulska et al. found significantly prolonged lower esophageal transit times suggestive of dysfunctional esophageal peristalsis in agreement with the findings of Suttrup et al. [77].

4.2. Stomach Dysfunction

Symptoms of gastroparesis are commonly associated with PD but the results from studies of objective gastroparesis are conflicting and methodological differences make individual studies difficult to compare [60].

Solid meal scintigraphy is considered the gold standard for estimating gastric emptying time (GET) [74]. After ingestion of a standardized meal containing ^{99m}Tc the emitted gamma radiation is measured by serial images recorded by a gamma camera (Figure 1) [78].

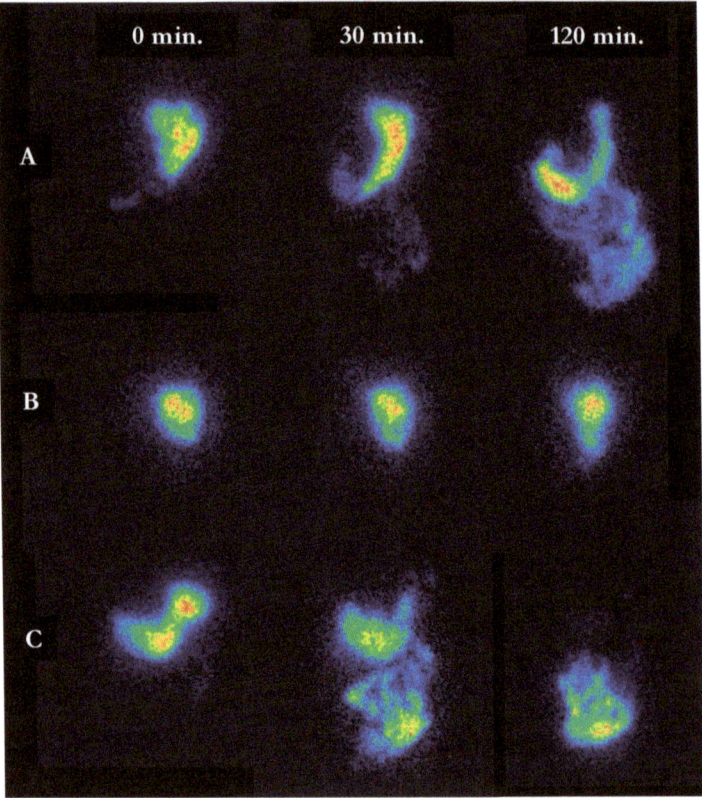

Figure 1. Gastric scintigraphy images at 0, 30 and 120 min after ingestion of a radioactive solid meal. (**A**). Healthy control with normal gastric emptying time. (**B**). Parkinson's disease (PD) patient with severely delayed gastric emptying time compatible with gastroparesis. (**C**). PD patient with rapid gastric emptying suggestive of "gastric dumping" (compare the image taken at 30 min. to the image from A taken at 120 min.).

A meta-analysis of studies using gastric scintigraphy in PD found a non-significant trend towards prolonged GET in PD patients [60]. However, the trend reached statistical significance after post-hoc exclusion of one outlier study.

Scintigraphy requires specialized facilities and exposes the patient to radiation but provides a reliable biomechanical measure of gastric emptying rate. Alternatively, a breath test using a meal containing ^{13}C-sodium octanoate is an indirect measure of gastric emptying based on the subsequent measurements of expired $^{13}CO_2$ [61]. This estimate is dependent not only on gastric emptying but also on small intestinal absorption and hepatic metabolism of the tracer [60]. This notion is supported by a comparative study of healthy individuals which found that the results of the breath test could not simply be adjusted to fit the results of the scintigraphy even though both methods are reproducible within each subject [79]. Theoretically, small intestinal dysmotility and malabsorption, bacterial overgrowth, and changes in liver metabolism can all interfere with results of the breath test [60]. In this light, it is worth noting that most studies using the breath test reported prolonged GET in PD patients compared to controls [60].

Interestingly, the breath test has been used to study a broader spectrum of disease stages. Unger et al. found prolonged GET estimates in untreated PD but not in iRBD [80] whereas Epprecht et al. found no difference between early-stage PD patients in the off-state and controls [81]. Collectively, this suggests that the disturbances giving rise to pathological parameter estimates on breath tests are not a feature of prodromal PD but develops at later disease stages.

The GET may also be influenced by anti-Parkinson medications, and administration of levodopa to healthy individuals have been shown to delay GET [82,83]. A solid meal scintigraphy study by Hardoff et al. found no difference in GET between mild and moderate disease stage PD patients and likewise, no difference between treated and untreated PD patients [84]. However, studies investigating the association between GET and motor fluctuations in PD patients treated with levodopa have yielded conflicting results [84,85]. In a study using breath tests to compare GET before and 3 months following initiation of deep brain stimulation in the subthalamic nucleus (STN-DBS) found no significant difference when comparing the pre-operative, off medication condition with the pre-operative on medication condition—indicating that levodopa administration does not affect GET [86]. However, a marked decrease in GET was demonstrated in the post-postoperative on medication-on stimulation condition compared to the pre-operative on medication condition suggesting a positive effect of STN-DBS on gastric emptying.

Whether the heterogenicity in gastric emptying time is influenced by more distal dysfunction has not been investigated, but chronic rectal distension due to defecatory disturbances could induce a cologastric reflex causing a delay in GET. To our knowledge, this has only been demonstrated in individuals without PD [87,88].

Novel methods to study stomach dysfunction in PD have introduced new measures of dysfunction and shown promising results. An MRI-based imaging study observed decreased emptying of gastric volume in PD patients with early satiety and dyspepsia. Additionally, decreased total gastric volume and decreased gastric motility was reported in patients with dyspepsia [89]. Another study used an electromagnetic capsule system to study gastric motility in PD patients and found prolonged GET compared to controls but similar frequency of gastric contractions indicating normal functioning of the intestinal cells of Cajal [90]. These methods are yet to be validated in PD but offer the possibility of repeated measurements in the same individuals without exposure to radiation.

In summary, it is not possible to make firm conclusions about the frequency and magnitude of gastric dysmotility in PD, since the seemingly compelling results from ^{13}C-sodium octanoate breath tests are prone to measuring other disturbances different from gastric emptying per se. However, the disturbances underlying these findings are noteworthy and further studies are needed to shed light on the association with symptoms and small intestinal dysfunction.

4.3. Small Intestinal Dysfunction

In comparison to the stomach and colon, very few studies have explored small intestinal dysfunction in PD.

Bacterial overgrowth of the small intestines is most often defined as above 10^5 colony forming units (CFU) per milliliter of jejunal fluid acquired by endoscopic aspiration [61]. Alternatively, breath tests can demonstrate the presence of bacteria in small intestine by measuring the concentration of H_2 in expired air following the intake of glucose or lactulose. Breath test provides a lower sensitivity (60–70%) and specificity (40–80%) when compared to jejunal aspiration [91] but are non-invasive and therefore used very frequently. However, the interpretation of breath test results is an area of ongoing discussion and the method is not fully validated [61].

In a study of PD patients, the prevalence of SIBO was investigated using both glucose and lactulose breath tests. Here, the SIBO prevalence was 54.5% in PD patients and 20% in controls with most cases being positive on only one of the two tests [92]. Another study used only glucose breath tests but reported a similar prevalence among PD patients and a prevalence of 8% among controls [93]. Interestingly, the former study found a higher frequency of delayed-on and increased daily off times [92] in patients with SIBO suggesting that SIBO could contribute to abnormal absorption of levodopa. Furthermore, a study by

Tan et al. found the presence of SIBO to be associated with worse motor symptoms [94]. A possible contributing factor to this is the finding that small intestinal enterococcus species may inactivate levodopa via decarboxylases [95,96]. Along the same line, infection with *helicobacter pylori* (HP) is associated with worse motor symptoms [97,98] and in epidemiological studies, HP infection has been linked to development of PD later in life [99]. Substantially improved motor function has been observed after eradication [98,100], but a recent randomized, controlled trial of HP eradication in infected PD patients did not find any improvement of motor or nonmotor symptoms at weeks 12 and 52 following eradication [101].

Small intestinal transit has been investigated using different ambulatory systems comprised of an ingestible capsule and a wireless data receiver [102–104]. These studies reported a delay in small intestinal transit time in PD compared to matched controls, although the magnitude of delayed transit was less marked than that seen in the colon. In support, studies of colonic transit time which uses ingested radiopaque plastic markers (ROM) sometimes report the presence of ROM in the small intestine 24 h after ingestion of the last capsule [105]. Such findings are a clear indication that upper GI tract transit can be severely impaired in some PD patients.

4.4. Colonic and Anorectal Dysfunction

Mechanistically, constipation can be separated into slow transit constipation due to prolonged colonic transit time (CTT) and outlet obstruction caused by dyssynergia of rectal muscles [106]. Presumably, outlet constipation is related to anorectal symptoms such as straining and incomplete emptying while prolonged colonic transit may be closer related to decreased frequency of bowel movements.

Objective measures of CTT are widely available and the most commonly used technique is based on the visualization of ingested radio-opaque markers (ROM) using abdominal x-ray (Figure 2) [107]. Typically, one capsule containing 10 ROMs is ingested for 6 consecutive days (a total of 60 markers) followed by an abdominal x-ray on day 7 revealing the number of retained markers. When this protocol was used with a cut-off of 25 markers for males and 29 markers for females, 80% of Parkinson's patients had prolonged CTT [105]. Specifically, the retention of markers is predominantly in the rectosigmoid part of the colon suggesting that outlet obstruction is a substantial contributor to the finding of CTT in PD [108,109]. Importantly, the correlation between objectively prolonged CTT and subjective symptoms as measured by questionnaires is generally poor [105,110,111]. Notably, the frequency of bowel movements seems to be a worse predictor of prolonged CTT than other symptoms such as bloating and use of an enema or manual evacuation of feces [109].

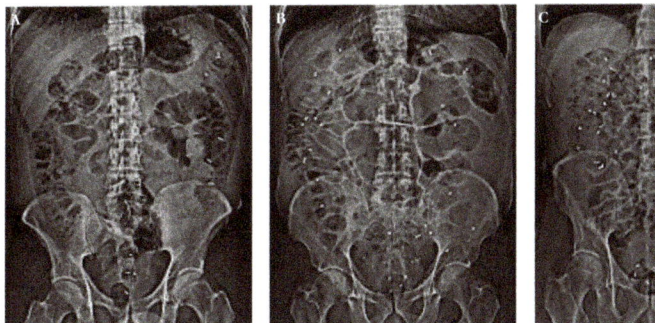

Figure 2. Abdominal x-ray topograms visualizing the retention of radio-opaque markers in the gastrointestinal tract as an objective measure of colonic transit time (CTT). (**A**). Healthy control with an estimated CTT within the normal range. (**B**). Parkinson's disease (PD) patient with an estimated CTT near the mean for PD patients. (**C**). PD patient with severely prolonged CTT.

Similarly, a study using a magnetic 3D-Transit system found no correlation between constipation and neither small intestinal nor colonic transit times, although both measures of intestinal transit were prolonged in the PD group compared to controls [102]. Evaluation of total and regional colonic volumes is possible when an abdominal CT-scan is performed, and with this method increased total colonic volume was demonstrated in a group of 22 iRBD cases compared to 26 controls [68]. Notably, the difference in total colonic volume was statistically stronger than the corresponding difference in colonic transit times as measured by radio-opaque markers as well as magnetic 3D-Transit capsule. The robustness of colonic volumetric measures was also utilized in a study comparing newly diagnosed PD patients. Here, a highly significant increase in colonic volume was detected in PD patients with RBD when comparing to PD patients without RBD [45].

Anorectal dysfunction in isolation or in combination with prolonged CTT is probably a major contributor to constipation in PD. Several approaches have been utilized to study different aspects of anorectal dysfunction including defecography, electromyography (EMG), balloon distension tests, and rectal manometry. Generally, studies of anorectal dysfunction in PD have used heterogeneous methods, small sample sizes, and often without control groups. In brief, incomplete emptying with dysfunction of the puborectalis muscles and paradoxical contraction of the external anal sphincter or lack of inhibition has been demonstrated by defecography and manometry, respectively [112,113]. Paradoxical sphincter contraction on defecation together with incomplete emptying have also been demonstrated in another study using rectoanal videomanometry [108]. Rectal sensitivity of urge was found to be normal in a study of unselected PD patients [113,114], while another study points to the possibility of rectal hypersensitivity in constipated PD patients [110]. Balloon expulsion tests in 35 PD patients, who did not fulfill the ROME-III criteria for defecatory dysfunction (DD), demonstrated abnormal expulsion in 27 of 35 cases compared to 24 of 35 in otherwise healthy adults fulfilling the criteria for DD [115]. Once again, these findings highlight the often poor correlation between subjective symptoms and objective measures [62]. Interestingly, no differences were found on manometry between early and late PD patients suggesting that significant dysfunction is present early in the disease [115]. In support, another study used manometry and reported a similar prevalence of pelvic floor dyssynergia of approximately 60% in early as well as in late PD [114].

Recent studies used ^{11}C-donepezil PET/CT (Figure 3) to measure cholinergic denervation in the GI tract of PD patients and reported decreased cholinergic signal in the small intestine and particularly in the colon [116,117]. Interestingly, similar magnitudes of decreased colonic signal are seen in iRBD patients, suggesting that cholinergic denervation is already manifest in the prodromal phase [44]. Although 70% of enteric neurons are cholinergic, the loss of cholinergic PET signal in the intestines is best compatible with parasympathetic denervation, since it is known that the DMV shows severe pathology and cell loss in PD, whereas no significant loss of enteric neurons has been detected [118].

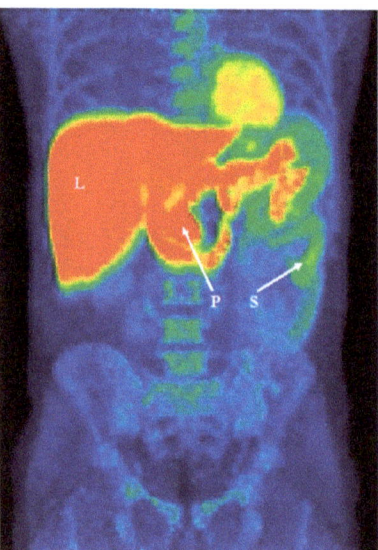

Figure 3. ^{11}C-Donepezil PET illustrating the summed signal of gastrointestinal organs (L liver, P pancreas, S small intestine).

It is well documented that PD patients show very dramatic sympathetic denervation of the heart [119,120]. Nearly all iRBD patients show the same profound loss of cardiac sympathetic signal, signifying that this subtype of prodromal PD show involvement of the autonomic system before the brain is markedly affected [45,121–123]. However, the importance of sympathetic denervation for gastrointestinal dysfunction is presently unclear and no studies have documented sympathetic denervation of the intestines in PD.

5. Treatment of Gastrointestinal Symptoms in PD

Recent review papers have provided detailed recommendations for treatment of gastrointestinal symptoms in PD [124,125]. Thus, treatment strategies will only be briefly summarized here.

For the treatment of drooling, behavioral modifications such as chewing gum have been suggested [54] as this may increase the rate of swallowing. An anticholinergic such as glycopyrrolate may give or exacerbate constipation and urinary retention, and local treatment options including oral atropine solutions and hyoscine patches as well as parotid and submandibular botulinum toxin injections are therefore often favored [124,125]. Other medications with anticholinergic properties might also be useful although evidence of their efficacy is limited.

For oropharyngeal dysphagia, the positive effects of optimized anti-Parkinson treatment on symptom severity is well established [55–57]. If symptoms persist, a speech and language therapist may initiate swallowing treatment with the use of methods aimed at the individual patient's difficulties—often based on objective evaluations such as fiberoptic endoscopic evaluation of swallowing [50].

Treatment of gastroparesis in PD is complex as the diagnosis cannot be made from symptoms alone and since pharmacological treatment is associated with a substantial risk of adverse effects. The prokinetic dopamine receptor antagonist domperidone is possibly useful for treatment of nausea and delayed gastric emptying in PD, since it does not cross the blood-brain barrier in contrast to metoclopramide [124]. Future treatment options might include the use of a gastric pacemaker as this has shown promising results in scintigraphy-confirmed gastroparesis caused by diabetic neuropathy [126].

SIBO is treatable with antibiotics and can lead to a reduction in motor fluctuations in some patients [61,92]. Eradication of SIBO using empirical antibiotic treatment has been demonstrated in populations without PD although recurrence rates of up to 44% after 9 months have been reported [61]. Theoretically, antibiotic treatments of SIBO impose a risk of generating resistant gastrointestinal infections and disturbance of colonic microbiota [61]. Clearly, there is a need for further studies evaluating the effects of SIBO eradication in PD.

For constipation, lifestyle modifications such as exercise and gradually increased fiber and fluid intake are often advised for the general population with functional constipation [127]. Although this has not been specifically investigated in PD patients, it is often recommended for this population as well [124]. Several studies have investigated the effects of pharmacological treatments of constipation in PD [124] and support the use of the bulk-forming psyllium [110], PEG (Macrogol) containing osmotic laxatives, and the chloride channel activator Lubiprostone [124]. Recently, a randomized controlled trial investigated the effects of a daily capsule containing a multi-strain probiotic supplement in PD patients and demonstrated an increase in spontaneous bowel movements in the treated group [128]. Furthermore, the patient-reported treatment satisfaction was 65.6% in the treated group compared to 21.6% in the placebo group supporting not only the feasibility of probiotic supplements in PD but also the possible interconnection between the microbiome and constipation. Specifically aimed at outlet constipation, biofeedback therapy has shown promising results in other patient populations [129,130] and ultimately, botulinum toxin injections into the puborectalis muscle have been found to be effective in PD patients with outlet constipation [131,132].

6. Conclusions

In conclusion, subjective gastrointestinal symptoms are common in PD and the prevalence of objectively measured dysfunction is even higher. Oropharyngeal dysphagia is often asymptomatic during the early stages, and since it improves with levodopa treatment, it is often viewed as a motor symptom. The prevalence and magnitude of delayed gastric emptying is unclear since findings in solid meal scintigraphy studies indicate that gastric emptying is only marginally delayed in early-to-moderate stage PD. Breath test studies generally report a more significant delay in gastric emptying of PD patients, but further studies are needed to clarify the extent to which small intestinal dysfunction and perturbed liver metabolism contribute to these observations.

Small intestinal bacterial overgrowth and altered microbiome in PD patients are active fields of investigation and highlight the complex interplay between microbiota and gastrointestinal dysfunction. Constipation is among the most common non-motor symptoms in PD, but research in this field is hampered by a lack of standardization and the symptoms of anorectal dysfunction are often missed. Additionally, the prevalence of objective colonic dysfunction in terms of delayed colonic transit and anorectal dysfunction far exceeds the reported frequency of subjective constipation and indicates that the gut is affected in the vast majority of PD patients.

Looking forward, studies of prodromal cases such as those with iRBD may provide important insights into the sequence of events behind the development and progression of PD. Additionally, further clinical trials are needed that specifically test tailored treatments of gastrointestinal symptoms in well characterized groups of PD patients.

Author Contributions: Conceptualization, C.S., P.B.; methodology, C.S., P.B., K.K., J.H.; writing—original draft preparation, C.S., P.B., K.K., J.H.; writing—review and editing, C.S., P.B., K.K., J.H.; visualization, C.S., P.B., K.K., J.H.; supervision, P.B.; project administration, P.B.; funding acquisition, P.B. All authors have read and agreed to the published version of the manuscript.

Funding: This research received no external funding.

Institutional Review Board Statement: Not applicable.

J. Clin. Med. **2021**, *10*, 493

Informed Consent Statement: Not applicable.

Data Availability Statement: Not applicable.

Acknowledgments: Publication costs for this review article was covered by a grant from Coloplast™. The authors have no financial relationships to the funding entity.

Conflicts of Interest: The authors declare no conflict of interest.

References

1. Poewe, W.; Seppi, K.; Tanner, C.M.; Halliday, G.M.; Brundin, P.; Volkmann, J.; Schrag, A.E.; Lang, A.E. Parkinson disease. *Nat. Rev. Dis. Primers* **2017**, *3*, 17013. [CrossRef] [PubMed]
2. Postuma, R.B.; Berg, D.; Stern, M.; Poewe, W.; Olanow, C.W.; Oertel, W.; Obeso, J.; Marek, K.; Litvan, I.; Lang, A.E.; et al. MDS clinical diagnostic criteria for Parkinson's disease. *Mov. Disord.* **2015**, *30*, 1591–1601. [CrossRef] [PubMed]
3. Schapira, A.H.V.; Chaudhuri, K.R.; Jenner, P. Non-motor features of Parkinson disease. *Nat. Rev. Neurosci.* **2017**, *18*, 435–450. [CrossRef] [PubMed]
4. Fasano, A.; Visanji, N.P.; Liu, L.W.; Lang, A.E.; Pfeiffer, R.F. Gastrointestinal dysfunction in Parkinson's disease. *Lancet Neurol.* **2015**, *14*, 625–639. [CrossRef]
5. Adams-Carr, K.L.; Bestwick, J.P.; Shribman, S.; Lees, A.; Schrag, A.; Noyce, A.J. Constipation preceding Parkinson's disease: A systematic review and meta-analysis. *J. Neurol. Neurosurg. Psychiatry* **2016**, *87*, 710–716. [CrossRef]
6. Braak, H.; Rub, U.; Gai, W.P.; Del Tredici, K. Idiopathic Parkinson's disease: Possible routes by which vulnerable neuronal types may be subject to neuroinvasion by an unknown pathogen. *J. Neural Transm. (Austria 1996)* **2003**, *110*, 517–536. [CrossRef]
7. Stokholm, M.G.; Danielsen, E.H.; Hamilton-Dutoit, S.J.; Borghammer, P. Pathological α-synuclein in gastrointestinal tissues from prodromal Parkinson disease patients: α-Synuclein in Prodromal PD. *Ann. Neurol.* **2016**, *79*, 940–949. [CrossRef]
8. Svensson, E.; Horváth-Puhó, E.; Thomsen, R.W.; Djurhuus, J.C.; Pedersen, L.; Borghammer, P.; Sørensen, H.T. Vagotomy and subsequent risk of Parkinson's disease. *Ann. Neurol.* **2015**, *78*, 522–529. [CrossRef]
9. Liu, B.; Fang, F.; Pedersen, N.L.; Tillander, A.; Ludvigsson, J.F.; Ekbom, A.; Svenningsson, P.; Chen, H.; Wirdefeldt, K. Vagotomy and Parkinson disease: A Swedish register-based matched-cohort study. *Neurology* **2017**, *88*, 1996–2002. [CrossRef]
10. Van Den Berge, N.; Ferreira, N.; Gram, H.; Mikkelsen, T.W.; Alstrup, A.K.O.; Casadei, N.; Tsung-Pin, P.; Riess, O.; Nyengaard, J.R.; Tamgüney, G.; et al. Evidence for bidirectional and trans-synaptic parasympathetic and sympathetic propagation of alpha-synuclein in rats. *Acta Neuropathol.* **2019**, *138*, 535–550. [CrossRef]
11. Pan-Montojo, F.; Anichtchik, O.; Dening, Y.; Knels, L.; Pursche, S.; Jung, R.; Jackson, S.; Gille, G.; Spillantini, M.G.; Reichmann, H.; et al. Progression of Parkinson's disease pathology is reproduced by intragastric administration of rotenone in mice. *PLoS ONE* **2010**, *5*, e8762. [CrossRef] [PubMed]
12. Holdorff, B. Friedrich Heinrich Lewy (1885–1950) and his work. *J. Hist. Neurosci.* **2002**, *11*, 19–28. [CrossRef]
13. Braak, H.; Tredici, K.D.; Rüb, U.; de Vos, R.A.I.; Jansen Steur, E.N.H.; Braak, E. Staging of brain pathology related to sporadic Parkinson's disease. *Neurobiol. Aging* **2003**, *24*, 197–211. [CrossRef]
14. Gai, W.P.; Blumbergs, P.C.; Geffen, L.B.; Blessing, W.W. Age-related loss of dorsal vagal neurons in Parkinson's disease. *Neurology* **1992**, *42*, 2106–2111. [CrossRef] [PubMed]
15. Eadie, M.J. The pathology of certain medullary nuclei in parkinsonism. *Brain* **1963**, *86*, 781–792. [CrossRef]
16. Hopkins, D.A.; Bieger, D.; deVente, J.; Steinbusch, W.M. Vagal efferent projections: Viscerotopy, neurochemistry and effects of vagotomy. *Prog. Brain Res.* **1996**, *107*, 79–96. [CrossRef]
17. Beach, T.G.; Adler, C.H.; Sue, L.I.; Vedders, L.; Lue, L.; White Iii, C.L.; Akiyama, H.; Caviness, J.N.; Shill, H.A.; Sabbagh, M.N.; et al. Multi-organ distribution of phosphorylated alpha-synuclein histopathology in subjects with Lewy body disorders. *Acta Neuropathol* **2010**, *119*, 689–702. [CrossRef]
18. Gelpi, E.; Navarro-Otano, J.; Tolosa, E.; Gaig, C.; Compta, Y.; Rey, M.J.; Marti, M.J.; Hernandez, I.; Valldeoriola, F.; Rene, R.; et al. Multiple organ involvement by alpha-synuclein pathology in Lewy body disorders. *Movement Disorders* **2014**, *29*, 1010–1018. [CrossRef]
19. Visser, M.; Marinus, J.; Stiggelbout, A.M.; Van Hilten, J.J. Assessment of autonomic dysfunction in Parkinson's disease: The SCOPA-AUT. *Mov. Disord. Off. J. Mov. Disord. Soc.* **2004**, *19*, 1306–1312. [CrossRef]
20. Damian, A.; Adler, C.H.; Hentz, J.G.; Shill, H.A.; Caviness, J.N.; Sabbagh, M.N.; Evidente, V.G.; Beach, T.G.; Driver-Dunckley, E. Autonomic function, as self-reported on the SCOPA-autonomic questionnaire, is normal in essential tremor but not in Parkinson's disease. *Parkinsonism Relat. Disord.* **2012**, *18*, 1089–1093. [CrossRef]
21. Svensson, E.; Henderson, V.W.; Borghammer, P.; Horváth-Puhó, E.; Sørensen, H.T. Constipation and risk of Parkinson's disease: A Danish population-based cohort study. *Parkinsonism Relat. Disord.* **2016**, *28*, 18–22. [CrossRef] [PubMed]
22. Hawkes, C.H.; Del Tredici, K.; Braak, H. Parkinson's disease: A dual-hit hypothesis. *Neuropathol. Appl. Neurobiol.* **2007**, *33*, 599–614. [CrossRef] [PubMed]
23. Hawkes, C.H.; Del Tredici, K.; Braak, H. Parkinson's disease: The dual hit theory revisited. *Ann. N. Y. Acad. Sci.* **2009**, *1170*, 615–622. [CrossRef] [PubMed]

24. Lebouvier, T.; Neunlist, M.; Bruley des Varannes, S.; Coron, E.; Drouard, A.; N'Guyen, J.M.; Chaumette, T.; Tasselli, M.; Paillusson, S.; Flamand, M.; et al. Colonic biopsies to assess the neuropathology of Parkinson's disease and its relationship with symptoms. *PLoS ONE* **2010**, *5*, e12728. [CrossRef]

25. Pouclet, H.; Lebouvier, T.; Coron, E.; des Varannes, S.B.; Rouaud, T.; Roy, M.; Neunlist, M.; Derkinderen, P. A comparison between rectal and colonic biopsies to detect Lewy pathology in Parkinson's disease. *Neurobiol. Dis.* **2012**, *45*, 305–309. [CrossRef]

26. Sanchez-Ferro, A.; Rabano, A.; Catalan, M.J.; Rodriguez-Valcarcel, F.C.; Fernandez Diez, S.; Herreros-Rodriguez, J.; Garcia-Cobos, E.; Alvarez-Santullano, M.M.; Lopez-Manzanares, L.; Mosqueira, A.J.; et al. In vivo gastric detection of alpha-synuclein inclusions in Parkinson's disease. *Mov. Disord. Off. J. Mov. Disord. Soc.* **2015**, *30*, 517–524. [CrossRef]

27. Gray, M.T.; Munoz, D.G.; Gray, D.A.; Schlossmacher, M.G.; Woulfe, J.M. Alpha-synuclein in the appendiceal mucosa of neurologically intact subjects. *Mov. Disord.* **2014**, *29*, 991–998. [CrossRef]

28. Svensson, E.; Horváth-Puhó, E.; Stokholm, M.G.; Sørensen, H.T.; Henderson, V.W.; Borghammer, P. Appendectomy and risk of Parkinson's disease: A nationwide cohort study with more than 10 years of follow-up: Appendectomy and Risk of PD. *Mov. Disord.* **2016**, *31*, 1918–1922. [CrossRef]

29. Killinger, B.A.; Madaj, Z.; Sikora, J.W.; Rey, N.; Haas, A.J.; Vepa, Y.; Lindqvist, D.; Chen, H.; Thomas, P.M.; Brundin, P.; et al. The vermiform appendix impacts the risk of developing Parkinson's disease. *Sci. Transl. Med.* **2018**, *10*, eaar5280. [CrossRef]

30. Marras, C.; Lang, A.E.; Austin, P.C.; Lau, C.; Urbach, D.R. Appendectomy in mid and later life and risk of Parkinson's disease: A population-based study. *Mov. Disord.* **2016**, *31*, 1243–1247. [CrossRef]

31. Beach, T.G.; Corbille, A.G.; Letournel, F.; Kordower, J.H.; Kremer, T.; Munoz, D.G.; Intorcia, A.; Hentz, J.; Adler, C.H.; Sue, L.I.; et al. Multicenter Assessment of Immunohistochemical Methods for Pathological Alpha-Synuclein in Sigmoid Colon of Autopsied Parkinson's Disease and Control Subjects. *J. Parkinsons Dis.* **2016**, *6*, 761–770. [CrossRef] [PubMed]

32. Corbille, A.G.; Letournel, F.; Kordower, J.H.; Lee, J.; Shanes, E.; Neunlist, M.; Munoz, D.G.; Derkinderen, P.; Beach, T.G. Evaluation of alpha-synuclein immunohistochemical methods for the detection of Lewy-type synucleinopathy in gastrointestinal biopsies. *Acta Neuropathol. Commun.* **2016**, *4*, 35. [CrossRef] [PubMed]

33. Johnson, M.E.; Stecher, B.; Labrie, V.; Brundin, L.; Brundin, P. Triggers, Facilitators, and Aggravators: Redefining Parkinson's Disease Pathogenesis. *Trends Neurosci.* **2019**, *42*, 4–13. [CrossRef] [PubMed]

34. Chen, S.G.; Stribinskis, V.; Rane, M.J.; Demuth, D.R.; Gozal, E.; Roberts, A.M.; Jagadapillai, R.; Liu, R.; Choe, K.; Shivakumar, B.; et al. Exposure to the Functional Bacterial Amyloid Protein Curli Enhances Alpha-Synuclein Aggregation in Aged Fischer 344 Rats and Caenorhabditis elegans. *Sci. Rep.* **2016**, *6*, 34477. [CrossRef] [PubMed]

35. Sampson, T.R.; Debelius, J.W.; Thron, T.; Janssen, S.; Shastri, G.G.; Ilhan, Z.E.; Challis, C.; Schretter, C.E.; Rocha, S.; Gradinaru, V.; et al. Gut Microbiota Regulate Motor Deficits and Neuroinflammation in a Model of Parkinson's Disease. *Cell* **2016**, *167*, 1469–1480.e1412. [CrossRef] [PubMed]

36. Lubomski, M.; Tan, A.H.; Lim, S.Y.; Holmes, A.J.; Davis, R.L.; Sue, C.M. Parkinson's disease and the gastrointestinal microbiome. *J. Neurol.* **2020**, *267*, 2507–2523. [CrossRef] [PubMed]

37. Houser, M.C.; Chang, J.; Factor, S.A.; Molho, E.S.; Zabetian, C.P.; Hill-Burns, E.M.; Payami, H.; Hertzberg, V.S.; Tansey, M.G. Stool Immune Profiles Evince Gastrointestinal Inflammation in Parkinson's Disease. *Mov. Disord. Off. J. Mov. Disord. Soc.* **2018**, *33*, 793–804. [CrossRef]

38. Schwiertz, A.; Spiegel, J.; Dillmann, U.; Grundmann, D.; Burmann, J.; Fassbender, K.; Schafer, K.H.; Unger, M.M. Fecal markers of intestinal inflammation and intestinal permeability are elevated in Parkinson's disease. *Parkinsonism Relat. Disord.* **2018**, *50*, 104–107. [CrossRef]

39. Forsyth, C.B.; Shannon, K.M.; Kordower, J.H.; Voigt, R.M.; Shaikh, M.; Jaglin, J.A.; Estes, J.D.; Dodiya, H.B.; Keshavarzian, A. Increased intestinal permeability correlates with sigmoid mucosa alpha-synuclein staining and endotoxin exposure markers in early Parkinson's disease. *PLoS ONE* **2011**, *6*, e28032. [CrossRef]

40. Villumsen, M.; Aznar, S.; Pakkenberg, B.; Jess, T.; Brudek, T. Inflammatory bowel disease increases the risk of Parkinson's disease: A Danish nationwide cohort study 1977–2014. *Gut* **2019**, *68*, 18. [CrossRef]

41. Postuma, R.B.; Iranzo, A.; Hu, M.; Hogl, B.; Boeve, B.F.; Manni, R.; Oertel, W.H.; Arnulf, I.; Ferini-Strambi, L.; Puligheddu, M.; et al. Risk and predictors of dementia and parkinsonism in idiopathic REM sleep behaviour disorder: A multicentre study. *Brain* **2019**, *142*, 744–759. [CrossRef] [PubMed]

42. Heinzel, S.; Berg, D.; Gasser, T.; Chen, H.; Yao, C.; Postuma, R.B. Update of the MDS research criteria for prodromal Parkinson's disease. *Mov. Disord. Off. J. Mov. Disord. Soc.* **2019**, *34*, 1464–1470. [CrossRef] [PubMed]

43. Leclair-Visonneau, L.; Clairembault, T.; Coron, E.; Le Dily, S.; Vavasseur, F.; Dalichampt, M.; Pereon, Y.; Neunlist, M.; Derkinderen, P. REM sleep behavior disorder is related to enteric neuropathology in Parkinson disease. *Neurology* **2017**, *89*, 1612–1618. [CrossRef] [PubMed]

44. Knudsen, K.; Fedorova, T.D.; Hansen, A.K.; Sommerauer, M.; Otto, M.; Svendsen, K.B.; Nahimi, A.; Stokholm, M.G.; Pavese, N.; Beier, C.P.; et al. In-vivo staging of pathology in REM sleep behaviour disorder: A multimodality imaging case-control study. *Lancet Neurol.* **2018**, *17*. [CrossRef]

45. Horsager, J.; Andersen, K.B.; Knudsen, K.; Skjærbæk, C.; Fedorova, T.D.; Okkels, N.; Schaeffer, E.; Bonkat, S.K.; Geday, J.; Otto, M.; et al. Brain-first versus body-first Parkinson's disease: A multimodal imaging case-control study. *Brain* **2020**, *143*. [CrossRef]

46. Rodriguez-Blazquez, C.; Forjaz, M.J.; Frades-Payo, B.; de Pedro-Cuesta, J.; Martinez-Martin, P. Independent validation of the scales for outcomes in Parkinson's disease-autonomic (SCOPA-AUT). *Eur. J. Neurol.* **2010**, *17*, 194–201. [CrossRef]

47. Chaudhuri, K.R.; Martinez-Martin, P.; Brown, R.G.; Sethi, K.; Stocchi, F.; Odin, P.; Ondo, W.; Abe, K.; Macphee, G.; Macmahon, D.; et al. The metric properties of a novel non-motor symptoms scale for Parkinson's disease: Results from an international pilot study. *Mov. Disord. Off. J. Mov. Disord. Soc.* **2007**, *22*, 1901–1911. [CrossRef]

48. Van Wamelen, D.J.; Martinez-Martin, P.; Weintraub, D.; Schrag, A.; Antonini, A.; Falup-Pecurariu, C.; Odin, P.; Ray Chaudhuri, K. The Non-Motor Symptoms Scale in Parkinson's disease: Validation and use. *Acta Neurol. Scand.* **2020**, *143*. [CrossRef]

49. Chaudhuri, K.R.; Martinez-Martin, P.; Schapira, A.H.; Stocchi, F.; Sethi, K.; Odin, P.; Brown, R.G.; Koller, W.; Barone, P.; MacPhee, G.; et al. International multicenter pilot study of the first comprehensive self-completed nonmotor symptoms questionnaire for Parkinson's disease: The NMSQuest study. *Mov. Disord. Off. J. Mov. Disord. Soc.* **2006**, *21*, 916–923. [CrossRef]

50. Suttrup, I.; Warnecke, T. Dysphagia in Parkinson's Disease. *Dysphagia* **2016**, *31*, 24–32. [CrossRef]

51. Carneiro, D.; das Graças Wanderley de Sales Coriolano, M.; Belo, L.R.; de Marcos Rabelo, A.R.; Asano, A.G.; Lins, O.G. Quality of Life Related to Swallowing in Parkinson's Disease. *Dysphagia* **2014**, *29*, 578–582. [CrossRef] [PubMed]

52. Kalf, J.G.; de Swart, B.J.M.; Bloem, B.R.; Munneke, M. Prevalence of oropharyngeal dysphagia in Parkinson's disease: A meta-analysis. *Parkinsonism Relat. Disord.* **2012**, *18*, 311–315. [CrossRef] [PubMed]

53. Lam, K.; Lam, F.K.; Lau, K.K.; Chan, Y.K.; Kan, E.Y.; Woo, J.; Wong, F.K.; Ko, A. Simple clinical tests may predict severe oropharyngeal dysphagia in Parkinson's disease. *Mov. Disord. Off. J. Mov. Disord. Soc.* **2007**, *22*, 640–644. [CrossRef] [PubMed]

54. Srivanitchapoom, P.; Pandey, S.; Hallett, M. Drooling in Parkinson's disease: A review. *Parkinsonism Relat. Disord.* **2014**, *20*, 1109–1118. [CrossRef]

55. Müller, B.; Assmus, J.; Larsen, J.P.; Haugarvoll, K.; Skeie, G.O.; Tysnes, O.-B. Autonomic symptoms and dopaminergic treatment in de novo Parkinson's disease. *Acta Neurol. Scand.* **2013**, *127*, 290–294. [CrossRef]

56. Monte, F.S.; da Silva-Júnior, F.P.; Braga-Neto, P.; Nobre e Souza, M.A.; de Bruin, V.M. Swallowing abnormalities and dyskinesia in Parkinson's disease. *Mov. Disord. Off. J. Mov. Disord. Soc.* **2005**, *20*, 457–462. [CrossRef]

57. Warnecke, T.; Hamacher, C.; Oelenberg, S.; Dziewas, R. Off and on state assessment of swallowing function in Parkinson's disease. *Parkinsonism Relat. Disord.* **2014**, *20*, 1033–1034. [CrossRef]

58. Verbaan, D.; Marinus, J.; Visser, M.; van Rooden, S.M.; Stiggelbout, A.M.; van Hilten, J.J. Patient-reported autonomic symptoms in Parkinson disease. *Neurology* **2007**, *69*, 333–341. [CrossRef]

59. Martinez-Martin, P. The importance of non-motor disturbances to quality of life in Parkinson's disease. *J. Neurol. Sci.* **2011**, *310*, 12–16. [CrossRef]

60. Knudsen, K.; Szwebs, M.; Hansen, A.K.; Borghammer, P. Gastric emptying in Parkinson's disease—A mini-review. *Parkinsonism Relat. Disord.* **2018**, *55*. [CrossRef]

61. Quigley, E.M.M.; Murray, J.A.; Pimentel, M. AGA Clinical Practice Update on Small Intestinal Bacterial Overgrowth: Expert Review. *Gastroenterology* **2020**, *159*, 1526–1532. [CrossRef] [PubMed]

62. Knudsen, K.; Krogh, K.; Østergaard, K.; Borghammer, P. Constipation in parkinson's disease: Subjective symptoms, objective markers, and new perspectives. *Mov. Disord.* **2017**, *32*, 94–105. [CrossRef] [PubMed]

63. Rome Foundation. Guidelines—Rome III Diagnostic Criteria for Functional Gastrointestinal Disorders. *J. Gastrointest. Liver Dis.* **2006**, *15*, 307–312.

64. Palsson, O.S.; Whitehead, W.E.; van Tilburg, M.A.L.; Chang, L.; Chey, W.; Crowell, M.D.; Keefer, L.; Lembo, A.J.; Parkman, H.P.; Rao, S.S.C.; et al. Development and Validation of the Rome IV Diagnostic Questionnaire for Adults. *Gastroenterology* **2016**, *150*, 1481–1491. [CrossRef] [PubMed]

65. Agachan, F.; Chen, T.; Pfeifer, J.; Reissman, P.; Wexner, S.D. A constipation scoring system to simplify evaluation and management of constipated patients. *Dis. Colon Rectum* **1996**, *39*, 681–685. [CrossRef]

66. Ashraf, W.; Park, F.; Lof, J.; Quigley, E.M. An examination of the reliability of reported stool frequency in the diagnosis of idiopathic constipation. *Am. J. Gastroenterol.* **1996**, *91*, 26–32.

67. Serrano Falcón, B.; Barceló López, M.; Mateos Muñoz, B.; Álvarez Sánchez, A.; Rey, E. Fecal impaction: A systematic review of its medical complications. *BMC Geriatr.* **2016**, *16*, 4. [CrossRef]

68. Knudsen, K.; Fedorova, T.D.; Hansen, A.K.; Sommerauer, M.; Haase, A.-M.; Svendsen, K.B.; Otto, M.; Østergaard, K.; Krogh, K.; Borghammer, P. Objective intestinal function in patients with idiopathic REM sleep behavior disorder. *Parkinsonism Relat. Disord.* **2019**, *58*, 28–34. [CrossRef]

69. Nihei, Y.; Takahashi, K.; Koto, A.; Mihara, B.; Morita, Y.; Isozumi, K.; Ohta, K.; Muramatsu, K.; Gotoh, J.; Yamaguchi, K.; et al. REM sleep behavior disorder in Japanese patients with Parkinson's disease: A multicenter study using the REM sleep behavior disorder screening questionnaire. *J. Neurol.* **2012**, *259*, 1606–1612. [CrossRef]

70. Edwards, L.L.; Pfeiffer, R.F.; Quigley, E.M.; Hofman, R.; Balluff, M. Gastrointestinal symptoms in Parkinson's disease. *Mov. Disord. Off. J. Mov. Disord. Soc.* **1991**, *6*, 151–156. [CrossRef]

71. Leopold, N.A.; Daniels, S.K. Supranuclear control of swallowing. *Dysphagia* **2010**, *25*, 250–257. [CrossRef] [PubMed]

72. Jean, A. Brain stem control of swallowing: Neuronal network and cellular mechanisms. *Physiol. Rev.* **2001**, *81*, 929–969. [CrossRef] [PubMed]

73. Mu, L.; Sobotka, S.; Chen, J.; Su, H.; Sanders, I.; Adler, C.H.; Shill, H.A.; Caviness, J.N.; Samanta, J.E.; Beach, T.G. Altered pharyngeal muscles in parkinson disease. *J. Neuropathol. Exp. Neurol.* **2012**, *71*, 520–530. [CrossRef] [PubMed]

74. Mu, L.; Sobotka, S.; Chen, J.; Su, H.; Sanders, I.; Nyirenda, T.; Adler, C.H.; Shill, H.A.; Caviness, J.N.; Samanta, J.E.; et al. Parkinson disease affects peripheral sensory nerves in the pharynx. *J. Neuropathol. Exp. Neurol.* **2013**, *72*, 614–623. [CrossRef]

75. Pflug, C.; Bihler, M.; Emich, K.; Niessen, A.; Nienstedt, J.C.; Flügel, T.; Koseki, J.C.; Plaetke, R.; Hidding, U.; Gerloff, C.; et al. Critical Dysphagia is Common in Parkinson Disease and Occurs Even in Early Stages: A Prospective Cohort Study. *Dysphagia* **2018**, *33*, 41–50. [CrossRef]

76. Suttrup, I.; Suttrup, J.; Suntrup-Krueger, S.; Siemer, M.L.; Bauer, J.; Hamacher, C.; Oelenberg, S.; Domagk, D.; Dziewas, R.; Warnecke, T. Esophageal dysfunction in different stages of Parkinson's disease. *Neurogastroenterol. Motil.* **2017**, *29*. [CrossRef]

77. Potulska, A.; Friedman, A.; Królicki, L.; Spychala, A. Swallowing disorders in Parkinson's disease. *Parkinsonism Relat. Disord.* **2003**, *9*, 349–353. [CrossRef]

78. Abell, T.L.; Camilleri, M.; Donohoe, K.; Hasler, W.L.; Lin, H.C.; Maurer, A.H.; McCallum, R.W.; Nowak, T.; Nusynowitz, M.L.; Parkman, H.P.; et al. Consensus recommendations for gastric emptying scintigraphy: A joint report of the American Neurogastroenterol. Motil. Society and the Society of Nuclear Medicine. *J. Nucl. Med. Technol.* **2008**, *36*, 44–54. [CrossRef]

79. Choi, M.G.; Camilleri, M.; Burton, D.D.; Zinsmeister, A.R.; Forstrom, L.A.; Nair, K.S. [13C]octanoic acid breath test for gastric emptying of solids: Accuracy, reproducibility, and comparison with scintigraphy. *Gastroenterology* **1997**, *112*, 1155–1162. [CrossRef]

80. Unger, M.M.; Möller, J.C.; Mankel, K.; Schmittinger, K.; Eggert, K.M.; Stamelou, M.; Stiasny-Kolster, K.; Bohne, K.; Bodden, M.; Mayer, G.; et al. Patients with idiopathic rapid-eye-movement sleep behavior disorder show normal gastric motility assessed by the 13C-octanoate breath test. *Mov. Disord. Off. J. Mov. Disord. Soc.* **2011**, *26*, 2559–2563. [CrossRef]

81. Epprecht, L.; Schreglmann, S.R.; Goetze, O.; Woitalla, D.; Baumann, C.R.; Waldvogel, D. Unchanged gastric emptying and visceral perception in early Parkinson's disease after a high caloric test meal. *J. Neurol.* **2015**, *262*, 1946–1953. [CrossRef] [PubMed]

82. Robertson, D.R.; Renwick, A.G.; Wood, N.D.; Cross, N.; Macklin, B.S.; Fleming, J.S.; Waller, D.G.; George, C.F. The influence of levodopa on gastric emptying in man. *Br. J. Clin. Pharmacol.* **1990**, *29*, 47–53. [CrossRef] [PubMed]

83. Robertson, D.R.C.; Renwick, A.G.; Macklin, B.; Jones, S.; Waller, D.G.; George, C.F.; Fleming, J.S. The influence of levodopa on gastric emptying in healthy elderly volunteers. *Eur. J. Clin. Pharmacol.* **1992**, *42*, 409–412. [CrossRef] [PubMed]

84. Hardoff, R.; Sula, M.; Tamir, A.; Soil, A.; Front, A.; Badarna, S.; Honigman, S.; Giladi, N. Gastric emptying time and gastric motility in patients with Parkinson's disease. *Mov. Disord. Off. J. Mov. Disord. Soc.* **2001**, *16*, 1041–1047. [CrossRef] [PubMed]

85. Djaldetti, R.; Baron, J.; Ziv, I.; Melamed, E. Gastric emptying in Parkinson's disease: Patients with and without response fluctuations. *Neurology* **1996**, *46*, 1051–1054. [CrossRef]

86. Arai, E.; Arai, M.; Uchiyama, T.; Higuchi, Y.; Aoyagi, K.; Yamanaka, Y.; Yamamoto, T.; Nagano, O.; Shiina, A.; Maruoka, D.; et al. Subthalamic deep brain stimulation can improve gastric emptying in Parkinson's disease. *Brain* **2012**, *135*, 1478–1485. [CrossRef]

87. Tjeerdsma, H.C.; Smout, A.J.; Akkermans, L.M. Voluntary suppression of defecation delays gastric emptying. *Dig. Dis. Sci.* **1993**, *38*, 832–836. [CrossRef]

88. Youle, M.S.; Read, N.W. Effect of painless rectal distension on gastrointestinal transit of solid meal. *Dig. Dis. Sci.* **1984**, *29*, 902–906. [CrossRef]

89. Cho, J.; Lee, Y.J.; Kim, Y.H.; Shin, C.M.; Kim, J.M.; Chang, W.; Park, J.H. Quantitative MRI evaluation of gastric motility in patients with Parkinson's disease: Correlation of dyspeptic symptoms with volumetry and motility indices. *PLoS ONE* **2019**, *14*, e0216396. [CrossRef]

90. Heimrich, K.G.; Jacob, V.Y.P.; Schaller, D.; Stallmach, A.; Witte, O.W.; Prell, T. Gastric dysmotility in Parkinson's disease is not caused by alterations of the gastric pacemaker cells. *NPJ Parkinson's Dis.* **2019**, *5*, 15. [CrossRef]

91. Bohm, M.; Siwiec, R.M.; Wo, J.M. Diagnosis and management of small intestinal bacterial overgrowth. *Nutr. Clin. Pract.* **2013**, *28*, 289–299. [CrossRef] [PubMed]

92. Fasano, A.; Bove, F.; Gabrielli, M.; Petracca, M.; Zocco, M.A.; Ragazzoni, E.; Barbaro, F.; Piano, C.; Fortuna, S.; Tortora, A.; et al. The role of small intestinal bacterial overgrowth in Parkinson's disease. *Mov. Disord.* **2013**, *28*, 1241–1249. [CrossRef] [PubMed]

93. Gabrielli, M.; Bonazzi, P.; Scarpellini, E.; Bendia, E.; Lauritano, E.C.; Fasano, A.; Ceravolo, M.G.; Capecci, M.; Rita Bentivoglio, A.; Provinciali, L.; et al. Prevalence of small intestinal bacterial overgrowth in Parkinson's disease. *Mov. Disord. Off. J. Mov. Disord. Soc.* **2011**, *26*, 889–892. [CrossRef] [PubMed]

94. Tan, A.H.; Mahadeva, S.; Thalha, A.M.; Gibson, P.R.; Kiew, C.K.; Yeat, C.M.; Ng, S.W.; Ang, S.P.; Chow, S.K.; Tan, C.T.; et al. Small intestinal bacterial overgrowth in Parkinson's disease. *Parkinsonism Relat. Disord.* **2014**, *20*, 535–540. [CrossRef]

95. Van Kessel, S.P.; Frye, A.K.; El-Gendy, A.O.; Castejon, M.; Keshavarzian, A.; van Dijk, G.; El Aidy, S. Gut bacterial tyrosine decarboxylases restrict levels of levodopa in the treatment of Parkinson's disease. *Nat. Commun.* **2019**, *10*, 310. [CrossRef] [PubMed]

96. Maini Rekdal, V.; Bess, E.N.; Bisanz, J.E.; Turnbaugh, P.J.; Balskus, E.P. Discovery and inhibition of an interspecies gut bacterial pathway for Levodopa metabolism. *Science (NY)* **2019**, *364*, eaau6323. [CrossRef]

97. Tan, A.H.; Mahadeva, S.; Marras, C.; Thalha, A.M.; Kiew, C.K.; Yeat, C.M.; Ng, S.W.; Ang, S.P.; Chow, S.K.; Loke, M.F.; et al. Helicobacter pylori infection is associated with worse severity of Parkinson's disease. *Parkinsonism Relat. Disord.* **2015**, *21*, 221–225. [CrossRef]

98. Lee, W.Y.; Yoon, W.T.; Shin, H.Y.; Jeon, S.H.; Rhee, P.L. Helicobacter pylori infection and motor fluctuations in patients with Parkinson's disease. *Mov. Disord. Off. J. Mov. Disord. Soc.* **2008**, *23*, 1696–1700. [CrossRef]

99. Huang, H.K.; Wang, J.H.; Lei, W.Y.; Chen, C.L.; Chang, C.Y.; Liou, L.S. Helicobacter pylori infection is associated with an increased risk of Parkinson's disease: A population-based retrospective cohort study. *Parkinsonism Relat. Disord.* **2018**, *47*, 26–31. [CrossRef]

100. Hashim, H.; Azmin, S.; Razlan, H.; Yahya, N.W.; Tan, H.J.; Manaf, M.R.; Ibrahim, N.M. Eradication of Helicobacter pylori infection improves levodopa action, clinical symptoms and quality of life in patients with Parkinson's disease. *PLoS ONE* **2014**, *9*, e112330. [CrossRef]

101. Tan, A.H.; Lim, S.-Y.; Mahadeva, S.; Loke, M.F.; Tan, J.Y.; Ang, B.H.; Chin, K.P.; Mohammad Adnan, A.F.; Ong, S.M.C.; Ibrahim, A.I.; et al. Helicobacter pylori Eradication in Parkinson's Disease: A Randomized Placebo-Controlled Trial. *Mov. Disord.* **2020**, *35*. [CrossRef] [PubMed]

102. Knudsen, K.; Haase, A.-M.; Fedorova, T.D.; Bekker, A.C.; Østergaard, K.; Krogh, K.; Borghammer, P. Gastrointestinal Transit Time in Parkinson's Disease Using a Magnetic Tracking System. *J. Parkinson's Dis.* **2017**, *7*, 471–479. [CrossRef] [PubMed]

103. Dutkiewicz, J.; Szlufik, S.; Nieciecki, M.; Charzyńska, I.; Królicki, L.; Smektała, P.; Friedman, A. Small intestine dysfunction in Parkinson's disease. *J. Neural Transm. (Austria 1996)* **2015**, *122*, 1659–1661. [CrossRef] [PubMed]

104. Su, A.; Gandhy, R.; Barlow, C.; Triadafilopoulos, G. Utility of the wireless motility capsule and lactulose breath testing in the evaluation of patients with Parkinson's disease who present with functional gastrointestinal symptoms. *BMJ Open Gastroenterol.* **2017**, *4*, e000132. [CrossRef]

105. Knudsen, K.; Fedorova, T.D.; Bekker, A.C.; Iversen, P.; Østergaard, K.; Krogh, K.; Borghammer, P. Objective Colonic Dysfunction is Far more Prevalent than Subjective Constipation in Parkinson's Disease: A Colon Transit and Volume Study. *J. Parkinson's Dis.* **2017**, *7*, 359–367. [CrossRef]

106. Steele, S.R.; Mellgren, A. Constipation and obstructed defecation. *Clin. Colon Rectal Surg.* **2007**, *20*, 110–117. [CrossRef]

107. Abrahamsson, H.; Antov, S.; Bosaeus, I. Gastrointestinal and colonic segmental transit time evaluated by a single abdominal x-ray in healthy subjects and constipated patients. *Scand. J. Gastroenterol. Suppl.* **1988**, *152*, 72–80. [CrossRef]

108. Sakakibara, R.; Odaka, T.; Uchiyama, T.; Asahina, M.; Yamaguchi, K.; Yamaguchi, T.; Yamanishi, T.; Hattori, T. Colonic transit time and rectoanal videomanometry in Parkinson's disease. *J. Neurol. Neurosurg. Psychiatry* **2003**, *74*, 268–272. [CrossRef]

109. Wang, C.P.; Sung, W.H.; Wang, C.C.; Tsai, P.Y. Early recognition of pelvic floor dyssynergia and colorectal assessment in Parkinson's disease associated with bowel dysfunction. *Colorectal Dis.* **2013**, *15*, e130–e137. [CrossRef]

110. Ashraf, W.; Park, F.; Lof, J.; Quigley, E.M. Effects of psyllium therapy on stool characteristics, colon transit and anorectal function in chronic idiopathic constipation. *Aliment. Pharmacol. Ther.* **1995**, *9*, 639–647. [CrossRef]

111. De Pablo-Fernández, E.; Passananti, V.; Zárate-López, N.; Emmanuel, A.; Warner, T. Colonic transit, high-resolution anorectal manometry and MRI defecography study of constipation in Parkinson's disease. *Parkinsonism Relat. Disord.* **2019**, *66*. [CrossRef] [PubMed]

112. Mathers, S.E.; Kempster, P.A.; Swash, M.; Lees, A.J. Constipation and paradoxical puborectalis contraction in anismus and Parkinson's disease: A dystonic phenomenon? *J. Neurol. Neurosurg. Psychiatry* **1988**, *51*, 1503–1507. [CrossRef] [PubMed]

113. Stocchi, F.; Badiali, D.; Vacca, L.; D'Alba, L.; Bracci, F.; Ruggieri, S.; Torti, M.; Berardelli, A.; Corazziari, E. Anorectal function in multiple system atrophy and Parkinson's disease. *Mov. Disord. Off. J. Mov. Disord. Soc.* **2000**, *15*, 71–76. [CrossRef]

114. Bassotti, G.; Maggio, D.; Battaglia, E.; Giulietti, O.; Spinozzi, F.; Reboldi, G.; Serra, A.M.; Emanuelli, G.; Chiarioni, G. Manometric investigation of anorectal function in early and late stage Parkinson's disease. *J. Neurol. Neurosurg. Psychiatry* **2000**, *68*, 768–770. [CrossRef] [PubMed]

115. Yu, T.; Wang, Y.; Wu, G.; Xu, Q.; Tang, Y.; Lin, L. High-resolution Anorectal Manometry in Parkinson Disease With Defecation Disorder: A Comparison With Functional Defecation Disorder. *J. Clin. Gastroenterol.* **2016**, *50*, 566–571. [CrossRef]

116. Gjerløff, T.; Fedorova, T.; Knudsen, K.; Munk, O.L.; Nahimi, A.; Jacobsen, S.; Danielsen, E.H.; Terkelsen, A.J.; Hansen, J.; Pavese, N.; et al. Imaging acetylcholinesterase density in peripheral organs in Parkinson's disease with 11C-donepezil PET. *Brain J. Neurol.* **2015**, *138*, 653–663. [CrossRef]

117. Fedorova, T.D.; Seidelin, L.B.; Knudsen, K.; Schacht, A.C.; Geday, J.; Pavese, N.; Brooks, D.J.; Borghammer, P. Decreased intestinal acetylcholinesterase in early Parkinson disease: An 11 C-donepezil PET study. *Neurology* **2017**, *88*, 775–781. [CrossRef]

118. Annerino, D.M.; Arshad, S.; Taylor, G.M.; Adler, C.H.; Beach, T.G.; Greene, J.G. Parkinson's disease is not associated with gastrointestinal myenteric ganglion neuron loss. *Acta Neuropathol.* **2012**, *124*, 665–680. [CrossRef]

119. Chung, E.J.; Kim, S.J. (123)I-Metaiodobenzylguanidine Myocardial Scintigraphy in Lewy Body-Related Disorders: A Literature Review. *J. Mov. Disord.* **2015**, *8*, 55–66. [CrossRef]

120. Satoh, A.; Serita, T.; Seto, M.; Tomita, I.; Satoh, H.; Iwanaga, K.; Takashima, H.; Tsujihata, M. Loss of 123I-MIBG uptake by the heart in Parkinson's disease: Assessment of cardiac sympathetic denervation and diagnostic value. *J. Nucl. Med. Off. Publ. Soc. Nucl. Med.* **1999**, *40*, 371–375.

121. Miyamoto, T.; Miyamoto, M.; Inoue, Y.; Usui, Y.; Suzuki, K.; Hirata, K. Reduced cardiac 123I-MIBG scintigraphy in idiopathic REM sleep behavior disorder. *Neurology* **2006**, *67*, 2236–2238. [CrossRef] [PubMed]

122. Miyamoto, T.; Miyamoto, M.; Iwanami, M.; Hirata, K. Follow-up study of cardiac ^{123}I-MIBG scintigraphy in idiopathic REM sleep behavior disorder. *Eur. J. Neurol.* **2011**, *18*, 1275–1278. [CrossRef] [PubMed]

123. Kashihara, K.; Imamura, T.; Shinya, T. Cardiac ^{123}I-MIBG uptake is reduced more markedly in patients with REM sleep behavior disorder than in those with early stage Parkinson's disease. *Parkinsonism Relat. Disord.* **2010**, *16*, 252–255. [CrossRef] [PubMed]

124. Seppi, K.; Ray Chaudhuri, K.; Coelho, M.; Fox, S.H.; Katzenschlager, R.; Perez Lloret, S.; Weintraub, D.; Sampaio, C. Update on treatments for nonmotor symptoms of Parkinson's disease-an evidence-based medicine review. *Mov. Disord. Off. J. Mov. Disord. Soc.* **2019**, *34*, 180–198. [CrossRef]

125. Chung, K.A.; Pfeiffer, R.F. Gastrointestinal dysfunction in the synucleinopathies. *Clin. Auton. Res.* **2020**, 1–23. [CrossRef]

126. Shada, A.; Nielsen, A.; Marowski, S.; Helm, M.; Funk, L.M.; Kastenmeier, A.; Lidor, A.; Gould, J.C. Wisconsin's Enterra Therapy Experience: A multi-institutional review of gastric electrical stimulation for medically refractory gastroparesis. *Surgery* **2018**, *164*, 760–765. [CrossRef]

127. Aziz, I.; Whitehead, W.E.; Palsson, O.S.; Törnblom, H.; Simrén, M. An approach to the diagnosis and management of Rome IV functional disorders of chronic constipation. *Expert Rev. Gastroenterol. Hepatol.* **2020**, *14*, 39–46. [CrossRef]

128. Tan, A.H.; Lim, S.-Y.; Chong, K.K.; Azhan, A.; Manap, M.A.; Hor, J.W.; Lim, J.L.; Low, S.C.; Chong, C.W.; Mahadeva, S. Probiotics for constipation in Parkinson's disease: A randomized placebo-controlled study. *Neurology* **2020**. [CrossRef]

129. Farid, M.; El Monem, H.A.; Omar, W.; El Nakeeb, A.; Fikry, A.; Youssef, T.; Yousef, M.; Ghazy, H.; Fouda, E.; El Metwally, T.; et al. Comparative study between biofeedback retraining and botulinum neurotoxin in the treatment of anismus patients. *Int. J. Colorectal Dis.* **2009**, *24*, 115–120. [CrossRef]

130. Ahadi, T.; Madjlesi, F.; Mahjoubi, B.; Mirzaei, R.; Forogh, B.; Daliri, S.S.; Derakhshandeh, S.M.; Behbahani, R.B.; Raissi, G.R. The effect of biofeedback therapy on dyssynergic constipation in patients with or without Irritable Bowel Syndrome. *J. Res. Med. Sci* **2014**, *19*, 950–955.

131. Cadeddu, F.; Bentivoglio, A.R.; Brandara, F.; Marniga, G.; Brisinda, G.; Maria, G. Outlet type constipation in Parkinson's disease: Results of botulinum toxin treatment. *Aliment. Pharmacol. Ther.* **2005**, *22*, 997–1003. [CrossRef] [PubMed]

132. Albanese, A.; Brisinda, G.; Bentivoglio, A.R.; Maria, G. Treatment of outlet obstruction constipation in Parkinson's disease with botulinum neurotoxin A. *Am. J. Gastroenterol.* **2003**, *98*, 1439–1440. [CrossRef] [PubMed]

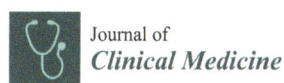

Journal of
Clinical Medicine

MDPI

Review

Neurogenic Bowel Dysfunction in Children and Adolescents

Giovanni Mosiello [1,*], Shaista Safder [2], David Marshall [3], Udo Rolle [4] and Marc A. Benninga [5]

[1] Department of Surgery, Division of Urology, Bambino Gesù Pediatric and Research Hospital, 00165 Rome, Italy
[2] College of Medicine, Center for Digestive, Health and Nutrition, Arnold Palmer Hospital for Children, Orlando, FL 32806, USA; shaista.safder@orlandohealth.com
[3] Department of Pediatric Surgery and Pediatric Urology, Royal Belfast Hospital for Sick Children, Belfast BT97AB, UK; david.marshall@belfasttrust.hscni.net
[4] Department of Pediatric Surgery and Pediatric Urology, Goethe-University Frankfurt, 60596 Frankfurt, Germany; udo.rolle@kgu.de
[5] Department of Pediatric Gastroenterology, Hepatology and Nutrition, Emma Children's Hospital, Amsterdam UMC, University of Amsterdam, 1105 AZ Amsterdam, The Netherlands; m.a.benninga@amsterdammumc.nl
* Correspondence: giovanni.mosiello@opbg.net; Tel.: +39-06-6859-2518

Citation: Mosiello, G.; Safder, S.; Marshall, D.; Rolle, U.; Benninga, M.A. Neurogenic Bowel Dysfunction in Children and Adolescents. *J. Clin. Med.* **2021**, *10*, 1669. https://doi.org/10.3390/jcm10081669

Academic Editor: Klaus Krough

Received: 21 February 2021
Accepted: 8 April 2021
Published: 13 April 2021

Publisher's Note: MDPI stays neutral with regard to jurisdictional claims in published maps and institutional affiliations.

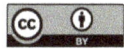

Copyright: © 2021 by the authors. Licensee MDPI, Basel, Switzerland. This article is an open access article distributed under the terms and conditions of the Creative Commons Attribution (CC BY) license (https://creativecommons.org/licenses/by/4.0/).

Abstract: Neurogenic/neuropathic bowel dysfunction (NBD) is common in children who are affected by congenital and acquired neurological disease, and negatively impacts quality of life. In the past, NBD received less attention than neurogenic bladder, generally being considered only in spina bifida (the most common cause of pediatric NBD). Many methods of conservative and medical management of NBD are reported, including relatively recently Transanal Irrigation (TAI). Based on the literature and personal experience, an expert group (pediatric urologists/surgeons/gastroenterologists with specific experience in NBD) focused on NBD in children and adolescents. A statement document was created using a modified Delphi method. The range of causes of pediatric NBD are discussed in this paper. The various therapeutic approaches are presented to improve clinical management. The population of children and adolescents with NBD is increasing, due both to the higher survival rate and better diagnosis. While NBD is relatively predictable in producing either constipation or fecal incontinence, or both, its various effects on each patient will depend on a wide range of underlying causes and accompanying comorbidities. For this reason, management of NBD should be tailored individually with a combined multidisciplinary therapy appropriate for the status of the affected child and caregivers.

Keywords: neurogenic bowel; bowel dysfunction; constipation; fecal incontinence; pediatric; children; adolescent; spina bifida; anorectal malformation; cerebral palsy

1. Introduction

Bowel dysfunction is reported in 0.7–29.6% of children and adolescents, and may be related to functional disorders or to congenital anatomical malformations or digestive tract and neurological causes [1–3]. Chronic constipation and fecal incontinence often coexist, sometimes with "overflow" diarrhea (where solid stool impacted higher up the rectum or colon only allows watery stool past it, which is then very difficult for even a neurologically intact anal sphincter to retain). This results in a frustrating situation for both patients and caregivers, especially in a neurogenic scenario, commonly defined as neurogenic or neuropathic bowel dysfunction (NBD) [4]. The term NBD implies autonomic and/or somatic denervation of the bowel. In pediatrics it is commonly thought of as being synonymous with spina bifida (SB) [5], without considering the wide range of other clinical conditions where NBD is present, such as in cerebral palsy, acquired brain and spinal cord injuries, transverse myelitis, etc. Globally, NBD in the pediatric population is still often not adequately considered or treated with the same standardized approach as neurogenic or neuropathic bladder dysfunction [6]. Yet addressing NBD is likely also to produce secondary benefits for the urinary tract, particularly improved functional bladder capacity (due to the rectum no longer compressing it, and reduction in the reflex detrusor overactivity that was promoted by rectal distension) and lower incidence of UTIs (thanks to improved bladder dynamics and the decrease in soiling of the perineum). Several approaches have been reported for managing NBD. However, it is common to observe many patients failing to respond to standard conservative and medical treatments such as dietary manipulation, manual evacuation, oral laxatives, suppositories, and/or enemas, with about half remaining fecally incontinent [7]. Before the introduction of a revised method of transanal irrigation (TAI) [8], many children were treated surgically with a Malone antegrade continence enema [7] or colostomy. TAI has transformed the management of NBD, and now is widely used in adults and children with SB [9–12]. Thanks to the improved survival of children with neurological conditions that were previously considered fatal, and better awareness and diagnostic techniques, the worldwide population of children and adolescents with NBD is growing. The aim of this paper, therefore, is to produce a statement regarding NBD in childhood and adolescent populations. We suggest to healthcare providers (HCPs) the clinical situations in childhood where NBD should be considered and investigated, and report recommendations for care, in order to improve the clinical outcome of management globally, as well as identifying issues for future research.

2. Methods

A group of specialists from different disciplines (pediatric gastroenterology, pediatric surgery, and pediatric urology) around the world (Europe and USA), with long-term experience in bowel management, was previously convened by Coloplast A/S, and was tasked to produce in 2017 best-practice recommendations for NBD management in pediatrics [13], an area of commercial interest for the company. A similar group decided to compile this follow-up report based on the current literature and personal experience, in order to offer a practical instrument for all HCPs involved in diagnosis and management of NBD in pediatrics, using a modified Delphi method [14]. Coloplast A/S, (Kokkedal, Denmark) sponsored the publication fee of this article through an educational grant, although its content was developed independently and was not in any way influenced by Coloplast A/S.

Three main topics were explored:

1. The causes and pathophysiology of NBD in children and adolescents
2. The conservative and medical management of NBD in children and adolescents
3. The surgical management of NBD in children and adolescents.

Panelists selected a topic of interest, then literature data were selected and reviewed independently. The validity assessment of the literature data was performed independently. Each participant produced their own draft document in their area of special interest that were then combined and revised to produce a preliminary team consensus. All panelists next reviewed the preliminary document, offering their final opinions and revisions. Changes were made accordingly to obtain this final unanimously agreed paper. There were no critical points of discordance.

Literature research was obtained using PUBMED and Cochrane database using the following keywords as search terms: transanal irrigation, bowel management in children/adolescents, neurogenic bowel in children/adolescents, neurogenic bowel in pediatrics/young adults, fecal incontinence in children/adolescents, constipation in children/adolescents, bowel management in anorectal malformation, bowel management in spinal dysraphism, surgery for bowel management. All identified papers were screened for relevance based on title and abstract in the English language.

3. Results

3.1. The Causes and Pathophysiology of NBD in Children and Adolescents

3.1.1. Causes

The causes and presentation of a neurogenic bowel dysfunction (NBD) in children and adolescents are different from adult forms. In most cases, pediatric NBD is caused by congenital problems such as spina bifida (SB). Acquired forms caused by trauma, infection, etc., are more similar to adult clinical pictures [15]. A range of etiologies are presented below, in approximate order of their pediatric relevance (determined by the prevalence of the cause in childhood and each cause's propensity to cause NBD in children).

Myelodysplasia

Commonly known as SB, myelodysplasia describes incomplete closure of the vertebral column and malformation of the embryonic neural tube. This term includes a group of neural tube defects (NTDs) ranging from spina bifida occulta to meningocele to myelomeningocele and lipo-myelomeningocele. Myelomeningocele (MMC) is one of the most common birth defects of the spine and brain, potentially involving any level of the spinal column (lumbo-sacral 47%, lumbar 26%, sacral 20%, thoracic 5%, and cervical spine 2%) [16]. The neurological lesions produced by SB are variable and contingent on the neural elements that protrude within the sac. In myelomeningocele, the neural roots or segments of the spinal cord herniate through the incompletely closed vertebrae, and so are exposed to damage antenatally (and/or postnatally, until the sac is surgically closed). However, the bony vertebral level correlates poorly with the neurological lesions produced. Moreover, during childhood from birth to puberty, different growth rates between the vertebral bodies and the elongating spinal cord can introduce a dynamic factor to the neurological lesion. Furthermore, scar tissue congenitally surrounding the cord at the site of the MMC, and/or acquired following surgical closure of the MMC, can produce primary and secondary tethering of the cord, leading to a changing neurological picture during periods of rapid growth.

Associated hydrocephalus (with an Arnold–Chiari, or Chiari type-II, malformation) is seen in 85% of children with MMC, often requiring ventriculo-peritoneal shunting of excess cerebrospinal fluid to reduce the impact of its pressure on the brain.

Widespread mandatory fortification of dietary staples with folic acid, and voluntary ingestion of folic acid prior to conception and during the first trimester of pregnancy, have significantly reduced the incidence of MMC and other neural tube defects [17]. The vast majority of cases of MMC affect the lumbar spinal cord and sacral roots that innervate the bladder, distal colon, and their respective sphincters, so some degree of neurogenic bladder and bowel dysfunction is almost universal in this population. The incidence of urethro-vesical dysfunction in myelomeningocele is not absolutely known, but most studies suggest it is very high (>90%). Similarly, anorectal dysfunction is very common [5].

By contrast, in meningocele the meninges protrude through a vertebral canal defect, but the neural elements of the cord remain confined within the canal and so generally are not damaged either antenatally or postnatally.

In occult myelodysplasia or occult spinal dysraphism or closed SB, the bony lesions are not open, so most cases have no evident signs of neurological lesion. Its incidental diagnosis is rising due to increasing use of spinal x-rays, ultrasonography and magnetic resonance imaging. In up to 90% of affected individuals, inspection reveals a cutaneous stigma overlying the lower spine such as a dimple, skin tag, hairy patch, hemangioma or subdermal lipoma. In some, subtle alterations may subsequently be found in the toes and feet, with discrepancies in lower extremity muscle size and strength, or abnormal gait. Back pain and an absence of perineal sensation are common symptoms in adolescents [18]. In symptomatic cases, the incidence of lower urinary tract dysfunction (e.g., urinary tract infection or urinary incontinence) is high, which is more commonly recognized as abnormal than are symptoms of NBD. Occult lesions may also become manifest with tethering of the cord later in life. This can lead to changes in bowel, bladder, sexual and lower extremity function [19].

Sacral Agenesis

Sacral agenesis (SA), or Caudal Regression Syndrome, is another neural tube defect, involving complete or partial absence of the lowest five vertebrae. Urinary and/or fecal incontinence are commonly described and recognized when the child fails toilet training on time. A careful inspection may reveal flattened buttocks [20,21], but a full physical examination should also include palpation of the spine to the tip of the coccyx (to exclude a bony defect), as well as neurological examination of the lower limbs and gait. SA is commonly associated with an anorectal malformation.

Anorectal Malformation

Anorectal malformation (ARM, previously referred to by the narrower term imperforate anus) has an estimated incidence ranging between 1 in 2000 and 1 in 5000 live births. It may occur as an isolated lesion or in conjunction with other congenital malformations, where spinal cord pathology occurs in 38% of cases [22]. The VATER or VACTERL association is a group of commonly coexisting abnormalities including Vertebral, Anorectal malformation, Cardiac, Tracheo-Esophageal fistula, Renal and Limb anomalies. ARM has previously been classified as high, intermediate, or low depending on whether the blind-ending rectum terminates above, at, or below the levator ani muscle. In the past, imperforate anus repair for high lesions involving a perineal approach to pull the rectum through to the anal verge frequently resulted in a pudendal nerve injury. With the innovation of the posterior sagittal anorectoplasty (PSARP) surgical approach this complication has been eliminated [23]. However, reports of spinal magnetic resonance imaging (MRI) reveal a 35–50% incidence of distal spinal cord abnormalities in children with ARM [22]. A complete pre-operative evaluation is recommended in all patients in order to detect early any spinal cord or bony malformation that may produce autonomic dysfunction [24], such as a low-lying conus medullaris (terminating below the normal L2 level). This can be more easily achieved by ultrasound scan in the first three months of life, before the spinal window ossifies [25]. It is also thought that pelvic nerves, both sensory and motor, may be affected at the same critical stage of fetal development as the anorectal region and the pelvic floor musculature. Therefore, the degree of long-term neuropathic bowel dysfunction in ARM depends not only on the extent of the congenital defect itself (both the intestinal anomaly and the associated congenital neuropathy), but also on possible iatrogenic damage by surgery and/or by potential secondary neuromuscular impact from inadequate medical evacuation of the rectum during infancy and childhood.

Cerebral Palsy

Cerebral palsy (CP) is defined as a congenital neurological condition due to non-progressive injury (typically presumed anoxic) or malformation of the brain occurring in the fetal or perinatal period [26]. The incidence of CP is about 1.5 per 1000 births, making it the most common neurological condition encountered in pediatrics. CP encompasses a group of disorders of differing degrees of the development of movement and posture. Up to 90% of the children with CP suffer from constipation and 47% fecal incontinence, though most to a minor extent [27]. These effects arise due to deranged higher-level control of the bowel and/or sphincter rather than a primary intrinsic neuropathy of these structures. About half of individuals with CP are intellectually disabled [28,29], which affects what treatment modalities for NBD are appropriate.

Muscular Dystrophies and Mitochondrial Disorders

Congenital muscular dystrophies (MD) are a wide group of muscle disorders that present with very early onset of muscular weakness. Affected individuals report symptoms of both bladder and bowel dysfunction. The most common bowel complaint is constipation, which in X-linked Duchenne Muscular Dystrophy (DMD) can become life-threatening, but generally the most disabling is fecal incontinence [30,31]. One series reported that in 47% of boys with DMD undergoing a colonic transit test, the radiopaque markers were retained in the recto-sigmoid, suggesting functional pelvic outlet obstruction [30]. According to Lo Cascio and colleagues, there is a substantial risk in patients with Duchenne Muscular Dystrophy of altered gastrointestinal (GI) transport and possible sensory impairment, due to expression of dystrophin isoform DP116 in peripheral nerve tissue and autosomal homologues of DP116 in sensory ganglia [30]. Also implicated in impaired GI tract motility are alterations of the myenteric plexus associated with reduced myo-electrical slow-wave activity (as shown in mice models), along with a reduced availability of nitric oxide (NO), due to the lack of dystrophin acting as an anchor for NO-synthase [30]. These direct effects on GI transit time are not helped by a decreased ability to strain voluntarily, and sometimes further exacerbated by the developmental delay seen in some forms of mitochondrial disorder.

Loss of the alpha-dystroglycan-laminin interaction, due to defective glycosylation of alpha-dystroglycan, underlies a group of congenital muscular dystrophies often associated with brain malformations, referred to as dystroglycanopathies, where NBD is reported [31]. Mitochondrial neurogastrointestinal encephalomyopathy (MNGIE) is frequently associated with chronic intestinal pseudo-obstruction. The pathophysiology resulting in impaired peristalsis and propulsion of intestinal contents relates to disturbed neuromuscular coordination due to myopathy (affecting intestinal contraction), neuropathy (affecting coordination of enteric reflexes), or mesenchymopathy (related to abnormalities of the interstitial cells of Cajal). Furthermore, mitochondrial abnormalities observed in MNGIE may contribute to disturbed homeostasis of gut microbiota, which may in turn be involved in the manifestation of gastrointestinal dysmotility seen in MNGIE [32].

Wolfram syndrome is a neuro-degenerative disorder characterized by childhood-onset diabetes mellitus, optic nerve atrophy, diabetes insipidus, hearing impairment, and commonly bowel and bladder dysfunction [33].

In all these muscle disorders, muscular dystrophies and mitochondrial cytopathy, NBD, and lower urinary tract symptoms can change over time with disease progression, so careful follow-up is required.

Acquired Brain Injury

Acquired brain injury (ABI) refers to a brain insult sustained after a period of normal development. ABI in children and adolescents is relatively common, with a heterogeneous group of underlying causes including vascular, oncological, and trauma (e.g., road traffic or sport). ABI represents the leading cause of death and neurologic disability in children after infancy. In the aftermath of more serious physical injuries, bladder and bowel dysfunction are often considered of secondary importance and managed with continence pads only until a delayed diagnosis and definitive management [34]. However, urinary retention and constipation often produce long-term urinary and fecal incontinence. Today survivors of ABI are increasing and comprise a large proportion of the work of a neurorehabilitation department. Functional impairments (motor, behavioral, educational, and cognitive) are common and can endure for life.

Acquired Pelvic Injury

NBD can occur from damage to the nerves innervating the pelvic organs, anywhere in the course of these nerves from the cauda equina, the spinal nerve roots, the sacral plexus, or to the various individual nerves that arise from the plexus. Most injuries to these nerves are iatrogenic, but rarely can occur as a result of high-impact trauma. Any pelvic surgery in infants and children for anorectal malformation (to mobilize the blind-ending rectum from the urinary tract, if necessary, and then to open it and bring it to the center of the anal sphincter complex) or Hirschsprung's disease (to pull through normally ganglionated bowel to the anus) [35,36], neuroblastoma, ganglioneuroma, sacrococcygeal teratoma, and aorto-iliac surgery is theoretically able to damage the pelvic parasympathetic nerves to the rectum, anus, bladder, and genitalia. Additionally, pelvic irradiation can cause damage to adjacent nerve fibers, resulting in altered function, as can certain cytotoxic drugs [35]. Bowel, voiding, and erectile dysfunction can result. Iatrogenic fecal incontinence can also be caused by sphincter damage caused during childbirth (including in post-pubertal teenagers), and surgery for anorectal problems such as trauma, fistulae, and abscesses. Vaginal delivery can damage not only the anal sphincteric muscle, but also the neurons innervating the anal sphincter, especially in younger individuals [37].

Acquired Spinal Cord Injury

The relative flexibility of childhood tissues compared to adults confers a degree of protection against traumatic spinal cord injury (SCI). However, voluntary control of defecation requires rectal sensation, peristalsis, and adequate anorectal sphincter function and coordination. Neurological defects in patients with spinal lesions may affect one or more of these components, resulting in various types of defecation disorders: fecal incontinence, chronic constipation, or both [38].

NBD is common among pediatric patients with acquired SCI [39]. According to electromyography (EMG) of the external anal sphincter, 25–33% had bilateral or unilateral muscle action abnormalities during defecation, and 88.5% showed pelvic floor dysfunction. The mean rectal volume to generate the first sensation was significantly higher in SCI patients.

The level of spinal injury dictates two distinct clinical patterns of NBD [40], although both feature constipation. Injuries above the conus medullaris result in an upper motor neuron pattern of hyperreflexic bowel where inhibitory input is lost; this is characterized by increased colonic and anal sphincter tone, often resulting in stool retention and constipation. In upper motor neuron lesions, there is preservation of reflex coordination (such as the gastrocolic response), hypertonia (with consequent reduced rectal compliance), and hyperreflexia distal to the splenic flexure (resulting in reflex defecation and incontinence). In contrast, injuries at the conus medullaris or cauda equina result in a lower motor neuron pattern of areflexic bowel, with loss of centrally mediated motor activity leading to slow bowel transit and an atonic external anal sphincter; these patients may experience constipation yet also a significant risk of fecal incontinence. Lesions within the conus or in the cauda equina (where excitatory sacral parasympathetic supply is lost) are associated with rectal hypotonia and hyporeflexia, predisposing to impaction and overflow incontinence. The degree of symptoms also depends on the grade of injury: complete SCI has been shown to result in the most severe form of NBD with loss of voluntary control of the external anal sphincter too [41].

Down's Syndrome

The secondary effects of Down's Syndrome (DS) on the bowel and bladder have, until recently, often been dismissed as an inevitable reflection of the severely disabling primary condition, or simply behavioral. It is now increasingly recognized that DS is associated with significant lower urinary tract symptoms (LUTS) in children, which can even require surgical intervention [42,43]. It is believed this typically results from the child's inability to relax their pelvic floor appropriately, leading to voiding dysfunction, fecal impaction, and secondary overflow incontinence. This bladder and bowel dysfunction in DS is undoubtedly multifactorial, but is often regarded as non-neurogenic neurogenic (as in Hinman bladder). However, the underlying neurological condition means it may have at least a neurogenic etiological component.

Autism

Similarly, it has historically been commonly assumed that inability to toilet-train is an unavoidable consequence of autism and its behavioral traits. Again, it is thought this bladder and bowel dysfunction is typically due to the child's over-reliance on their pelvic floor muscles, and this often persists into adulthood [44]. While the cause of this dysfunction is presumably multifactorial, the underlying neurological condition suggests it is at least partially neurogenic.

Transverse Myelitis

Transverse myelitis (TM) is a rare immune-mediated process leading to neural injury in the spinal cord. TM is reported to have an incidence of 1–4 new cases per million, with bi-modal peaks between the ages of 10–19 years and 30–39 years, and is commonly para-infectious [45]. TM can clinically be divided into acute or sub-acute, affecting motor, sensory and/or autonomic nerves, so presentation can be varied with weakness, sensory alterations and, virtually always, autonomic dysfunction of storage and emptying of the bladder and bowel [46,47]. Approximately 20% of cases of acute TM occur in children, in whom one of the most common initial symptoms is pain (60%). Other common symptoms in children include motor deficits, numbness, ataxic gait, and loss of bowel or bladder control. Constipation can be severe and may present in children as increased irritability with fullness in the left lower quadrant. Long-term autonomic sphincter dysfunction is reported in different series in between 22–80% of children [48].

Guillain–Barré Syndrome

Guillain–Barré syndrome (GBS) has become the most common cause for acute, flaccid paralysis in many parts of the world [49]. It presents as a rapidly progressing ascending areflexic motor paralysis, with or without sensory and autonomic dysfunction. The initial acute progressive phase, which generally reaches a nadir within four weeks, is typically followed by a plateau phase and finally a recovery phase.

GBS affects children and adults of all ages and both sexes. Bowel dysfunction, seen in up to 15% of patients, occurs much less commonly than cardiovascular or limb dysfunction [50,51], so it is not often encountered by pediatric surgeons.

Cauda Equina Syndrome

The spinal cord terminates at the lower border of the L1 vertebra, and the nerve roots of L2 to S4 below form a tightly packed bundle, the so-called cauda equina ("horse's tail"). Damage to these nerve roots produces a characteristic pattern of symptoms called the cauda equina syndrome (CES), where the predominant findings are bladder, bowel, and sexual dysfunction along with sensory loss of the perineum [52,53].

Central lumbar disc prolapse is rare in childhood, but can compress sacral nerve fibers to and from the bladder, the large bowel, the anal and urethral sphincters, and the pelvic floor, producing low-back pain, bilateral sciatica, saddle anesthesia, urinary retention, and constipation. Other causes include trauma, tumor, spinal canal stenosis, spinal AV malformation, and iatrogenic (during spinal surgery or spinal anesthesia) [54].

Multiple Sclerosis

Multiple sclerosis (MS) is the most common progressive neurological disorder in young people, with a mean age at onset of 30 years, and a prevalence of 40–220 cases per 100,000 people in Europe [55], with similar rates in North America [56]. The incidence of pediatric onset of MS is low at 0.3–0.9/100,000. The prevalence of pediatric MS is 5–10% of all cases of MS [57,58].

Bowel effects are common in patients who have MS and can have a significant impact on quality of life (QoL) [59]. Symptoms were found in 45 to 68% of cases and can be defined as "retentive" (constipation, seen in 31% to 54% of patients) or "irritant" (including diarrhea and false urges to defecate, with a prevalence of 6–20%) [60]. Data reported mainly refer to adult populations, although teenagers are included.

Acute Disseminated Encephalomyelitis and Meningitis-Retention Syndrome

Acute disseminated encephalomyelitis (ADEM), also known as postinfectious encephalomyelitis, is a rare demyelinating disorder of the central nervous system. It follows an exanthematous infection or, occasionally, vaccination [61], suggesting a para-infectious or autoimmune origin [62]. ADEM is characterized by an inflammatory reaction and demyelination in the brain and spinal cord. Lesions observed on MRI of the brain are usually confined to the white matter. Lesions in the spinal cord involving the conus are also seen [63]. The early symptoms of ADEM are similar to an acute relapse of multiple sclerosis (MS) and can cause diagnostic confusion in adolescents and young adults. Presence of symptoms such as fever and headache, along with a combination of signs of encephalitis (disturbance of consciousness, epilepsy, and hemi-paresis) and of myelitis (sensory disturbance below the level of the lesion, spastic paraplegia), may help differentiate this condition. Bowel and lower urinary tract dysfunction are common in ADEM [61–64].

Meningitis retention syndrome (MRS), a rare and very mild form of ADEM, has been recognized as a specific condition in its own right [63]. The frequency of NBD in pediatric MRS is not clear since it has a benign and self-remitting course (with a duration of 2–10 weeks). For the same reason, the effectiveness of immune treatments (steroid therapy) remains unclear, although such treatments may shorten the duration.

Spinal Canal Stenosis

While rarely arising in childhood, patients with spinal canal stenosis (SCS) may present with bladder and/or bowel involvement. To demonstrate narrowing of the lumbar canal with compression of the cauda equina by bony or soft tissue, CT or MRI is often recommended [65].

About half of the patients with intractable leg pain in spinal canal stenosis also have bladder and bowel symptoms from effects on the cauda equina. Schkrohowsky et al. [66] reported that one-third of patients with achondroplasia developed SCS, especially at the lumbar level. SCS is reported in Klippel–Feil and other syndromes [67]. Signs and symptoms of compressive neuropathy of multiple lumbar and sacral roots is an indication for surgical decompression, which usually improves the condition.

Other Rare Pediatric Neurological Disease

Motor neuron diseases or disorders (MNDs) are rare neurological conditions affecting the anterior horn cells of the motor neurons that control voluntary skeletal muscle activity (i.e., the external anal sphincter rather than the bowel itself, although they can also indirectly affect bowel function due to weakened abdominal musculature and immobility). MNDs are associated with a very poor prognosis since they are often progressive and currently no known cure is available (treatment being limited to symptomatic relief and supporting primary vital functions like breathing and feeding). MNDs can be classified according to the part of the body affected and the pattern of nerve involvement (upper or lower motor neurons, or both), and include spinal muscular atrophy (SMA), amyotrophic lateral sclerosis (ALS), progressive muscular atrophy (PMA), progressive bulbar palsy (PBP), and primary lateral sclerosis (PLS). While most of these are adult conditions, SMA is inherited and usually becomes symptomatic in childhood, with the earlier presentations seen in the more severe forms. Werdnig–Hoffmann disease is the most common and most severe form of SMA, type 1, whereas SMA-2 is an intermediate form compared to SMA-3; the mildest form, SMA-4, usually presents in early adulthood. The poor prognosis in MNDs such as SMA-1, means that NBD, although usually present, is often under-recognized [68].

In the most common disorder of the neuromuscular junction, myasthenia gravis, intestinal pseudo obstruction is reported [69].

X-linked adrenoleukodystrophy (ALD) is a neurometabolic disorder caused by mutations in the ABCD1 gene resulting in a defect in peroxisomal degradation of very long-chain fatty acids (VLCFAs) with their accumulation in plasma and tissues, affecting both spinal cord and brain. Bowel dysfunction and lower urinary tract symptoms have been described [70].

Menkes disease is an X-linked recessive disorder of copper metabolism due to a mutation in the ATP7A gene that leads to copper deficiency, culminating in a severe progressive neurodegenerative disease including bowel and bladder dysfunction [71].

In theory, any congenital or acquired medical condition that affects neurological and/or cognitive development and behavior can also produce secondary effects on the bowel (and bladder) of a child or adolescent.

Summary

NBD is commonly experienced in children and adolescents, often associated with neurogenic dysfunction of the bladder. In some neurological diseases, NBD has been more fully evaluated and early management is generally instituted. However, it is often missed, neglected, or undertreated in other conditions, both rare and common. Therefore, NBD must be considered in all children with special needs due to common congenital conditions like cerebral palsy and Down's Syndrome, as well as all forms of rare acquired neurological damage such as post-trauma, Guillain–Barré syndrome, transverse myelitis, etc. Future research must address these clinical situations in order to define tailored diagnostic pathways and management.

3.1.2. Pathophysiology

The term 'neurogenic bowel' encompasses the manifestations of bowel dysfunction resulting from sensory and/or motor disturbances due to central neurological disease or damage [72].

The gastrointestinal tract has a complex control that relies on coordinated interaction between muscular contractions and neuronal impulses [73]. Constipation and/or fecal incontinence occur when there is a problem with the normal bowel functioning; this could be for a variety of reasons. The usual defecation pathway involves contractions of the colon to help mix the contents, absorb water, and propel the contents along the intestine. This results in the feces moving through the colon to the rectum [74]. The presence of stool in the rectum causes a reflex relaxation of the internal anal sphincter (rectoanal inhibitory reflex, RAIR), allowing the contents of the rectum to move into the anal canal. This produces the conscious feeling of the need to defecate. At a socially suitable time, the brain sends nerve signals causing the voluntary external anal sphincter and puborectalis muscles to relax and this allows defecation to take place [15,74].

There are two main types of nervous system within the lower gastrointestinal (GI) tract: the intrinsic enteric nervous system (located within the wall of the gut) and the extrinsic nervous system (comprising sympathetic and parasympathetic innervation) [73]. The intrinsic enteric nervous system controls gut motility directly, whereas the extrinsic nerve pathways influence gut contractility indirectly by modifying this intrinsic enteric response [73]. In almost all cases of neurogenic bowel dysfunction, it is the extrinsic nervous supply that is affected while the intrinsic enteric nervous supply remains intact.

Defecation involves conscious and subconscious processes and, when the extrinsic nervous system is damaged, either of these can be affected. Conscious processes are controlled by the somatic nervous system; these are voluntary movements, for example the contraction of the striated muscle of the external anal sphincter is instructed by the brain, which activates the neurons innervating this muscle [75,76]. Subconscious processes are controlled by the autonomic nervous system; these are involuntary movements such as contraction of the smooth muscle of the colon or the internal anal sphincter. The autonomic nervous system also provides sensory information; this could be about the degree of distension within the colon or rectum [75,76].

Neurogenic bowel dysfunction (NBD) is generally related to spinal cord lesions in pediatric patients, mainly represented by open or closed neural tube defects (spina bifida) resulting from antenatal developmental neurological events.

Patients with spinal cord lesions, either congenital or acquired, have an anatomically intact rectal ampulla, anal canal, and sphincter but experience constipation and/or incontinence due to damage of their enteric nervous system, reduced sensation, and limited mobility. In these children, anal squeeze pressure, anorectal sensitivity, and anal resting pressure may also be impaired, while rectal compliance may be reduced due to hyperreactivity of the rectum [5,77], impacting colorectal motility, transit time and bowel emptying, which often leads to constipation, fecal incontinence, or a combination of both.

Bowel dysfunction occurs in children with spina bifida because, while their spinal rectoanal inhibitory reflex (RAIR) is generally maintained, their defecation urge is not present. When the internal sphincter relaxes, bowel soiling occurs. Constipation results from an increased colonic transit time and a lack of sphincter relaxation with rectal distension [77,78]. Additional factors leading to bowel dysfunction in children with spinal cord issues are a general decrease in activity and, depending on the level of the spinal lesion, abdominal muscle weakness resulting in a reduced ability to push out stool [79]. Most children develop constipation, typically passing frequent, small, and hard stools.

Impact of Anatomical Location of Nerve Damage

Damage to the spinal cord or brain can interrupt neural pathways. The location and severity of such damage are the key factors in determining colorectal function and the nature and extent of subsequent symptoms. However, it should be kept in mind that symptoms are not always easy to determine and can change with time. For instance, in spinal cord injury, the precise level of injury is often not clear during the early stages due to spinal shock, which can last up to six weeks. Moreover, the nervous system, being a complex entity, does not always present a fixed clinical pattern even in the same disease or trauma patterns.

Broadly, neurogenic bowel symptoms are divided into two patterns depending upon the level of disease or injury in relation to the conus medullaris:

1. Supraconal disorder—"upper motor neuron bowel syndrome" or "hyperreflexic bowel", or "spastic bowel"

This pattern is seen in patients who have disease/injury above the conus medullaris and involves loss of supraspinal inhibitory input resulting in hypertonia of the colorectum. The increase in tone of the colonic wall, pelvic floor, and anus results in reduced colonic compliance, overactive segmental peristalsis, and underactive propulsive peristalsis [80–82]. As the peristaltic and haustral movements become less effective, the transit slows down throughout the colon [75,76]. The spastic constricted state of the external anal sphincter (EAS) worsens the situation further by causing retention of stool. The combination of these physiological responses to supraconal injury makes constipation the dominant gut symptom. When the anal sphincter cannot be voluntarily relaxed, signals between the colon and the brain become disrupted: the reflex that triggers a bowel movement still works, but the child may not feel it coming, resulting in a sudden unplanned passage of stool whenever the rectum is full. These disorders are characterized by high resting anal tone, anal/anocutaneous reflex present (reflex contraction of anus in response to stroking of perianal skin), and bulbospongiosus/bulbocavernosus reflex present (reflex contraction of anus in response to squeezing the glans penis or clitoris).

2. Infraconal disorder—"lower motor neuron type" or "areflexic bowel"

A flaccid bowel may follow a lower spinal cord injury. Infraconal lesions are a consequence of disruption of autonomic motor nerves due to damage to parasympathetic cell bodies in the conus medullaris or their axons in the cauda equina. This is characterized by loss of colorectal tone and reduced amplitude of rectoanal inhibitory reflex (RAIR), resulting in a cyclical pattern of insensate rectal filling and progressive rectal distension eventually leading to fecal incontinence. Furthermore, the incontinence is not helped by a reduction in resting and squeeze anal pressures due to flaccid anal sphincters and laxity of pelvic floor muscles which allows excessive descent of pelvic contents, reducing the anorectal angle and opening the rectal lumen [82]. In a flaccid bowel situation, there is reduced movement in the colon, less peristalsis, and the anal sphincter is more relaxed than normal. This can lead to constipation with frequent leaking of stool. Typically, these patients have no or low resting anal tone, and absence of the anal/anocutaneous and bulbospongiosus/bulbocavernosus reflexes.

Tools for Assessment of NBD

Important questions must first be asked during a thorough medical history regarding current stool frequency, consistency, and amounts. It is helpful to use a bowel diary to record the time(s) of the day when a bowel movement occurs and the presence of awareness or urge [83–87]. An accurate history should be obtained of both facilitators and barriers to success in any bowel management programs that have previously been attempted. Medications should be recorded, especially those that have the intended consequence or known side-effects of either constipation (since anticholinergics are commonly used for associated neurogenic bladder, or constipating-agents may deliberately have been used in an attempt to reduce soiling) or diarrhea. Indeed, in a situation of "overflow" diarrhea, sometimes antidiarrheal medication is unwittingly prescribed, which obviously only compounds the problem. Any previous surgery (especially abdominal and perineal) should be documented.

A full physical examination should include abdominal palpation for evidence of fecal loading, which would suggest that chronic constipation may be the cause of (overflow) fecal incontinence. Palpation is also used to assess for sensation, discomfort, tenderness, abdominal muscle tone and non-fecal masses. Percussion and auscultation of bowel sounds can suggest constipation, obstruction or pseudo obstruction. The perianal region should next be inspected for soiling, dermatitis, anal fissures, patulous anus, anal prolapse, or external hemorrhoids (although the latter are quite rare in children). Assessment should be made of perianal sensation and the corresponding reflex response of the anal sphincter. In obese individuals, fecal loading can be more accurately determined by judicious rectal examination, which can additionally provide evidence of the patient's ability to produce voluntary contraction of the EAS and puborectalis muscles [88].

Various diagnostic tests can supplement the above clinical findings. In children with obesity or distorted body habitus (e.g., due to scoliosis associated with SB), abdominal x-ray can confirm fecal loading, although this does not always correlate well with symptoms [89], but it can provide useful evidence to convince skeptical parents or caregivers. Colonic transit time can be estimated by means of an abdominal x-ray taken a specified time after the child has swallowed small radio-opaque markers [90]. Anorectal manometry is a useful test to measure anorectal function and define NBD [91]. An endo-anal ultrasound can identify an external or internal anal sphincter defect, and barium enema or dynamic magnetic resonance (MR) proctogram can diagnose paradoxical sphincter contractions. Electromyography can test the electrical activity of the muscles around the anus and rectum. MRI or CT scan of brain and/or spinal cord may also be helpful in defining NBD. If clinical or radiological assessment raises a concern, it is important to exclude the rare possibility of a colonic stricture, if necessary by colonoscopy, before proceeding to any surgical treatment for symptoms that have been assumed to be caused by NBD.

3.2. The Conservative and Pharmacological Management of NBD in Children and Adolescents

Since NBD interferes with the normal voluntary control of defecation, the aim of all bowel management strategies is to allow emptying of as much as possible of the colon in the bathroom at a socially convenient time for the patient (and family), so that there is little or no possibility of fecal incontinence or constipation occurring whenever school, work, sport and hobbies, social activities, travel, or sleep preclude visiting the toilet at short notice. This target should be delivered with the minimum of time, fuss, discomfort/pain, side-effects, and expense. How exactly that is best achieved varies from child to child (and family), so treatment must be individualized and regularly reviewed to ensure it continues to meet this objective as the child grows and the degree of NBD perhaps alters with time.

3.2.1. Starting a Bowel Management Program

The goal of establishing or maintaining a bowel management routine is to prevent constipation, optimize continence, maintain skin integrity [92], and maximize independence. When deciding on a treatment plan, it is essential first to undertake a thorough medical history and clinical examination (as outlined in Section Tools for Assessment of NBD above). This information will help providers to recommend a program most likely to succeed in the long term.

It is vital to establish from the offset whether an individual has a hyperreflexic or areflexic bowel, to help tailor their management accordingly. Patients with a hyperreflexic bowel have an intact reflex arc between the spinal cord and colon/anorectum and, as such, stimulation of the rectum (chemically or mechanically) results in evacuation of any rectal stool. The aim in hyperreflexic bowel is to attain a relatively soft stool consistency to encourage evacuation. In these patients, stool softeners and stimulant laxatives with mechanical stimulation of the anorectum may provide relief of stool.

On the other hand, individuals with areflexic bowel may require abdominal muscle exercises, gentle Valsalva maneuvers, and/or manual evacuation of stool. In these patients, who have low resting anal sphincter tone, more formed stool can help reduce incontinence episodes, so overuse of stool softeners and stimulant laxatives should generally be avoided.

In those with a neurological level at T_6 or above, any treatment that produces rapid emptying of the rectum carries a threat of precipitating life-threatening autonomic dysreflexia [93]. At-risk patients or caregivers must be made aware of this danger and issued with advice on and supplies of appropriate emergency rescue strategies (such as nifedipine).

As previously proposed by this group (see modification in Figure 1), interventions should generally be considered in a stepwise manner, with the aim of finding the least invasive intervention that balances stool consistency and frequency, thus optimizing continence [13]. Treatments should be implemented for a minimum of two weeks consistently before considering altering the program further.

Tailoring treatment to the individual, considering whether they have upper or lower motor neuron bowel dysfunction, is important in the success of the bowel program [83,86]. In working with school-age children, consideration should also be given to the use of school staff to aid in tracking. The school nurse plays a vital role in assisting the child to reach their educational goals at the same time as managing their health concerns [81].

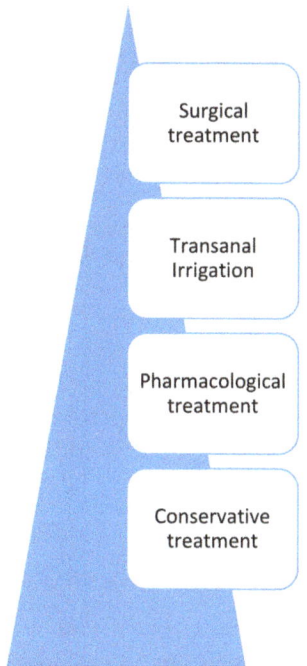

Figure 1. Pyramid of treatment recommendations for neurogenic bowel dysfunction, adapted from Mosiello et al. [13].

3.2.2. The Pediatric Neurogenic Bowel Dysfunction Score

The Pediatric Neurogenic Bowel Dysfunction Score (PNBDS) is used widely by healthcare professionals managing children and adolescents with NBD. It is a validated standardized symptom-based measure of bowel function in patients who have neurogenic bowel. Such a scoring system was originally intended for use among adult patients with spinal cord injury and other neurological disorders and was initially validated in patients from 8 to 88 years old [94]. Thereafter, it was validated in the pediatric population ranging from 6 to 18 years old [95]. The PNBDS is derived from a 15-item questionnaire, covering bowel frequency, bowel continence, independence with bowel management, and impact on QoL of bowel symptoms and treatment. Scores are weighted based on QoL and can range from 0 to 41. A score <8 is considered to represent no bowel dysfunction, while higher scores are indicative of more severe NBD. Prior research has shown good measures of validity and reliability, making it useful as a monitoring tool to evaluate the efficacy of current bowel management regimens.

3.2.3. Conservative Treatments
Dietary Patterns, Particularly Fiber

Changing diet to include higher fiber content is usually recommended as a first step in a bowel management program. For simplicity and safety, recommended minimal daily fiber intake (g/day) for children and adolescents from 3 to 20 years of age is calculated by the formula: age plus 5 g (e.g., 8 g/d at age 3 years, 15 g/d at age 10 years, and 25 g/d at age 20), and thereafter following adult guidelines of 25 to 35 g/d [96]. A well-balanced diet should be encourages, which includes fruits, vegetables, and plenty of water, and constipating foods such as cheese and white rice should be limited. Fiber supplements, which are often recommended for managing constipation for people with neurotypical bowel innervation, can cause constipation and discomfort for those with

J. Clin. Med. **2021**, *10*, 1669

NBD and are not routinely recommended. However, it is important to understand the difference between soluble and insoluble fiber. Soluble fiber is hydrophilic; by attracting water, it removes excess fluid from the feces, making the stool more formed and decreasing liquid stool. Insoluble fiber, on the other hand, does not dissolve in water, so it stays intact as it moves through the digestive system, adding substance to the stool and so acts as a bulk-forming laxative. Soluble fiber includes plant pectins and gums commonly found in foods like lentils, peas, oats, barley, apples, and citrus foods. Insoluble fiber includes plant cellulose and hemicellulose including whole wheat or bran products, green beans, potatoes, cauliflower, and nuts. The fluid/fiber ratio is also important: inadequate fluid intake with the fiber can make constipation worse. A systematic review looking at non-neurogenic chronic idiopathic constipation concluded that, although few studies have shown benefit from using soluble fiber in this patient group, the evidence for using insoluble fiber is conflicting [97].

Similar results were reported by Markland et al. in their review of more than 10,000 adults, where they found a beneficial effect of increasing intake of fluid but not of fiber or exercise in managing constipation [98]. Looking specifically at individuals with NBD, a case series of 11 adults with SCI reported an increase in colonic transit time (i.e., constipation), rather than an improvement, with the use of insoluble fiber [99].

Consumption of a very high-fiber diet without proper advice on fluid intake may worsen constipation symptoms in certain patients who are fluid-sensitive. An individualized approach should be used with the use of insoluble fiber as a bulk-forming agent and factoring in fluid intake to optimize stool consistency [100–103].

Oral Fluid Intake

Good hydration is an important component of successful bowel management. Adequate fluid intake optimizes the effect of osmotic laxatives and fiber and is also necessary for bowel health overall. Fiber absorbs large amounts of water in the intestine, so a high-fiber diet can cause constipation if plenty of fluids are not also taken. Based on a normal child's weight, their recommended daily fluid intake is as follows: 5–10 kg: 2–4 US cups (~500–1000 mL); 10–20 kg: 4–6 cups (~1000–1500 mL); 20–30 kg: 6–7 cups (~1500–1750 mL); 30–40 kg: 7–8 cups (~1750–2000 mL); 40–50 kg: 8–9 cups (~2000–2250 mL); >50 kg: 9–10 US cups (~2250–2500 mL) of water per day [104].

Physical Activity

Similar to diet, there is no unanimous opinion about the effects of increased physical activity on managing constipation, as there are a few studies in favor of it [105–107] and a few against it [108–110]. Despite the absence of a strong evidence base for these conservative interventions, they have been found to be useful in patients with NBD. Regular activity can help reduce constipation by stimulating the bowel's peristaltic motility. It is important to encourage the young person to establish and continue a daily exercise program, which may include tailored wheelchair activities such as push-ups and transfers if necessary. A physical therapist can help develop such an exercise program, which is unlikely to do any harm and will have other health benefits for the child, even if bowel effects cannot be guaranteed.

Scheduled Defecation

We support the aim of establishing a pattern of scheduled defecation and exhausting the conservative interventions of dietary and lifestyle modification before moving on to pharmacological interventions. In general, to benefit from the diurnal "body clock," scheduled defecation should be attempted once per day at approximately the same time every day (or, if not possible, on alternate days).

Maximizing the Gastrocolic Reflex

Another point to consider while setting the regimen is that the bowel contractions are maximal on waking up and after a meal or warm drink (the gastrocolic reflex). Although there is no strong evidence for its use in NBD [111,112], patients are still advised to make use of gastrocolic reflex by attempting to empty their bowels 10–30 min after eating or drinking [113]. For maximum effect, this can be combined with the scheduled defecation mentioned above.

Positioning

Several physical positions can encourage the passage of a bowel movement: placing the knees higher than hips, or the knees and hips bent in a typical squatting position. While no scientific studies exist on the use of specific commercially designed stools (e.g., Squatty Potty ®, LLC, St. George, UT, USA) the authors emphasize maximizing the squat position and adaptive seating to promote defecation. Additionally, in order to relax the pelvic floor muscles when sitting on the toilet, the feet should always be comfortably supported on a foot-stool, a customized orthopedic support, or the floor.

Abdominal Massage

Abdominal massage was used as a treatment for chronic constipation in the late 1800 s when there was a belief that it stimulated peristalsis [114]. Over the intervening years it fell out of favor but, with growing evidence in both children and adults, it has started regaining its popularity and it has reportedly been used beneficially by 22–30% of patients with NBD [4,115]. In a study of 24 adult patients with SCI, adding abdominal massage to the standard bowel program led to a significant reduction in colonic transit time (90.60 ± 32.67 h versus 72 ± 34.10 h, $p = 0.035$), abdominal distension (45.8% versus 12.5%, $p = 0.008$), and fecal incontinence (41.7% versus 16.7%, $p = 0.031$), while increasing the frequency of defecation (4.61 ± 2.17 versus 3.79 ± 2.15, $p = 0.006$) [116].

Despite the evidence showing this to be an effective technique, its mechanism of action is not entirely clear. Several observations have been noted and theories proposed, including activation of intestinal stretch receptors, which causes an increase in intestinal and rectal contraction [117], elicitation of measurable waves of rectal muscle contraction [118], decrease in colonic transit time [116], stimulation of the parasympathetic nervous system, thereby leading to an increase in gut secretions and motility and relaxing sphincters in the digestive tract [119]. In thin individuals, there may also be a direct mechanical effect. Whatever the mechanism, abdominal massage has a clear advantage of being non-invasive and risk-free, which is especially attractive to children, as well as repeatable and inexpensive. Abdominal massage in children is typically performed starting in the right iliac fossa, using a gentle, compressive, kneading motion in an upside-down "U" direction around the top of the umbilicus to the left iliac fossa, and then deep into the suprapubic region in order to help to move gas and stool along the course of the colon towards the rectum [114,120,121].

Digital Anorectal Stimulation

Digital anal/rectal stimulation [109,111–113] is a well-established technique used in individuals with NBD to help facilitate bowel evacuation. It requires the patient or caregiver to insert a gloved, lubricated finger into the rectum and move it in a rotatory pattern. This works by dilating the anal canal and relaxing the puborectalis muscle, which leads to a reduction in the anorectal angle. Both these effects lead to a reduction in resistance to the passage of stool, thereby assisting bowel emptying. Shafik et al. [122] in their study on 11 patients, noted left colonic contractions upon rectal distension which were absent after anesthetizing the rectum and anal canal. They therefore named this the rectocolic reflex [122], and it has been found to be useful in initiating bowel movement in individuals with supraconal disorders, but not in those with infraconal lesions. Overall, digital anorectal stimulation is a safe and effective intervention, with the main precaution advised to be gentle to avoid rectal mucosa injuries [122], especially if fingernails are long. This technique of digital stimulation is quite distinct from digital/manual evacuation, where the stool is extracted directly by the finger and which is generally not appropriate as a regular treatment for an older child.

Biofeedback and Physiotherapy

Biofeedback has anecdotally become quite popular in the treatment of various forms of fecal and urinary incontinence, including in children. In the early eighties, small case studies suggested a long-lasting beneficial effect of biofeedback in children aged 5–17 years with fecal incontinence secondary to myelomeningocele; in more than 50% of these children, fecal incontinence disappeared without the need for enemas or suppositories [123,124]. Larger controlled trials, however, showed insufficient effect of biofeedback alone in children with fecal incontinence due to spina bifida; patients allocated to behavior modification alone (defecation immediately after the evening meal each day, receiving a reward for defecating in the toilet without an enema or suppository, and undergoing an enema if unsuccessful for two consecutive days) showed a similar clinical improvement to patients allocated to behavior modification plus biofeedback [125,126] suggesting that the previous uncontrolled studies had overestimated the value of biofeedback in this population. Furthermore, biofeedback did not improve anal squeeze pressures or rectal sensation in these children [126]. Currently, therefore, it appears that there is no long-term advantage in adding biofeedback training to the conventional treatment of NBD in children, although there is limited evidence showing a short-term benefit in functional constipation [127].

Similarly, while (non-biofeedback) pelvic floor physiotherapy may be useful in some cases of functional constipation or bladder problems, there appears to be no literature justifying its routine use in children with NBD.

Non-invasive Electrical Stimulation

Normal bowel function depends on the passage of electrical impulses in sensory neurons from the rectum to the higher centers and returning via motor neurons to the anorectal muscles. Since this natural two-way communication process is interrupted in neuropathic conditions, investigators have attempted to restore the electrical milieu by providing replacement artificial electrical signals. Initial experimental treatment of neurogenic bladder/sphincter in adults and then children has been followed more recently by application of similar techniques to various bowel pathologies. Clearly, non-invasive techniques are preferable to surgical approaches, especially in children, but may not deliver the same potential therapeutic benefit.

Transcutaneous Electrical Nerve Stimulation

Non-invasive nerve stimulation such as transcutaneous electrical nerve stimulation (TENS) is widely used for bowel dysfunction in children: Veiga at al. in 2013 showed a 85.7% improvement in constipation in patients treated with para-sacral TENS [128]. TENS is well-accepted, safe, and studies suggest significant improvement in bowel function [129,130], although few have included a placebo-controlled group (essential for symptoms that are very open to psychological modification). Unfortunately, no specific data are presently available for NBD.

Posterior Tibial Nerve Stimulation

Posterior tibial nerve stimulation (PTNS) has reportedly improved the bowel dysfunction score in SCI [131], but no data or analysis have been presented specifically for neurogenic patients [132]

Other Electrostimulation

Other modalities of electrical stimulation have been suggested for NBD: transrectal and intravesical [133,134]. The limited experience reported does not yet permit these to be considered in daily clinical practice.

3.2.4. Pharmacological Treatments

Probiotics

There is no specific evidence for the use of probiotics in children with NBD. However, the use of a probiotic can be considered for a general improvement in gut health and microbiome biodiversity. Probiotics can result in increased bowel frequency and improved bowel consistency in adults. When the probiotic *Lactobacillus reuteri* was administered to infants older than six months, there was improved bowel frequency [135].

Oral Laxatives

Oral laxatives are the next step up the ladder in the management of NBD. High-quality data exist in the form of several RCTs confirming the beneficial effect of laxatives in individuals with NBD. Polyethylene glycol (PEG)/macrogol has been found to be superior to lactulose in one RCT involving pediatric NBD [136], leading to higher bowel frequency ($p < 0.01$). Other commonly used oral laxatives include bisacodyl and senna (colonic stimulants), docusate (stool softener), and ispaghula husk (Fybogel, bulk-forming). While osmotic and stimulant laxatives form the mainstay of treatment in pediatrics, several different categories of oral laxatives are used. Lubricants such as mineral oil can also be used to help with passage of hard stool.

Osmotic laxatives used to improve the consistency of hard stool (types 1 or 2 on the Bristol Stool Chart [137]:

Lactulose (10 g/15 mL suspension)—response may take 24–48 h.

Polyethylene glycol (PEG)/macrogol 3350 (powder mixed with water) 0.2–1.5 g/kg/day; onset of action is 24–96 h.

There is no recommendation from the literature on the optimum number of doses per day of lactulose and PEG. However, compliance with any laxative improves if prescribed only once per day [138]. On the other hand, PEG involves a large volume of liquid to be ingested (typically 125 mL per adult sachet, or half of this per pediatric sachet), so many doctors dose at least twice per day.

Milk of Magnesia:

- 2–5 years old: 0.4–1.2 g/day, in 1 or more doses;
- 6–11 years old: 1.2–2.4 g/day, in 1 or more doses;
- 12–18 years old: 2.4–4.8 g/day, in 1 or more doses.

Stimulant Laxatives Used to Increase Frequency of Bowel Movements Through Intestinal Contraction:

Bisacodyl:

- 2–10 years old: 5 mg once per day;
- 10–18 years old: 5–10 mg once per day.

Sennosides (Docusate Sodium oral suspension or Sennosides tablets)—onset of action is 6–10 h:

- 2–6 years old: 2.5–5 mg/day in 1–2 doses;
- 6–12 years old: 7.5–10 mg/day in 1–2 doses;
- 12–18 years old: 15–20 mg/day in 1–2 doses.

Initial laxative doses suggested to families are intended only as a guide: the response of pediatric neurogenic bowel to laxatives can be quite variable, so parents or caregivers need to be advised to titrate up or down the starting doses of osmotic and stimulant laxatives separately every few days until their child achieves just the right stool consistency and frequency respectively. Similarly variable can be the timing between ingestion and action of an oral laxative in children with NBD so that, especially for those with poor anal sphincter control, it can be difficult to ensure that the resulting evacuation does not occur at a socially inconvenient time such as during school. This tends to limit the usefulness of oral laxatives in children with NBD.

Suppositories

If digital stimulation is not effective in providing the desired symptomatic relief, or rectal lesion occurred [139] it can be augmented by the use of laxative suppositories glycerin(e)/glycerol and bisacodyl are the commonly used suppositories, with the former mild enough to be used in infants, but often ineffective in older children with NBD. The latter is a stimulant laxative that has either hydrogenated vegetable oil or polyethylene glycol (PEG) as a base; three studies (including one good-quality randomized controlled trial, RCT) have reported better results with PEG-based suppositories [140–142]. Sodium bicarbonate (Lecicarbon) is a newer effervescent suppository, releasing bubbles of carbon dioxide to stimulate reflex rectal activity, which has a quicker onset of action than fat-based bisacodyl suppositories (15–20 min compared to 30–40 min) but similar efficacy [143].

In children with a patulous anus (often seen in spina bifida), the suppository sometimes falls out before it has had a chance to work. This can often be resolved by holding the buttocks together and/or encouraging the child to lie prone and stay relatively still until they feel contractions or start to stool.

Enemas

An enema is an instillation of liquid into the rectum to evacuate stool. Although enemas are often used for acute constipation in people with neurotypical bowels, regular enemas can form part of an effective bowel management program for people with NBD. They are generally used in the event of suppositories being unproductive.

The two main approaches are to either deliver a relatively large volume of water or saline into the colon to produce a mechanical flush, or to use commercially available micro-enema tubes, usually containing 5 mL of a strong stimulant laxative to act locally. The former approach will be considered below as transanal irrigation. In the latter category, docusate sodium mini-enema has been shown to be more effective in NBD than glycerine or bisacodyl suppositories [140]. The other commonly used micro-enemas are sodium citrate and sorbitol. Sodium phosphate enemas, on the other hand, contain a medium volume of laxative (60 mL for ages 5–11 years, and 120 mL for ages 12+), so can be convenient and effective in occasional acute cases of fecal impaction in an otherwise well child. However, phosphate enemas are not routinely used on a regular basis as part of a bowel program, as they can be messy, and risk dehydration and electrolyte abnormalities secondary to inadvertent retention of the medication if they do not produce a stool within 10 min (a particular risk in children with megacolon or with renal compromise due to an associated neurogenic bladder); long-term use can also cause colitis due to chronic irritation, sometimes leading to diarrhea secondary to a narrow hyperactive colon [142]. However, this complication has recently been reported in both children and adults using other antegrade and retrograde enema irrigants too [143].

The tip of any enema tube can injure the fragile rectal mucosa, especially in a child. As with suppositories, the liquid medication in an enema can also sometimes dribble out prematurely past a lax anus, reducing its efficacy.

Transanal Irrigation

When a micro-enema tube is not being used, there are various options for delivery of a larger volume of liquid into the rectum and colon:

a. Bulb syringe enemas are used for smaller volume enemas in older infants and young toddlers. The bulb is inserted through the anus and 60–90 mL of warm water can be instilled.

b. Balloon enemas use a 24 Fr Foley catheter to administer a high-volume rectal enema. To have the enema administered, the patient must usually lie down, with the catheter's balloon inflated inside the lower rectum to create a leak-proof seal above the anal canal. The individual must then transfer to the toilet to deflate the balloon and evacuate at the appropriate time, all of which can be quite challenging for a child who may have other disabilities.

c. Cone enemas involve insertion of the tip of a graduated silicone cone until it occludes the anus (whether patulous or not) with a water-tight seal. This is simpler, less cumbersome, and somewhat less invasive than a balloon catheter and so may better suit younger children. The cone is connected to enema tubing in a similar manner to balloon enemas. Afterwards, the cone and tubing can easily be washed and re-used, making it relatively inexpensive compared to balloon enemas and specifically designed kits.

d. Commercially available transanal irrigation (TAI) systems were designed to speed up the colonic washout process and increase independence in bowel management compared to the previous generic balloon catheter and cone techniques. All incorporate either a customized bag or chamber from where the irrigant solution drains along a tube ending in either a catheter or a cone that is passed through the anus to administer high-volume enemas over several minutes that have been shown on scintigraphy to clear far enough up the colon to render someone reliably clean for a few days [144].

In balloon catheter TAI systems, a rectal catheter is intended to stay in place without assistance while the enema fluid is released via a pump operated either manually (e.g., Peristeen by Coloplast® A/S (Kokkedal, Denmark) or IrriSedo Klick by Qufora® (Allerod, Denmark) or electrically (e.g., Navina by Wellspect®, Molndal, Sweden). However, those patients with a lax anal sphincter generally find the washout is interrupted prematurely when the balloon is inadvertently expelled intact (whether by gravity, recoil, or rectal contraction). Therefore, they depend on the catheter being held in place manually. Younger children, and those whose neurological condition also affects their balance or manual dexterity, are generally unable to achieve this for themselves, so require a caregiver to be present throughout the few minutes when the fluid is being administered.

In cone TAI systems, the silicone cone tip, where the irrigation fluid meets the body, must be held inside the anus throughout the delivery of the irrigant in order to plug the fluid from being expelled prematurely. In patients with a patulous anus, the graduated shape of the cone tends to achieve a more effective seal than a balloon catheter, but again a carer is often required to hold the cone in place. The various cone systems use gravity (e.g., Assura by Coloplast®), a manual pump (e.g., IrriSedo Cone by Qufora® or Peristeen Cone by Coloplast®), or an electric pump (e.g., IryPump by B Braun® Melsungen, Germany) to drive the irrigation.

Either way, the washout can be performed completely on the toilet (or on a commode or shower-chair in a suitable wet-room) or may involve transferring from the floor/bench to the toilet before its onset of action a few minutes later. Complete emptying of all the irrigant and the accompanying stool takes up to one hour on the toilet, depending on the volume of fluid used, which determines how far proximally the colon is cleared, and so how many days the child can remain clean for afterwards. This emptying process can be augmented by abdominal massage (see Section Abdominal Massage above).

This method of irrigation has been used clinically starting in 1987 to treat constipation and fecal incontinence in children [145]. In children with NBD who do not respond to conservative or medical treatments, TAI is an increasingly accepted treatment [13]. There are studies demonstrating improved QoL and outcomes with children utilizing TAI for functional incontinence and functional constipation, and some authors recommend TAI should be mandated prior to considering any invasive surgical intervention [146]. A summary publication of TAI use in children incorporated a literature review comprising 27 studies with 1040 patients whose average age was 8 years old [13]. Of these children, 78–84% had improved bowel continence, and 95% had improved QoL, after starting TAI. There are undoubtedly some children who, even as adults, will never achieve independence with TAI, particularly due to their body shape and neurological function. However, in some units TAI has largely replaced the traditional surgical approach for individuals who fail to respond to escalating conservative and medical treatments, as it has proven to be as effective as surgery without the additional morbidity.

Whatever the mode of delivery, the irrigant solutions used will vary based on individual needs. The vast majority of prescribing clinicians in Europe and North America recommend tap water as the irrigant of choice. However, this introduces the possibility of the hypotonic water being absorbed by the colon, producing a theoretical risk of iatrogenic hyponatremia. The number of published reports of successful and safe colonic irrigation including TAI using simple tap water suggest that such concerns are probably unfounded. Nonetheless, to counter this risk, some units instead irrigate with normal (0.9%) saline, either commercially prepared or approximated at home by adding 9 g (1.5 teaspoons) of standard table salt (but not low-salt/low-sodium preparations) to each one liter of tap-water. However, this approach carries its own risk of errors in parental understanding and titration. Water or saline alone may be sufficient for an enema program but, if not successful, relatively gentle additives can make the enema more effective. Examples include baby soap (contains glycerine as an ingredient), USP-grade glycerin (used as a stimulant laxative), Castile soap (considered "stronger" than glycerin or baby soap), or PEG in the enema fluid (instead of, or in addition to, taking PEG orally). For those patients preferring a longer interval between washouts, and willing to accept a longer sit on the toilet or the possibility of increased abdominal cramps, a larger volume of irrigant (up to 20 mL/kg body weight) can be instilled and/or a stronger stimulant laxative such as bisacodyl can be added to the liquid. Conversely, for other children and families their priority is as short a TAI session as possible, so they use a smaller volume of liquid every day.

Summary

Many therapeutic approaches exist for the management of NBD in children and adolescents. Treatment must be tailored to the needs and circumstances of the individual child and their caregivers. Although isolated strategies may act as a starting point, more often than not, the management becomes multidimensional, involving different treatment modalities. To be maximally effective, a bowel management program in pediatric NBD must also be multidisciplinary, involving close and long-term teamwork between the child with their parents or caregivers and a wide range of specialists including continence nurse specialists/uro-therapists, school and community nurses, family doctor, physical therapist, pediatricians, pediatric gastroenterologists, pediatric clinical psychologists, radiologists, pediatric surgeons/urologists, and pediatric anesthesiologists.

3.3. The Surgical Management of NBD in Children and Adolescents
3.3.1. Sacral Nerve Modulation

Sacral nerve modulation (SNM) is a step up from transcutaneous electrostimulation techniques, involving invasive implantation of electrodes along sacral nerve roots, which brings more targeted effects (i.e., it is possible to focus on either the rectum or the anal sphincter or both) but this is balanced by higher risks of nerve damage and introducing infection. SNM was initially developed to control lower urinary tract symptoms, primarily in neuropathic conditions, and has more recently been used for bowel dysfunction too. SNM works by stimulating the somatic and autonomic nervous systems, although the exact mode of action is not completely understood [147,148] and few studies have proposed its effect on the central nervous system [138]. Its impact in cases of constipation has been suggested to be due to an increased frequency and amplitude of antegrade pressure sequences, but whether these are mediated via a central or peripheral mode of action remains unclear. In adults, randomized controlled trials of SNM in chronic constipation have not shown benefit [149], so it is currently indicated only for fecal incontinence. In children and young adults with refractory functional constipation, SNM has shown some sustained benefit, although it is debatable whether this is enough to justify the risks and high costs [150]. However, SNM is not FDA-approved in the USA for bowel dysfunction in children under the age of 18 (nor under the age of 16 for bladder dysfunction). Furthermore, it may not be technically feasible for the more common causes of NBD which involve anatomical abnormality of the spinal cord, such as spina bifida and spinal cord injury. The role of SNM in neurogenic patients has been evaluated in a few studies and improvement has been reported in SCI [151].

3.3.2. Bowel Surgery

Surgical management of NBD is regarded as a valuable option in selected cases [152]. With respect to the treatment pyramid of pediatric NBD, chronic constipation and/or fecal incontinence that was previously proposed by our group (see modification in Figure 1), surgical methods for bowel management are usually utilized only after failure of the full range of conventional conservative and pharmacological medical treatments, which now includes transanal irrigation (TAI) [13]. Nevertheless, a recent survey showed that, in order to achieve fecal control, surgery is required (due to failure of medical treatment) in about 40% of pediatric and adult patients with NBD secondary to myelomeningocele [153]. Several studies show that surgical treatment of NBD can be successful in providing an improved QoL if appropriately indicated and with patients carefully selected. The aim of surgery for NBD, just as with its conservative and pharmacological management, is to evacuate the colon at a time and place of the child and family's choosing, in order to reduce the prospect of soiling at times when the child is unable to visit the toilet. It should also minimize the average time the child needs to spend in the bathroom every week.

So far, most reports on surgical treatment of NBD deal with adult patients and very little has been published on children and adolescents on this topic. However, most of the benefits and drawbacks of surgery in these patients apply to all age groups. Nevertheless, it is important to remember that young patients are still growing (physically and emotionally), and probably need to continue for life with the surgical established method for emptying their colon. The proposed surgical options also have to respect the pediatric patient's developmental age and any comorbidities, as well as the family dynamics and environment, in order to produce an appropriate individualized solution that allows optimum social integration with their age-appropriate peers [154].

The surgical approach for NBD in children primarily involves creating artificial "upstream" access for antegrade administration of colonic irrigation enemas, either by Malone's antegrade continence enema (ACE) procedure, or by tube cecostomy. This might be especially advantageous in patients with stool impaction due to NBD [155] or in those who, due to comorbidities, lack the balance, manual dexterity, or motivation to self-administer retrograde washouts by TAI [13]. Many teenagers can administer their antegrade enemas independently via an intermittently inserted catheter or an indwelling tube. The final surgical alternative in children is a colostomy (fecal diversion), but Malone´s ACE procedure is by far the most utilized method [156]. Unfortunately, some other reconstructive techniques available to adults with NBD, such as artificial anal sphincter implantation [157], are generally not appropriate for the growing child.

Malone Antegrade Continence Enema Procedure

Malone´s ACE procedure has been shown to be a safe surgical method, with minimal mortality but several minor complications [158]. The successful use of the Malone antegrade continence enema (MACE) via a neo-appendicostomy has increased QoL in 80% of adult patients [159]. The MACE has also been successfully implemented in children with spina bifida and resulted in a significant improvement in fecal continence and QoL scores [160,161].

The current standard in situ appendicostomy for the MACE produces a continent catheterizable appendiceal channel to the cecum by creating a valve mechanism at the cecal end (to reduce leakage of feces onto the skin) and bringing the decapitated end of the appendix up to a convenient site on the abdominal wall such as the umbilicus or hidden under a cosmetic skin-flap elsewhere that also serves to reduce the risk of stomal stenosis. Beside this technique, other open surgical modifications have been performed in the pediatric age group such as the cecal extension (when the appendix is not long enough), the Yang-Monti ileo-cecostomy (using a short section of detubularized retubularized ileum to create an alternative channel when a suitable appendix is not available) and cecal or colon flap channels (again if an adequate appendix is not available) [161]. MACE channels are often constructed at the same time as urinary reconstructive surgery such as a Mitrofanoff procedure for associated neurogenic bladder. If the appendix is not long enough, or cannot be extended sufficiently, to create both channels, this may give rise to surgical dilemmas regarding the optimum use of the appendix, and the need to use such modifications. However, the rate of surgical revisions required after some of these modifications appears to be higher than for a standard MACE [162]. In the subsequent laparoscopic adaptation, there is usually no attempt at the technically difficult creation of a valve mechanism, yet the rates of fecal leakage via such stomas are still surprisingly low [163,164].

If investigation such as a colonic transit study suggests mega-rectum and/or distal colonic delay with feces impacting in the recto-sigmoid, then a "distal ACE" (e.g., in the transverse or descending colon) can produce a more effective evacuation of feces and reduce the risk of retention of the irrigant compared to the conventional cecal ACE [165].

Tube Cecostomy

Another modification of the MACE is the utilization of a Chait® (Cook Medical LLC, IN, USA) cecostomy tube, or a "button" device, placed as either a percutaneous endoscopic cecostomy (PEC), under fluoroscopic guidance, or via laparoscopy. It has been proven significantly to improve fecal continence and QoL in patients with NBD [166]. The disadvantage is that any such tube needs to be replaced at regular intervals, and sooner if it blocks, dislodges, or breaks.

As with a conventional ACE, in cases of slow colonic transit the Chait® tube or button device can instead be placed more distally in the colon (e.g., at the descending/sigmoid junction) as a percutaneous endoscopic colostomy [167].

Outcomes of MACE and tube cecostomy are comparable in children with spina bifida (SB) [154]. Nonetheless, both procedures, however performed, carry the important potential risk of jeopardizing the critical ventriculo-peritoneal shunt in children with hydrocephalus associated with spina bifida [168].

Bowel Diversion

A colostomy involves bringing part of the large intestine to the abdomen's surface to form a stoma. Stool is collected in an external bag worn by the patient over the stoma. Perhaps the main barrier to performing a bowel stoma in any age group is the reluctance of the patient to accept it from a psychological perspective. This is particularly relevant in the pediatric population, where children and parents may fear leakage of feces, flatus, or smell, its impact on bodily integrity and self-image, and the possibility of teasing or bullying by peers. However, ostomy (either colostomy or ileostomy) as a bowel diversion produces similar or even superior outcomes in selected patients in regard to QoL compared to conservative bowel management strategies in NBD. For those individuals who prefer their stoma to act at a convenient time, the upstream colon can be irrigated retrogradely in a similar fashion to TAI (see Section Transanal Irrigation.). Nevertheless, a relevant number of postoperative complications has been reported. The main advantage of diversion is the reduction of time taken to empty the bowel. Patients who undergo ostomy surgery, often as a "last resort," are usually very satisfied with the resulting improvement, and a significant proportion of patients afterwards report a desire to have been counselled about this option earlier [169] rather than reserving it for supposed failure of care [170,171]. Furthermore, adult series of colostomy in fecal incontinence showed a reduced number of hospitalizations [172]. Colostomy formation early after spinal cord injury has also been shown to improve independence and increase acceptability of bowel management [173,174].

Occasionally ostomy is mandated in order to divert the fecal stream from the perineum so that chronic decubitus pressure-sores may heal without being soiled.

Bowel Resection

Bowel resection has been proposed for selected cases of functional constipation and/or fecal incontinence after failed conservative treatment [175,176]. Outcomes in these children were reported to be favorable in most (up to 80%) of the cases [177]. However, bowel resection does not play a role in the surgical treatment of NBD apart from occasional limited resections during creation of MACE or ostomy [178]. Some authorities recommend routine consideration of bowel resection at the time of MACE creation to encourage faster and more complete bowel evacuation. On the other hand, others suggest that bowel resection should be reserved for the few individual cases where there is a strong indication. However, while this is controversial topic, currently there is no common consensus to resect bowel at the time of MACE creation.

Summary

For children born with NBD, fecal continence can be achieved in about 50% with conservative and medical treatment, although the advent of more user-friendly versions of TAI promises to raise this proportion. The vast majority of the remaining patients should also reach fecal continence by undergoing one of several possible surgical interventions, most often the MACE. Nevertheless, all surgical procedures carry a risk of postoperative complications and revisionary surgery, which can be especially difficult to deal with for children and adolescents and their families. Therefore, surgical treatment in pediatric NBD should be offered only on an individually indicated basis [158].

4. Discussion

Today the majority of pediatric patients with NBD can theoretically achieve social fecal continence and treat chronic constipation, reducing their need for pads and time spent in the bathroom, enriching their QoL and social relationships, improving their productivity in school/work, and reducing the incidence of related urinary tract infections. In the past, this goal has often only been achieved by resorting to surgical procedures such as the Malone ACE, or even ostomy. Such traditional surgical continence procedures can indeed be highly effective in carefully selected patient groups [155], but they carry a relatively high risk of surgical complications and an increased risk of anesthesiology procedures. The advent of TAI changed traditional bowel management for the significant numbers who do not respond to conservative and pharmacological approaches alone, permitting successful treatment of a large population of pediatric and adolescent patients with NBD, without requiring surgery. TAI can be frustratingly time-consuming for impatient children, but has been shown to reduce total time spent in the bathroom dealing with the effects of constipation and/or incontinence. Of course, TAI must be tailored to different patient populations and individual requirements in order to obtain a good outcome for the child and their caregivers [13]. Indeed, TAI may not be feasible for certain individuals with reduced hand control, poor balance, or distorted spines who wish to be independent in their bowel evacuation. In those circumstances, surgery instead can be life-enhancing. However, TAI now forms part of a thorough bowel management program that must first include a range of conventional conservative measures (such as physical activity, correct fluid intake and diet, probiotics, etc.), followed by the addition of laxative medication administered orally and/or per rectum. All the therapeutic strategies for bowel management must be individually tailored to each different child and family, considering the pathophysiology of their neurogenic bowel dysfunction, their primary disease and associated comorbidities, emotional, educational, or mental status, manual dexterity, as well as the fears, motivation, and compliance of the child and caregivers. Today invasive surgical treatment is usually postponed and used only in case of failure of conservative, pharmacological and mini-invasive (i.e., TAI) treatment applied in a stepwise approach as recommended by our group [13] and by the International Children's Continence Society [18]. For this reason, the indignity of NBD must be addressed in all pediatric populations with neurological conditions, including patients with severe disabilities such as cerebral palsy, acquired brain injury for trauma, tumor, vascular injury or systemic disease that, until now, have not been afforded the same therapeutic attention as spina bifida or traumatic spinal injury.

5. Conclusions

NBD today should be considered, investigated, and treated in all children and adolescents with any congenital or acquired neurological disease, with a high expectation of success. Bowel management should be tailored to the individual needs and circumstances of each patient and their family, and all conventional conservative and medical treatments must be exhausted before considering proceeding to a surgical approach. A structured but aggressive approach to the treatment of NBD should improve distressing symptoms, enhance QoL for the child and their caregivers, and will decrease hospital readmissions. TAI seems a very effective bridge between conservative/medical management, that is only effective in about half of affected children, and definitive surgery that is much more effective for most but carries unwanted risks.

Author Contributions: Conceptualization: G.M., S.S., D.M., U.R., M.A.B.; methodology, G.M.; validation, G.M., S.S., D.M., U.R., M.A.B.; formal analysis: G.M., S.S., D.M., U.R., M.A.B.; resources, G.M., S.S., D.M., U.R., M.A.B.; writing—original draft preparation, G.M., S.S., D.M., U.R., M.A.B.; —review and editing G.M., D.M.; supervision, M.A.B. All authors have read and agreed to the published version of the manuscript.

Funding: This research received no external funding.

Informed Consent Statement: Not applicable.

Acknowledgments: The authors are grateful to Coloplast A/S for sponsoring the publication fee of this article through an educational grant (although the content was not in any way influenced by Coloplast A/S).

Conflicts of Interest: The authors are all current members of a Pediatric Global Advisory Board convened by Coloplast A/S, and receive payment for attending meetings arranged by Coloplast A/S, although the work for this article was not in any way influenced nor paid for by Coloplast A/S.

References

1. Mugie, S.M.; Benninga, M.A.; Di Lorenzo, C. Epidemiology of constipation in children and adults: A systematic review. *Best Pract. Res. Clin. Gastroenterol.* **2011**, *25*, 3–18. [CrossRef]
2. Rajindrajith, S.; Devanarayana, N.M.; Benninga, M.A. Review article: Faecal incontinence in children: Epidemiology, pathophysiology, clinical evaluation and management. *Aliment. Pharmacol. Ther.* **2013**, *37*, 37–48. [CrossRef]
3. Mugie, S.M.; Di Lorenzo, C.; Benninga, M.A. Constipation in childhood. *Nat. Rev. Gastroenterol. Hepatol.* **2011**, *8*, 502–511. [CrossRef] [PubMed]
4. Coggrave, M. Neurogenic continence. Part 3: Bowel management strategies. *Br. J. Nurs* **2008**, *17*, 962–968. [CrossRef] [PubMed]
5. Krogh, K.; Lie, H.R.; Bilenberg, N.; Laurberg, S. Bowel function in Danish children with myelomeningocele. *APMIS Suppl.* **2003**, *109*, 81–85.
6. Midrio, P.; Mosiello, G.; Ausili, E.; Gamba, P.; Marte, A.; Lombardi, L.; Iacobelli, B.D.; Caponcelli, E.; Marrello, S.; Meroni, M.; et al. Peristeen ® transanal irrigation in paediatric patients with anorectal malformations and spinal cord lesions: A multicentre Italian study. *Colorectal. Dis.* **2016**, *18*, 86–93. [CrossRef] [PubMed]
7. Malone, P.S.; Wheeler, R.A.; Williams, J.E. Continence in patients with spina bifida: Long term results. *Arch. Dis. Child.* **1994**, *70*, 107–110. [CrossRef]
8. Shandling, B.; Gilmour, R.F. The enema continence catheter in spina bifida: Successful bowel management. *J. Pediatr. Surg.* **1987**, *22*, 271–273. [CrossRef]
9. Emmanuel, A.V.; Krogh, K.; Bazzocchi, G.; Leroi, A.M.; Bremers, A.; Leder, D.; van Kuppevelt, D.; Mosiello, G.; Vogel, M.; Perrouin-Verbe, B.; et al. Consensus review of best practice of transanal irrigation in adults. *Spinal Cord* **2013**, *51*, 732–738. [CrossRef]
10. Bray, L.; Sanders, C. An evidence-based review of the use of transanal irrigation in children and young people with neurogenic bowel. *Spinal Cord* **2013**, *51*, 88–93. [CrossRef]

11. Faaborg, P.M.; Christensen, P.; Kvitsau, B.; Buntzen, S.; Laurberg, S. Long-term outcome and safety of transanal colonic irrigation for neurogenic bowel dysfunction. *Spinal Cord* **2009**, *47*, 545–549. [CrossRef]
12. Ausili, E.; Marte, A.; Brisighelli, G.; Midrio, P.; Mosiello, G.; La Pergola, E.; Lombardi, L.; Iacobelli, B.D.; Caponcelli, E.; Meroni, M.; et al. Short versus mid-long-term outcome of transanal irrigation in children with spina bifida and anorectal malformations. *Childs Nerv. Syst.* **2018**, *34*, 2471–2479. [CrossRef]
13. Mosiello, G.; Marshall, D.; Rolle, U.; Cretolle, C.; Santacruz, B.G.; Frischer, J.; Benninga, M.A. Consensus review of best practice of transanal irrigation in children. *J. Pediatr. Gastroenterol. Nutr.* **2017**, *64*, 343–352. [CrossRef]
14. Fink, A.; Kosecoff, J.; Chassin, M.; Brook, R.H. Consensus methods: Characteristics and guidelines for use. *Am. J. Public Health* **1984**, *74*, 979–983. [CrossRef] [PubMed]
15. Krogh, K.; Christensen, P.; Laurberg, S. Colorectal symptoms in patients with neurological diseases. *Acta Neurol. Scand.* **2001**, *103*, 335–343. [CrossRef] [PubMed]
16. Northrup, H.; Volcik, K.A. Spina bifida and other neural tube defects. *Curr. Probl. Pediatr.* **2000**, *30*, 313–332. [CrossRef]
17. Bauer, S.B. The management of the myelodysplastic child: A paradigm shift. *BJU Int.* **2003**, *92*, 23–28. [CrossRef] [PubMed]
18. Capitanucci, M.L.; Rivosecchi, M.; Silveri, M.; Lucchetti, M.C.; Mosiello, G.; De Gennaro, M. Neurovesical dysfunction due to spinal dysraphism in anorectal anomalies. *Eur. J. Pediatr. Surg.* **1996**, *6*, 159–162. [CrossRef]
19. Rawashdeh, Y.F.; Austin, P.; Siggaard, C.; Bauer, S.B.; Franco, I.; de Jong, T.P.; Jorgensen, T.M. International Children's Continence Society's recommendations for therapeutic intervention in congenital neuropathic bladder and bowel dysfunction in children. *Neurourol. Urodyn.* **2012**, *31*, 615–620. [CrossRef]
20. Guzman, L.; Bauer, S.B.; Hallett, M.; Khoshbin, S.; Colodny, A.H.; Retik, A.B. Evaluation and management of children with sacral agenesis. *Urology* **1983**, *22*, 506–510. [CrossRef]
21. Borrelli, M.; Spinola, R.; Bruschini, H.; Walligora, M.; Nahas, W.C.; Freire, G.C.; Figueiredo, J.A.; De Goes, G.M.; Prado, M.J. Sacral agenesis: Why is it so frequently misdiagnosed? *Urology* **1985**, *26*, 351–355. [CrossRef]
22. Mosiello, G.; Capitanucci, M.L.; Gatti, C.; Adorisio, O.; Lucchetti, M.C.; Silveri, M.; Schingo, P.S.M.; De Gennaro, M. How to investigate neurovesical dysfunction in children with anorectal malformations. *J. Urol.* **2003**, *170*, 1610–1613. [CrossRef]
23. Peña, A. Posterior sagittal approach for the correction of anorectal malformations. *Adv. Surg.* **1986**, *19*, 69–100. [PubMed]
24. Emir, H.; Soylet, Y. Neurovesical dysfunction in patients with anorectal malformations. *Eur. J. Pediatr. Surg.* **1998**, *8*, 95–97. [CrossRef] [PubMed]
25. Fitzgerald, K. Ultrasound examination of the neonatal spine. *Australas J. Ultrasound. Med.* **2011**, *14*, 39–41. [CrossRef]
26. Richards, C.L.; Malouin, F. Cerebral palsy: Definition, assessment and rehabilitation. *Handb. Clin. Neurol.* **2013**, *111*, 183–195. [CrossRef] [PubMed]
27. Ozturk, M.; Oktem, F.; Kisloglu, N.; Demirci, M.; Altuntas, I.; Kutluhan, S.; Dogan, M. Bladder and bowel control in children with cerebral palsy. *Croat. Med. J.* **2006**, *47*, 264–270.
28. Von Wendt, L.; Similä, S.; Niskanen, P.; Järvelin, M.R. Development of bowel and bladder control in the mentally retarded. *Dev. Med. Child Neurol.* **1990**, *32*, 515–518. [CrossRef]
29. Bohmer, C.J.; Taminiau, J.A.; Klinkenberg-Knol, E.C.; Meuwissen, S.G. The prevalence of constipation in institutionalized people with intellectual disability. *J. Intellect. Disabil. Res.* **2001**, *45*, 212–218. [CrossRef] [PubMed]
30. Lo Cascio, C.M.; Goetze, O.; Latshang, T.D.; Bluemel, S.; Frauenfelder, T.; Bloch, K.E. Gastrointestinal Dysfunction in Patients with Duchenne Muscular Dystrophy. *PLoS ONE* **2016**, *11*, e0163779. [CrossRef]
31. Crockett, C.D.; Bertrand, L.A.; Cooper, C.S.; Rahhal, R.M.; Liu, K.; Zimmerman, M.B.; Moore, S.A.; Mathews, K.D. Urologic and gastrointestinal symptoms in the dystroglycanopathies. *Neurology* **2015**, *84*, 532–539. [CrossRef] [PubMed]
32. Yadak, R.; Breur, M.; Bugiani, M. Gastrointestinal Dysmotility in MNGIE: From thymidine phosphorylase enzyme deficiency to altered interstitial cells of Cajal. *Orphanet J. Rare Dis.* **2019**, *14*, 33. [CrossRef]
33. Barrett, T.G.; Scott-Brown, M.; Seller, A.; Bednarz, A.; Poulton, K.; Poulton, J. The mitochondrial genome in Wolfram syndrome. *J. Med. Genet.* **2000**, *37*, 463–466. [CrossRef]
34. Chiminello, R.; Mosiello, G.; Castelli, E. Bladder and bowel dysfunctions in children with cerebral palsy and acquired brain injury: Are we able to define incidence and to predict them? *Eur. Urol. Suppl.* **2018**, *17*, e1179–e1180. [CrossRef]
35. Berger, M.; Heinrich, M.; Lacher, M.; Hubertus, J.; Stehr, M.; von Schweinitz, D. Postoperative bladder and rectal function in children with sacro-coccygeal teratoma. *Pediatr. Blood Cancer* **2011**, *56*, 397–402. [CrossRef] [PubMed]
36. Mosiello, G.; Gatti, C.; De Gennaro, M.; Capitanucci, M.; Silveri, M.; Inserra, A.; Milano, G.; De Laurentis, C.; Boglino, C. Neurovesical dysfunction in children after treating pelvic neoplasms. *BJU Int.* **2003**, *92*, 289–292. [CrossRef]
37. Fitzpatrick, M.; O'Brien, C.; O'Connell, P.R.; O'Herlihy, C. Patterns of abnormal pudendal nerve function that are associated with postpartum fecal incontinence. *Am. J. Obstet. Gynecol.* **2003**, *189*, 730–735. [CrossRef]
38. Ng, C.; Prott, G.; Rutkowski, S.; Li, Y.; Hansen, R.; Kellow, J.; Malcolm, A. Gastrointestinal symptoms in spinal cord injury: Relationships with level of injury and psychologic factors. *Dis. Colon Rectum* **2005**, *48*, 1562–1568. [CrossRef]
39. Silveri, M.; Salsano, L.; Pierro, M.M.; Mosiello, G.; Capitanucci, M.L.; De Gennaro, M. Pediatric spinal cord injury: Approach for urological rehabilitation and treatment. *J. Pediatr. Urol.* **2006**, *2*, 10–15. [CrossRef]
40. Valles, M.; Vidal, J.; Clave, P.; Mearin, F. Bowel dysfunction in patients with motor complete spinal cord injury: Clinical, neurological, and pathophysiological associations. *Am. J. Gastroenterol.* **2006**, *101*, 2290–2299. [CrossRef] [PubMed]
41. Qi, Z.; Middleton, J.W.; Malcolm, A. Bowel Dysfunction in Spinal Cord Injury. *Curr. Gastroenterol. Rep.* **2018**, *20*, 47. [CrossRef]

42. Bhatt, N.R.; Murchison, L.; Yardy, G.; Kulkarni, M.; Mathur, A.B. Bladder bowel dysfunction in children with Down's syndrome. *Pediatr. Surg. Int.* **2020**, *36*, 763–772. [CrossRef] [PubMed]

43. Handel, L.N.; Barqawi, A.; Checa, G.; Furness, P.D., 3rd; Koyle, M.A. Males with Down's syndrome and nonneurogenic neurogenic bladder. *J. Urol.* **2003**, *169*, 646–649. [CrossRef]

44. Gubbiotti, M.; Balboni, G.; Bini, V.; Elisei, S.; Bedetti, C.; Marchiafava, M.; Giannantoni, A. Bladder and Bowel Dysfunction, Adaptive Behaviour, and Psychiatric Profiles in Adults Affected by Autism Spectrum Disorders. *Neurourol. Urodyn.* **2019**, *38*, 1866–1873. [CrossRef] [PubMed]

45. Pidcock, F.S.; Krishnan, C.; Crawford, T.O.; Salorio, C.F.; Trovato, M.; Kerr, D.A. Acute transverse myelitis in childhood: Center-based analysis of 47 cases. *Neurology* **2007**, *68*, 1474–1480. [CrossRef] [PubMed]

46. Kalra, V.; Sharma, S.; Sahu, J.; Sankhyan, N.; Chaudhry, R.; Dhawan, B.; Mridula, B. Childhood acute transverse myelitis: Clinical profile, outcome, and association with antiganglioside antibodies. *J. Child Neurol.* **2009**, *24*, 466–471. [CrossRef] [PubMed]

47. Miyazawa, R.; Ikeuchi, Y.; Tomomasa, T.; Ushiku, H.; Ogawa, T.; Morikawa, A. Determinants of prognosis of acute transverse myelitis in children. *Pediatr. Int.* **2003**, *45*, 512–516. [CrossRef]

48. Wolf, V.L.; Lupo, P.J.; Lotze, T.E. Pediatric transverse myelitis. *J. Child Neurol.* **2012**, *27*, 1426–1436. [CrossRef]

49. Hughes, R.A.; Cornblath, D.R. Guillain-Barre syndrome. *Lancet* **2005**, *366*, 1653–1666. [CrossRef]

50. Sawai, S.; Sakakibara, R.; Uchiyama, T.; Liu, Z.; Yamamoto, T.; Ito, T.; Kuwabara, S.; Kanai, K.; Asahina, M.; Yamanaka, T.; et al. Acute motor axonal neuropathy presenting with bowel, bladder, and erectile dysfunction. *J. Neurol.* **2007**, *254*, 250–252. [CrossRef]

51. Zochodne, D.W. Autonomic involvement in Guillain-Barre syndrome: A review. *Muscle Nerve* **1994**, *17*, 1145–1155. [CrossRef]

52. McCarthy, M.J.; Aylott, C.E.; Grevitt, M.P.; Hegarty, J. Cauda equina syndrome: Factors affecting long-term functional and sphincteric outcome. *Spine* **2007**, *32*, 207–216. [CrossRef]

53. Podnar, S. Bowel dysfunction in patients with cauda equina lesions. *Eur. J. Neurol.* **2006**, *13*, 1112–1117. [CrossRef]

54. Podnar, S. Epidemiology of cauda equina and conus medullaris lesions. *Muscle Nerve* **2007**, *35*, 529–531. [CrossRef] [PubMed]

55. Kingwell, E.; Marriott, J.J.; Jette, N.; Pringsheim, T.; Makhani, N.; Morrow, S.A.; Fisk, J.D.; Evans, C.; Béland, S.G.; Kulaga, S.; et al. Incidence and prevalence of multiple sclerosis in Europe: A systematic review. *BMC Neurol.* **2013**, *13*, 128. [CrossRef] [PubMed]

56. Evans, C.; Beland, S.G.; Kulaga, S.; Wolfson, C.; Kingwell, E.; Marriott, J.; Koch, M.; Makhani, N.; Morrow, S.; Fisk, J.; et al. Incidence and prevalence of multiple sclerosis in the Americas: A systematic review. *Neuroepidemiology* **2013**, *40*, 195–210. [CrossRef]

57. Mah, J.K.; Thannauser, J.E. Management of multiple sclerosis in adolescents, current treatment options and related adherence issues. *Adolesc. Health Med. Ther.* **2010**, *1*, 31–43. [CrossRef] [PubMed]

58. Kuntz, N.; Chabas, D.; Weinstock-Guttman, B.; Chitnis, T.; Yeh, E.A.; Krupp, L.; Ness, J.; Rodriguez, M.; Waubant, E. Treatment of multiple sclerosis in children and adolescents. *Expert Opin. Pharmacother.* **2010**, *11*, 505–520. [CrossRef]

59. Nortvedt, M.W.; Riise, T.; Frugard, J.; Mohn, J.; Bakke, A.; Skar, A.B. Prevalence of bladder, bowel and sexual problems among multiple sclerosis patients two to five years after diagnosis. *Mult. Scler.* **2007**, *13*, 106–112. [CrossRef]

60. Munteis, E.; Andreu, M.; Tellez, M.J.; Mon, D.; Ois, A.; Roquer, J. Anorectal dysfunction in multiple sclerosis. *Mult. Scler.* **2006**, *12*, 215–218. [CrossRef] [PubMed]

61. Tenembaum, S.; Chitnis, T.; Ness, J.; Hahn, J.S. International Pediatric MSSG. Acute disseminated encephalomyelitis. *Neurology* **2007**, *68* (Suppl. S2), S23–S36. [CrossRef]

62. Schwarz, S.; Mohr, A.; Knauth, M.; Wildemann, B.; Storch-Hagenlocher, B. Acute disseminated encephalomyelitis: A follow-up study of 40 adult patients. *Neurology* **2001**, *22*, 1313–1318. [CrossRef]

63. Sakakibara, R.; Uchiyama, T.; Liu, Z.; Yamamoto, T.; Ito, T.; Uzawa, A.; Suenaga, T.; Kanai, K.; Awa, Y.; Sugiyama, Y.; et al. Meningitis-retention syndrome. An unrecognized clinical condition. *J. Neurol.* **2005**, *252*, 1495–1499. [CrossRef]

64. Wender, M. Acute disseminated encephalomyelitis (ADEM). *J. Neuroimmunol.* **2011**, *231*, 92–99. [CrossRef]

65. Goh, K.J.; Khalifa, W.; Anslow, P.; Cadoux-Hudson, T.; Donaghy, M. The clinical syndrome associated with lumbar spinal stenosis. *Eur. Neurol.* **2004**, *52*, 242–249. [CrossRef]

66. Schkrohowsky, J.G.; Hoernschemeyer, D.G.; Carson, B.S.; Ain, M.C. Early presentation of spinal stenosis in achondroplasia. *J. Pediatr. Orthop.* **2007**, *27*, 119–122. [CrossRef]

67. Tubbs, R.S.; Oakes, W.J.; Blount, J.P. Isolated atlantal stenosis in a patient with idiopathic growth hormone deficiency, and Klippel-Feil and Duane's syndromes. *Childs Nerv. Syst.* **2005**, *21*, 421–424. [CrossRef] [PubMed]

68. McDermott, C.J.; Shaw, P.J. Diagnosis and management of motor neurone disease. *BMJ* **2008**, *336*, 658–662. [CrossRef] [PubMed]

69. Szobor, A.; Máttyus, A.; Molnár, J. Myasthenia gravis in childhood and adolescence. Report on 209 patients and review of the literature. *Acta Paediatr. Hung.* **1988**, *29*, 299–312.

70. Silveri, M.; De Gennaro, M.; Gatti, C.; Bizzarri, C.; Mosiello, G.; Cappa, M. Voiding dysfunction in x-linked adrenoleukodystrophy: Symptom score and urodynamic findings. *J. Urol.* **2004**, *171*, 2651–2653. [CrossRef]

71. Kim, M.Y.; Kim, J.H.; Cho, M.H.; Choi, Y.H.; Kim, S.H.; Im, Y.J.; Park, K.; Kang, H.G.; Chae, J.H.; Cheong, H.I. Urological Problems in Patients with Menkes Disease. *J. Korean Med. Sci.* **2019**, *34*, e4. [CrossRef]

72. Chung, E.A.; Emmanuel, A.V. Gastrointestinal symptoms related to autonomic dysfunction following spinal cord injury. *Prog. Brain Res.* **2006**, *152*, 317–333. [CrossRef]

73. Brookes, S.J.; Dinning, P.G.; Gladman, M.A. Neuroanatomy and physiology of colorectal function and defaecation: From basic science to human clinical studies. *Neurogastroenterol. Motil.* **2009**, *21* (Suppl. S2), 9–19. [CrossRef]

74. Palit, S.; Lunniss, P.J.; Scott, S.M. The physiology of human defecation. *Dig. Dis. Sci.* **2012**, *57*, 1445–1464. [CrossRef] [PubMed]
75. Krogh, K.; Nielsen, J.; Djurhuus, J.C.; Mosdal, C.; Sabroe, S.; Laurberg, S. Colorectal function in patients with spinal cord lesions. *Dis. Colon Rectum* **1997**, *40*, 1233–1239. [CrossRef] [PubMed]
76. Leduc, B.E.; Giasson, M.; Favreau-Ethier, M.; Lepage, Y. Colonic transit time after spinal cord injury. *J. Spinal Cord Med.* **1997**, *20*, 416–421. [CrossRef] [PubMed]
77. Krogh, K.; Mosdal, C.; Laurberg, S. Gastrointestinal and segmental colonic transit times in patients with acute and chronic spinal cord lesions. *Spinal Cord* **2000**, *38*, 615–621. [CrossRef] [PubMed]
78. Di Lorenzo, C.; Benninga, M.A. Pathophysiology of pediatric fecal incontinence. *Gastroenterology* **2004**, *126* (Suppl. S1), S33–S40. [CrossRef] [PubMed]
79. Emmanuel, A.V.; Chung, E.A.; Kamm, M.A.F.; Middleton, F. Relationship between gut-specific autonomic testing and bowel dysfunction in spinal cord injury patients. *Spinal Cord* **2009**, *47*, 623–627. [CrossRef]
80. Banwell, J.G.; Creasey, G.H.; Aggarwal, A.M.; Mortimer, J.T. Management of the neurogenic bowel in patients with spinal cord injury. *Urol. Clin. N. Am.* **1993**, *20*, 517–526. [CrossRef]
81. Camilleri, M.; Bharucha, A.E. Gastrointestinal dysfunction in neurologic disease. *Semin. Neurol.* **1996**, *16*, 203–216. [CrossRef]
82. Stiens, S.A.; Bergman, S.B.; Goetz, L.L. Neurogenic bowel dysfunction after spinal cord injury: Clinical evaluation and rehabilitative management. *Arch. Phys. Med. Rehabil.* **1997**, *78* (Suppl. S3), S86–S102. [CrossRef]
83. Doolin, E. Bowel management for patients with myelodysplasia. *Surg. Clin. N. Am.* **2006**, *86*, 505–514. [CrossRef]
84. Garman, K.M.; Ficca, M. Managing encopresis in the elementary school setting: The school nurse's role. *J. Sch. Nurs.* **2012**, *28*, 175–180. [CrossRef] [PubMed]
85. McClurg, D.; Norton, C. What is the best way to manage neurogenic bowel dysfunction? *BMJ* **2016**, *354*, i3931. [CrossRef] [PubMed]
86. Velde, S.V.; Biervliet, S.V.; Bruyne, R.D.; Winckel, M.V. A systematic review on bowel management and the success rate of the various treatment modalities in spina bifida patients. *Spinal Cord* **2013**, *51*, 873–881. [CrossRef] [PubMed]
87. Wide, P.; Glad Mattsson, G.; Drott, P.; Mattsson, S. Independence does not come with the method—Treatment of neurogenic bowel dysfunction in children with myelomeningocele. *Acta Paediatr.* **2014**, *103*, 1159–1164. [CrossRef]
88. Benevento, B.T.; Sipski, M.L. Neurogenic bladder, neurogenic bowel, and sexual dysfunction in people with spinal cord injury. *Phys. Ther.* **2002**, *82*, 601–612. [CrossRef]
89. Benninga, M.A.; Tabbers, M.M.; van Rijn, R.R. How to use a plain abdominal radiograph in children with functional defecation disorders. *Arch. Dis. Child Educ. Pract. Ed.* **2016**, *101*, 187–193. [CrossRef] [PubMed]
90. Kim, E.R.; Rhee, P.L. How to interpret a functional or motility test—Colon transit study. *J. Neurogastroenterol. Motil.* **2012**, *18*, 94–99. [CrossRef] [PubMed]
91. Noviello, C.; Cobellis, G.; Papparella, A.; Amici, G.; Martino, A. Role of anorectal manometry in children with severe constipation. *Colorectal. Dis.* **2009**, *11*, 480–484. [CrossRef] [PubMed]
92. Baharestani, M.M.; Ratliff, C.R. Pressure ulcers in neonates and children: An NPUAP white paper. *Adv. Skin. Wound Care* **2007**, *20*, 208–220. [CrossRef]
93. Kewalramani, L.S. Autonomic dysreflexia in traumatic myelopathy. *Am. J. Phys. Med.* **1980**, *59*, 1–21.
94. Krogh, K.; Christensen, P.; Sabroe, S.; Laurberg, S. Neurogenic bowel dysfunction score. *Spinal Cord* **2006**, *44*, 625–631. [CrossRef] [PubMed]
95. Kelly, M.S.; Hannan, M.; Cassidy, B.; Hidas, G.; Selby, B.; Khoury, A.E.; McLorie, G. Development, reliability and validation of a neurogenic bowel dysfunction score in pediatric patients with spina bifida. *Neurourol. Urodynam.* **2016**, *35*, 212–217. [CrossRef]
96. Williams, C.L.; Dwyer, J.; Agostoni, C.; Hillemeier, C.; Kimm, S.Y.S.; Kwiterovich, P.O.; McClung, J.; Nicklas, T.A.; Saldanha, L. A Summary of Conference Recommendations on Dietary Fiber in Childhood. *Pediatrics* **1995**, *96*, 1023–1028.
97. Suares, N.C.; Ford, A.C. Systematic review: The effects of fibre in the management of chronic idiopathic constipation. *Aliment. Pharmacol. Ther.* **2011**, *33*, 895–901. [CrossRef] [PubMed]
98. Markland, A.D.; Palsson, O.; Goode, P.S.; Burgio, K.L.; Busby-Whitehead, J.; Whitehead, W.E. Association of low dietary intake of fiber and liquids with constipation: Evidence from the National Health and Nutrition Examination Survey. *Am. J. Gastroenterol.* **2013**, *108*, 796–803. [CrossRef]
99. Cameron, K.J.; Nyulasi, I.B.; Collier, G.R.; Brown, D.J. Assessment of the effect of increased dietary fibre intake on bowel function in patients with spinal cord injury. *Spinal Cord* **1996**, *34*, 277–283. [CrossRef] [PubMed]
100. Bischoff, A.; Levitt, M.A.; Bauer, C.; Jackson, L.; Holder, M.; Peña, A. Treatment of fecal incontinence with a comprehensive bowel management program. *J. Pediatr. Surg.* **2009**, *44*, 1278–1283. [CrossRef]
101. Choi, E.K.; Shin, S.H.; Im, Y.J.; Kim, M.J.; Han, S.W. The effects of transanal irrigation as a stepwise bowel management program on the quality of life of children with spina bifida and their caregivers. *Spinal Cord* **2013**, *51*, 384–388. [CrossRef]
102. Krassioukov, A.; Eng, J.J.; Claxton, G.; Sakakibara, B.M.; Shum, S. Neurogenic bowel management after spinal cord injury: A systematic review of the evidence. *Spinal Cord* **2010**, *48*, 718–733. [CrossRef]
103. Lemelle, J.L.; Guillemin, F.; Aubert, D.; Guys, J.M.; Lottmann, H.; Lortat-Jacob, S.; Moscovici, J.; Mouriquand, P.; Ruffion, A.; Schmitt, M. A multicentre study of the management of disorders of defecation in patients with spina bifida. *Neurogastroenterol. Motil.* **2006**, *18*, 123–128. [CrossRef] [PubMed]

104. Institute of Medicine. *Dietary Reference Intakes for Water, Potassium, Sodium, Chloride, and Sulfate*; The National Academies Press: Washington, DC, USA, 2005; p. 638.

105. Peters, H.P.; De Vries, W.R.; Vanberge-Henegouwen, G.P.; Akkermans, L.M. Potential benefits and hazards of physical activity and exercise on the gastrointestinal tract. *Gut* **2001**, *48*, 435–439. [CrossRef]

106. De Oliveira, E.P.; Burini, R.C. The impact of physical exercise on the gastrointestinal tract. *Curr. Opin. Clin. Nutr. Metab. Care* **2009**, *12*, 533–538. [CrossRef] [PubMed]

107. Speelman, A.D.; van de Warrenburg, B.P.; van Nimwegen, M.; Petzinger, G.M.; Munneke, M.; Bloem, B.R. How might physical activity benefit patients with Parkinson disease? *Nat. Rev. Neurol.* **2011**, *7*, 528–534. [CrossRef] [PubMed]

108. Meshkinpour, H.; Selod, S.; Movahedi, H.; Nami, N.; James, N.; Wilson, A. Effects of regular exercise in management of chronic idiopathic constipation. *Dig. Dis. Sci.* **1998**, *43*, 2379–2383. [CrossRef]

109. Wald, A. Constipation in the primary care setting: Current concepts and misconceptions. *Am. J. Med.* **2006**, *119*, 736–739. [CrossRef] [PubMed]

110. Robertson, G.; Meshkinpour, H.; Vandenberg, K.; James, N.; Cohen, A.; Wilson, A. Effects of exercise on total and segmental colon transit. *J. Clin. Gastroenterol.* **1993**, *16*, 300–303. [CrossRef]

111. Aaronson, M.J.; Freed, M.M.; Burakoff, R. Colonic myoelectric activity in persons with spinal cord injury. *Dig. Dis. Sci.* **1985**, *30*, 295–300. [CrossRef]

112. Menardo, G.; Bausano, G.; Corazziari, E.; Fazio, A.; Marangi, A.; Genta, V.; Marenco, G. Large-bowel transit in paraplegic patients. *Dis. Colon Rectum* **1987**, *30*, 924–928. [CrossRef] [PubMed]

113. Walter, S.A.; Morren, G.L.; Ryn, A.K.; Hallböök, O. Rectal pressure response to a meal in patients with high spinal cord injury. *Arch. Phys. Med. Rehabil.* **2003**, *84*, 108–111. [CrossRef]

114. Sinclair, M. The use of abdominal massage to treat chronic constipation. *J. Bodyw. Mov. Ther.* **2011**, *15*, 436–445. [CrossRef]

115. Han, T.R.; Kim, J.H.; Kwon, B.S. Chronic gastrointestinal problems and bowel dysfunction in patients with spinal cord injury. *Spinal Cord* **1998**, *36*, 485–490. [CrossRef]

116. Ayaş, S.; Leblebici, B.; Sözay, S.; Bayramoğlu, M.; Niron, E.A. The effect of abdominal massage on bowel function in patients with spinal cord injury. *Am. J. Phys. Med. Rehabil.* **2006**, *85*, 951–955. [CrossRef] [PubMed]

117. Brookes, S.J.; Chen, B.N.; Costa, M.; Humphreys, C.M. Initiation of peristalsis by circumferential stretch of flat sheets of guinea-pig ileum. *J. Physiol.* **1999**, *516*, 525–538. [CrossRef]

118. Liu, Z.; Sakakibara, R.; Odaka, T.; Uchiyama, T.; Yamamoto, T.; Ito, T.; Hattori, T. Mechanism of abdominal massage for difficult defecation in a patient with myelopathy (HAM/TSP). *J. Neurol.* **2005**, *252*, 1280–1282. [CrossRef]

119. Lämås, K.; Lindholm, L.; Stenlund, H.; Engström, B.; Jacobsson, C. Effects of abdominal massage in management of constipation— A randomized controlled trial. *Int. J. Nurs. Stud.* **2009**, *46*, 759–767. [CrossRef]

120. Choi, H.; Kim, S.J.; Oh, J.; Lee, M.N.; Kim, S.; Kang, K.A. The effects of massage therapy on physical growth and gastrointestinal function in premature infants: A pilot study. *J. Child Health Care* **2016**, *20*, 394–404. [CrossRef] [PubMed]

121. Turan, N.; Aşt, T.A. The Effect of Abdominal Massage on Constipation and Quality of Life. *Gastroenterol. Nurs.* **2016**, *39*, 48–59. [CrossRef] [PubMed]

122. Shafik, A. Recto-colic reflex: Role in the defecation mechanism. *Int. Surg.* **1996**, *81*, 292–294.

123. Whitehead, W.E.; Parker, L.H.; Masek, B.J.; Cataldo, M.F.; Freeman, J.M. Biofeedback treatment of fecal incontinence in patients with myelomeningocele. *Dev. Med. Child Neurol.* **1981**, *23*, 313–322. [CrossRef]

124. Wald, A. Use of biofeedback in treatment of fecal incontinence in patients with meningomyelocele. *Pediatrics* **1981**, *68*, 45–49. [CrossRef]

125. Whitehead, W.E.; Parker, L.; Bosmajian, L.; Morrill-Corbin, E.D.; Middaugh, S.; Garwood, M.; Cataldo, M.F.; Freeman, J. Treatment of fecal incontinence in children with spina bifida: Comparison of biofeedback and behavior modification. *Arch. Phys. Med. Rehabil.* **1986**, *67*, 218–224.

126. Loening-Baucke, V.; Desch, L.; Wolraich, M. Biofeedback training for patients with myelomeningocele and fecal incontinence. *Dev. Med. Child Neurol.* **1988**, *30*, 781–790. [CrossRef] [PubMed]

127. Rao, S.S.; Benninga, M.A.; Bharucha, A.E.; Chiarioni, G.; Di Lorenzo, C.; Whitehead, W.E. ANMS-ESNM position paper and consensus guidelines on biofeedback therapy for anorectal disorders. *Neurogastroenterol. Motil.* **2015**, *27*, 594–609. [CrossRef] [PubMed]

128. Veiga, M.L.; Lordêlo, P.; Farias, T.; Barroso, U., Jr. Evaluation of constipation after parasacral transcutaneous electrical nerve stimulation in children with lower urinary tract dysfunction—A pilot study. *J. Pediatr. Urol.* **2013**, *9*, 622–626. [CrossRef] [PubMed]

129. Ismail, K.A.; Chase, J.; Gibb, S.; Clarke, M.; Catto-Smith, A.G.; Robertson, V.J.; Hutson, J.M.; Southwell, B.R. Daily transabdominal electrical stimulation at home increased defecation in children with slow-transit constipation: A pilot study. *J. Pediatr. Surg.* **2009**, *44*, 2388–2392. [CrossRef]

130. Wright, A.J.; Haddad, M. Electroneurostimulation for the management of bladder bowel dysfunction in childhood. *Eur. J. Paediatr. Neurol.* **2017**, *21*, 67–74. [CrossRef]

131. Mentes, B.B.; Yüksel, O.; Aydin, A.; Tezcaner, T.; Leventoğlu, A.; Aytaç, B. Posterior tibial nerve stimulation for faecal incontinence after partial spinal injury: Preliminary report. *Tech. Coloproctol.* **2007**, *11*, 115–119. [CrossRef]

132. Leroi, A.M.; Siproudhis, L.; Etienney, I.; Damon, H.; Zerbib, F.; Amarenco, G.; Vitton, V.; Faucheron, J.L.; Thomas, C.; Mion, F.; et al. Transcutaneous electrical tibial nerve stimulation in the treatment of fecal incontinence: A randomized trial (CONSORT 1a). *Am. J. Gastroenterol.* **2012**, *107*, 1888–1896. [CrossRef]

133. Palmer, L.S.; Richards, I.; Kaplan, W.E. Transrectal electrostimulation therapy for neuropathic bowel dysfunction in children with myelomeningocele. *J. Urol.* **1997**, *157*, 1449–1452. [CrossRef]

134. Han, S.W.; Kim, M.J.; Kim, J.H.; Hong, C.H.; Kim, J.W.; Noh, J.Y. Intravesical electrical stimulation improves neurogenic bowel dysfunction in children with spina bifida. *J. Urol.* **2004**, *171*, 2648–2650. [CrossRef]

135. Coccorullo, P.; Strisciuglio, C.; Martinelli, M.; Miele, E.; Greco, L.; Staiano, A. Lactobacillus reuteri (DSM 17938) in infants with functional chronic constipation: A double-blind, randomized, placebo-controlled study. *J. Pediatr.* **2010**, *157*, 598–602. [CrossRef] [PubMed]

136. Rendeli, C.; Ausili, E.; Tabacco, F.; Focarelli, B.; Pantanella, A.; Di Rocco, C.; Genovese, O.; Fundarò, C. Polyethylene glycol 4000 vs. lactulose for the treatment of neurogenic constipation in myelomeningocele children: A randomized-controlled clinical trial. *Aliment. Pharmacol. Ther.* **2006**, *23*, 1259–1265. [CrossRef] [PubMed]

137. Lewis, S.J.; Heaton, K.W. Stool form scale as a useful guide to intestinal transit time. *Scand. J. Gastroenterol.* **1997**, *32*, 920–924. [CrossRef]

138. House, J.G.; Stiens, S.A. Pharmacologically initiated defecation for persons with spinal cord injury: Effectiveness of three agents. *Arch. Phys. Med. Rehabil.* **1997**, *78*, 1062–1065. [CrossRef]

139. Dunn, K.L.; Galka, M.L. A comparison of the effectiveness of Therevac SB and bisacodyl suppositories in SCI patients' bowel programs. *Rehabil. Nurs* **1994**, *19*, 334–338. [CrossRef] [PubMed]

140. Frisbie, J.H. Improved bowel care with a polyethylene glycol based bisacadyl suppository. *J. Spinal. Cord. Med.* **1997**, *20*, 227–229. [CrossRef] [PubMed]

141. Coggrave, M.; Emmanuel, A. Neurogenic bowel management. In *Pelvic Organ Dysfunction in Neurological Disease—Clinical Management and Rehabilitation*; Fowler, C., Panicker, J., Emmanuel, A., Eds.; Cambridge University Press: Cambridge, UK, 2010; pp. 138–152.

142. Bischoff, A.; Levitt, M.A.; Peña, A. Bowel management for the treatment of pediatric fecal incontinence. *Pediatr. Surg. Int.* **2009**, *25*, 1027–1042. [CrossRef] [PubMed]

143. Peña, A.; De La Torre, L.; Belkind-Gerson, J.; Lovell, M.; Ketzer, J.; Bealer, J.; Bischoff, A. Enema-Induced spastic left colon syndrome: An unintended consequence of chronic enema use. *J. Pediatr. Surg.* **2021**, *56*, 424–428. [CrossRef]

144. Christensen, P.; Olsen, N.; Krogh, K.; Bacher, T.; Laurberg, S. Scintigraphic assessment of retrograde colonic washout in fecal incontinence and constipation. *Dis. Colon Rectum* **2003**, *46*, 68–76. [CrossRef] [PubMed]

145. Ausili, E.; Focarelli, B.; Tabacco, F.; Murolo, D.; Sigismondi, M.; Gasbarrini, A.; Rendeli, C. Transanal irrigation in myelomeningo-cele children: An alternative, safe and valid approach for neurogenic constipation. *Spinal Cord* **2010**, *48*, 560–565. [CrossRef]

146. Kelly, M.S.; Dorgalli, C.; McLorie, G.; Khoury, A.E. Prospective evaluation of Peristeen® transanal irrigation system with the validated neurogenic bowel dysfunction score sheet in the pediatric population. *Neurourol. Urodyn.* **2017**, *36*, 632–635. [CrossRef]

147. Gourcerol, G.; Vitton, V.; Leroi, A.M.; Michot, F.; Abysique, A.; Bouvier, M. How sacral nerve stimulation works in patients with faecal incontinence. *Colorectal. Dis.* **2011**, *13*, e203–e211. [CrossRef]

148. Sheldon, R.; Kiff, E.S.; Clarke, A.; Harris, M.L.; Hamdy, S. Sacral nerve stimulation reduces corticoanal excitability in patients with faecal incontinence. *Br. J. Surg.* **2005**, *92*, 1423–1431. [CrossRef]

149. Patton, V.; Stewart, P.; Lubowski, D.Z.; Cook, I.J.; Dinning, P.G. Sacral Nerve Stimulation Fails to Offer Long-term Benefit in Patients With Slow-Transit Constipation. *Dis. Colon Rectum* **2016**, *59*, 878–885. [CrossRef] [PubMed]

150. Van der Wilt, A.A.; van Wunnik, B.P.W.; Sturkenboom, R.; Han-Geurts, I.J.; Melenhorst, J.; Benninga, M.A.; Baeten, C.G.M.I.; Breukink, S.O. Sacral neuromodulation in children and adolescents with chronic constipation refractory to conservative treatment. *Int. J. Colorectal. Dis.* **2016**, *31*, 1459–1466. [CrossRef]

151. Holzer, B.; Rosen, H.R.; Novi, G.; Ausch, C.; Hölbling, N.; Schiessel, R. Sacral nerve stimulation for neurogenic faecal incontinence. *Br. J. Surg.* **2007**, *94*, 749–753. [CrossRef] [PubMed]

152. Cotterill, N.; Madersbacher, H.; Wyndaele, J.J.; Apostolidis, A.; Drake, M.J.; Gajewski, J.; Heesakkers, J.; Panicker, J.; Radziszewski, P.; Sakakibara, R.; et al. Neurogenic bowel dysfunction: Clinical management recommendations of the Neurologic Incontinence Committee of the Fifth International Consultation on Incontinence 2013. *Neurourol. Urodyn.* **2018**, *37*, 46–53. [CrossRef]

153. Kelly, M.S.; Wiener, J.S.; Liu, T.; Patel, P.; Castillo, H.; Castillo, J.; Dicianno, B.E.; Jasien, J.; Peterson, P.; Routh, J.C.; et al. Neurogenic bowel treatments and continence in children and adults with myelomeningocele. *J. Pediatr. Rehabil. Med.* **2020**, *13*, 685–693. [CrossRef]

154. Ambartsumyan, L.; Rodriguez, L. Bowel management in children with spina bifida. *J. Pediatr. Rehabil. Med.* **2018**, *11*, 293–301. [CrossRef]

155. Gor, R.A.; Katorski, J.P.; Elliott, S.P. Medical and surgical management of neurogenic bowel. *Curr. Opin. Urol.* **2016**, *26*, 369–375. [CrossRef]

156. Johnston, A.W.; Wiener, J.S.; Purves, J.T. Pediatric neurogenic bladder and bowel dysfunction: Will my child ever be out of diapers? *Eur. Urol. Focus* **2020**, *6*, 838–867. [CrossRef]

157. Wong, D.W.; Jensen, L.L.; Bartolo, D.C.C.; Rothenberger, D.A. Artificial anal sphincter. *Dis. Colon Rectum* **1996**, *39*, 1345–1351. [CrossRef] [PubMed]

158. Griffiths, D.M.; Malone, P.S. The Malone antegrade continence enema (MACE). *J. Pediatr. Surg.* **1995**, *30*, 68–71. [CrossRef]
159. Ok, J.; Kurzrock, E.A. Objective measurement of quality of life changes after ACE Malone using FICQOL survey. *J. Pediatr. Urol.* **2011**, *7*, 389–393. [CrossRef]
160. Brinas, P.; Zalay, N.; Philis, A.; Castel-Lacanal, E.; Barrieu, M.; Portier, G. Use of Malone antegrade continence enemas in neurological bowel dysfunction. *J. Visc. Surg.* **2020**, *157*, 453–459. [CrossRef] [PubMed]
161. Bani-Hani, A.H.; Cain, M.P.; Kaefer, M.; Meldrum, K.K.; King, S.; Johnson, C.S.; Rink, R.C. The Malone Antegrade Continence Enema: Single Institutional Review. *J. Urol.* **2008**, *180*, 1106–1110. [CrossRef] [PubMed]
162. VanderBrink, B.A.; Cain, M.P.; Kaefer, M.; Meldrum, K.K.; Misseri, R.; Rink, R.C. Outcomes following Malone antegrade continence enema and their surgical revisions. *J. Pediatr. Surg.* **2013**, *48*, 2134–2139. [CrossRef] [PubMed]
163. Lynch, A.; Beasley, S.; Robertson, R.; Morreau, P.N. Comparison of results of laparoscopic and open antegrade continence enema procedures. *Pediatr. Surg. Int.* **1999**, *15*, 343–346. [CrossRef] [PubMed]
164. Kim, J.; Beasley, S.W.; Maoate, K. Appendicostomy Stomas and Antegrade Colonic Irrigation After Laparoscopic Antegrade Continence Enema. *J. Laparoendosc. Adv. Surg. Tech.* **2006**, *16*, 400–403. [CrossRef] [PubMed]
165. Malone, P.; Curry, J.; Osborne, A. The antegrade continence enema procedure why, when and how? *World J. Urol.* **1998**, *16*, 274–278. [CrossRef] [PubMed]
166. Bevill, M.D.; Bonnett, K.; Arlen, A.; Cooper, C.; Baxter, C.; Storm, D.W. Outcomes and satisfaction in pediatric patients with Chait cecostomy tubes. *J. Pediatr. Urol.* **2017**, *13*, 365–370. [CrossRef]
167. Rawat, D.J.; Haddad, M.; Geoghegan, N.; Clarke, S.; Fell, J.M. Percutaneous endoscopic colostomy of the left colon: A new technique for management of intractable constipation in children. *Gastrointest. Endosc.* **2004**, *60*, 39–43. [CrossRef]
168. Kelly, M.S. Malone antegrade continence enemas vs. cecostomy vs. transanal irrigation—What is new and how do we counsel patients? *Curr. Urol. Rep.* **2019**, *20*, 41. [CrossRef]
169. Beckers, G.M.A.; de Meij, T.G.J. Peritonitis After Endoscopic Caecostomy With a Chait Trapdoor Catheter: What Lessons Can Be Learned? *J. Pediatr. Gastroenterol. Nutr.* **2012**, *55*, 217–218. [CrossRef]
170. Hocevar, B.; Gray, M. Intestinal diversion (colostomy or ileostomy) in patients with severe bowel dysfunction following spinal cord injury. *J. Wound Ostomy Cont. Nurs.* **2008**, *35*, 159–166. [CrossRef]
171. Coggrave, M.; Ingram, R.M.; Gardner, B.P.; Norton, C.S. The impact of stoma for bowel management after spinal cord injury. *Spinal Cord* **2012**, *50*, 848–852. [CrossRef]
172. Branagan, G.; Tromans, A.; Finnis, D. Effect of stoma formation on bowel care and quality of life in patients with spinal cord injury. *Spinal Cord* **2003**, *41*, 680–693. [CrossRef] [PubMed]
173. Cooper, E.A.; Bonne Lee, B.; Muhlmann, M. Outcomes following stoma formation in patients with spinal cord injury. *Colorectal Dis.* **2019**, *21*, 1415–1420. [CrossRef] [PubMed]
174. Boucher, M.; Dukes, S.; Bryan, S.; Branagan, G. Early colostomy formation can improve independence following spinal cord injury and increase acceptability of bowel management. *Top. Spinal Cord Inj. Rehabil.* **2019**, *25*, 23–30. [CrossRef]
175. Gasior, A.; Reck, C.; Vilanova-Sanchez, A.; Diefenbach, K.A.; Yacob, D.; Lu, P.; Vaz, K.; Di Lorenzo, C.; Levitt, M.A.; Wood, R.J. Surgical management of functional constipation: An intermediate report of a new approach using laparoscopic sigmoid resection combined with Malone appendicostomy. *J. Pediatr. Surg.* **2018**, *53*, 1160–1162. [CrossRef] [PubMed]
176. Kilpatrick, J.A.; Zobell, S.; Leeflang, E.J.; Cao, D.; Mammen, L.; Rollins, M.D. Intermediate and long-term outcomes of a bowel management program for children with severe constipation or fecal incontinence. *J. Pediatr. Surg.* **2020**, *55*, 545–548. [CrossRef]
177. Halleran, D.R.; Sloots, C.E.J.; Fuller, M.K.; Diefenbach, K. Adjuncts to bowel management for fecal incontinence and constipation, the role of surgery; appendicostomy, cecostomy, neoappendicostomy, and colonic resection. *Sem. Pediatr. Surg.* **2020**, *29*, 150998. [CrossRef] [PubMed]
178. Siminas, S.; Losty, P.D. Current surgical management of pediatric idiopathic constipation: A systematic review of published studies. *Ann. Surg.* **2015**, *262*, 925–933. [CrossRef]

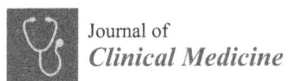

Journal of
Clinical Medicine

MDPI

Review

Faecal Microbiota in Patients with Neurogenic Bowel Dysfunction and Spinal Cord Injury or Multiple Sclerosis—A Systematic Review

Willemijn Faber [1,*], Janneke Stolwijk-Swuste [2], Florian van Ginkel [3], Janneke Nachtegaal [4], Erwin Zoetendal [5], Renate Winkels [6] and Ben Witteman [6]

[1] Heliomare Rehabilitation Centre, 1949 EC Wijk aan Zee, The Netherlands
[2] Center of Excellence for Rehabilitation Medicine, Brain Center Rudolf Magnus, University Medical Center Utrecht and De Hoogstraat Rehabilitation, Utrecht University, 3583 TM Utrecht, The Netherlands; j.stolwijk@dehoogstraat.nl
[3] Faculty of Medicine, Utrecht University, 3584 CG Utrecht, The Netherlands; f.vanginkel@students.uu.nl
[4] Heliomare Rehabilitation Center, Department of Research & Development, 1949 EC Wijk aan Zee, The Netherlands; J.Nachtegaal@heliomare.nl
[5] Laboratory of Microbiology, Wageningen University and Research, Wageningen University, 6708 PB Wageningen, The Netherlands; erwin.zoetendal@wur.nl
[6] Division of Human Nutrition and health, Wageningen University and Research, Wageningen University, 6708 PB Wageningen, The Netherlands; renate.winkels@wur.nl (R.W.); ben.witteman@wur.nl (B.W.)
* Correspondence: W.Faber@heliomare.nl; Tel.: +31-88-9208257

Citation: Faber, W.; Stolwijk-Swuste, J.; van Ginkel, F.; Nachtegaal, J.; Zoetendal, E.; Winkels, R.; Witteman, B. Faecal Microbiota in Patients with Neurogenic Bowel Dysfunction and Spinal Cord Injury or Multiple Sclerosis—A Systematic Review. *J. Clin. Med.* **2021**, *10*, 1598. https://doi.org/10.3390/jcm10081598

Academic Editor: Romain Coriat

Received: 11 February 2021
Accepted: 4 April 2021
Published: 9 April 2021

Publisher's Note: MDPI stays neutral with regard to jurisdictional claims in published maps and institutional affiliations.

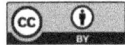

Copyright: © 2021 by the authors. Licensee MDPI, Basel, Switzerland. This article is an open access article distributed under the terms and conditions of the Creative Commons Attribution (CC BY) license (https://creativecommons.org/licenses/by/4.0/).

Abstract: Background: Neurogenic bowel dysfunction (NBD) frequently occurs in patients with spinal cord injury (SCI) and multiple sclerosis (MS) with comparable symptoms and is often difficult to treat. It has been suggested the gut microbiota might influence the course of NBD. We systematically reviewed the literature on the composition of the gut microbiota in SCI and MS, and the possible role of neurogenic bowel function, diet and antibiotic use. Methods: A systematic search was conducted in PubMed and Embase, which retrieved studies on the gut microbiota in SCI and MS. The Newcastle–Ottawa Quality Assessment Scale (NOS) was used to assess methodological quality. Results: We retrieved fourteen papers (four on SCI, ten on MS), describing the results of a total of 479 patients. The number of patients per study varied from 13 to 89 with an average of 34. Thirteen papers were observational studies and one study was an intervention study. The studies were case control studies in which the gut microbiota composition was determined by 16S rRNA gene sequencing. The methodological quality of the studies was mostly rated to be moderate. Results of two studies suggested that alpha diversity in chronic SCI patients is lower compared to healthy controls (HC), whereas results from five studies suggest that the alpha diversity of MS patients is similar compared to healthy subjects. The taxonomic changes in MS and SCI studies are diverse. Most studies did not account for possible confounding by diet, antibiotic use and bowel function. Conclusion: Based on these 14 papers, we cannot draw strong conclusions on the composition of the gut microbiota in SCI and MS patients. Putatively, alpha diversity in chronic SCI patients may be lower compared to healthy controls, while in MS patients, alpha diversity may be similar or lower compared to healthy controls. Future studies should provide a more detailed description of clinical characteristics of participants and of diet, antibiotic use and bowel function in order to make valid inferences on changes in gut microbiota and the possible role of diet, antibiotic use and bowel function in those changes.

Keywords: spinal cord injury; multiple sclerosis; neurogenic bowel dysfunction; gut microbiota

1. Introduction

Multiple sclerosis (MS) has been estimated to affect 2.3 million people globally and prevalence of spinal cord injury (SCI) ranges from 223 to 755 per million people globally [1,2]. Both numbers are increasing each year. One of the most often reported secondary complications in individuals with SCI is neurogenic bowel dysfunction (NBD) [3]. NBD is a severe disabling impairment and can be caused by SCI and MS. It is defined as a colonic and/or anorectal dysfunction resulting from a lack of central nervous control [4]. SCI and MS patients often suffer from the same symptoms and the etiology, dysfunction of the spinal cord, is compatible. Bowel management can reduce the impact on a person's quality of life (QOL) and can prevent faecal incontinence and constipation [5,6]. Current guidelines refer to a stepped-up pyramid tool for bowel management in individuals with MS and SCI [7]. The first step in the pyramid is optimizing dietary and fluid adjustments or the use of stool modulating agents (e.g., stool softeners, stimulant laxatives and bulking agents) [8,9]. The next steps are the use of more invasive techniques, such as the perianal/rectal stimulation technique, a manual removal of faeces or transanal irrigation [10]. Finally, the implantation of electrical stimulation systems, antegrade colonic enemas or the formation of a bowel stoma are all possible treatment options if problems persist.

Of the MS patients, 39–73% report neurogenic bowel problems [11]. There appears to be a correlation between bowel problems and the Expanded Disability Status Scale (EDSS) and disease duration, but not the type of MS [12–16]. Surprisingly, MS patients with a short period of time since onset and a low disability can also have bowel problems, with severe constipation having been reported as the first symptom of MS [17]. MS patients score their bowel problems as the third-most bothersome symptom. These problems are a major cause of not being able to participate in society and work and account for a significant part of the daily routine [11].

From research done in the SCI rehabilitation centres in the Netherlands, we know that 31% of the sub-acute SCI patients are not satisfied with their bowel functions at the moment of discharge from their first inpatient rehabilitation. NBD can result in faecal incontinence, abdominal bloating, and constipation [5,6]. In the chronic phase, this percentage increases up to 80% [4]. In a survey among 1334 people with SCI, for instance, 39% reported constipation, 36% haemorrhoids, and 31% abdominal distension [4]. Other issues that were reported included diarrhoea and incontinence [8]. NBD following SCI has a huge impact on the QOL [8]. In people with faecal incontinence, 62% reported a negative effect on the QOL compared to 8% in controls [18]. A questionnaire completed by members of the Dutch Spinal Cord Injury Patient Society, showed bowel problems as the second most important topic that, according to patients, should be studied more.

It is hard to achieve adequate bowel management in NBD as bowel management is influenced by many factors such as diet, level of mobility or pharmacological treatment [4]. One of the factors could be the gut microbiota. There is some evidence that alteration of the gut microbiota could result in better bowel function in the healthy population, patients with Irritable Bowel Syndrome or SCI [3,19,20].

The composition and activity of the gut microbiota co-develop with the host from birth and is subject to a complex interplay. There are numerous host factors, such as age, gender, and ethnicity, as well as environmental factors related to our lifestyle that can influence the gut microbiota [21–24].

A large Flemish/Dutch study on gut microbiota variation in the average, healthy population showed that of all measured factors, stool consistency has the largest effect size [25]. The increase of transit time, independent of other factors, may affect the composition and metabolism of the gut microbiota as well. The transit time is one of the factors that explain some of the modifications seen in the gut microbiota of the elderly, as well as in patients with slow transit time [26]. Several studies with SCI patients show longer colon transit time compared to uncompromised subjects [27].

Alterations in diet, primarily influenced by the consumption of dietary fiber from fruits, vegetables, and other plant components, have been associated with changes in the gut microbiota. It has been reported that even a short-term dietary shift can significantly change gut microbiota [28]. NBD and altered colonic transit time in SCI and MS patients might lead to a change in the composition of the gut microbiota that might be influenced by a diet change. Therefore, the first step in bowel management in SCI and MS patients with NBD could be a specific diet to target the gut microbiota in order to improve the intestinal complications in SCI and MS patients.

In addition to the impact of diet, treatment with most antibiotics, especially broad-spectrum antibiotics, have also been shown to affect the gut microbiota composition. Antibiotic therapies may affect not only the target microorganisms but also the host-associated microbial communities, particularly those in the intestine [29]. In MS and SCI patients, neurogenic lower urinary tract dysfunction, respiratory and skin problems frequently occur [30] and hence this population is at risk of developing infections that often require antibiotic treatment [31,32]. Therefore, they might also be at risk of altered gut microbiota composition.

The following research questions for this systematic review are based on the possible NBD of SCI and MS patients, their frequent use of antibiotics and the distinct impact of diet: What is the difference in the composition of the gut microbiota, with focus on bacteria, of patients with SCI or MS compared to HC? What is the possible role of neurogenic bowel function, diet and antibiotic use on the composition of the gut microbiota?

2. Methods

2.1. Information Sources

This review was performed in accordance with the Preferred Reporting Items for Systematic Reviews and Meta-Analyses (PRISMA) [33]. Studies were identified by searching the National Library of Medicine (PubMed) and Excerpta Medica (Embase) for available studies on the gut microbiota of patients with NBD due to SCI or MS. The search was performed on 8 July 2020. Figure 1 shows the flowchart of studies through the screening process. The search terms consisted of the following keywords including Medical Subject Headings (MeSH)terms, synonyms and acronyms: "multiple sclerosis", "spinal cord injury", "gastrointestinal microbiome", "dysbiosis" and "stool sample". The full syntax can be found in Table A1.

2.2. Eligibility Criteria

Two independent reviewers (WF and FG) screened the studies on eligibility for inclusion in the review using Rayyan [34]. Firstly, studies were screened by title to exclude studies that clearly did not meet the eligibility criteria. Then, the abstracts of the remaining studies were screened and finally, the full-text articles were screened. On top of the database searches, after screening the abstracts, the reference lists were also checked to prevent missing relevant studies. Differences between the reviewers in agreement to include a study were assessed at both stages and were discussed to reach consensus.

Studies that met the following criteria were included:

- Study on the gut microbiota of patients with SCI or MS.
- Study included a group of HC.
- Participants were aged 18 years and older.
- Gut microbiota composition was determined by 16S rRNA gene sequencing.
- Published as full-text article in English in a peer-reviewed journal.

Studies which focused on Neuromyelitis Optica were excluded.

2.3. Data Extraction and Outcome Measures

WF extracted the data from the full-text articles, which was checked by a second reviewer (JN).

Extracted data included: (1) authors and publication year, (2) objective of the study, (3) characteristics of the included study sample (sample size, mean age, disease characteristics) (4) study design (including number of faecal samples taken), (5) outcome variables and potential confounding factors including use of antibiotics, bowel function, and diet, (6) results.

The main outcome was the difference between the composition of the gut microbiota of patients with NBD due to SCI or MS and that of HC. Differences in gut microbiota are defined as differences in diversity and taxonomic differences. Alpha diversity provides a measure of the variety of the species represented within the sample.

In addition, an evaluation took place of which studies took into account the role of antibiotic use, diet, and bowel function on the gut microbiota.

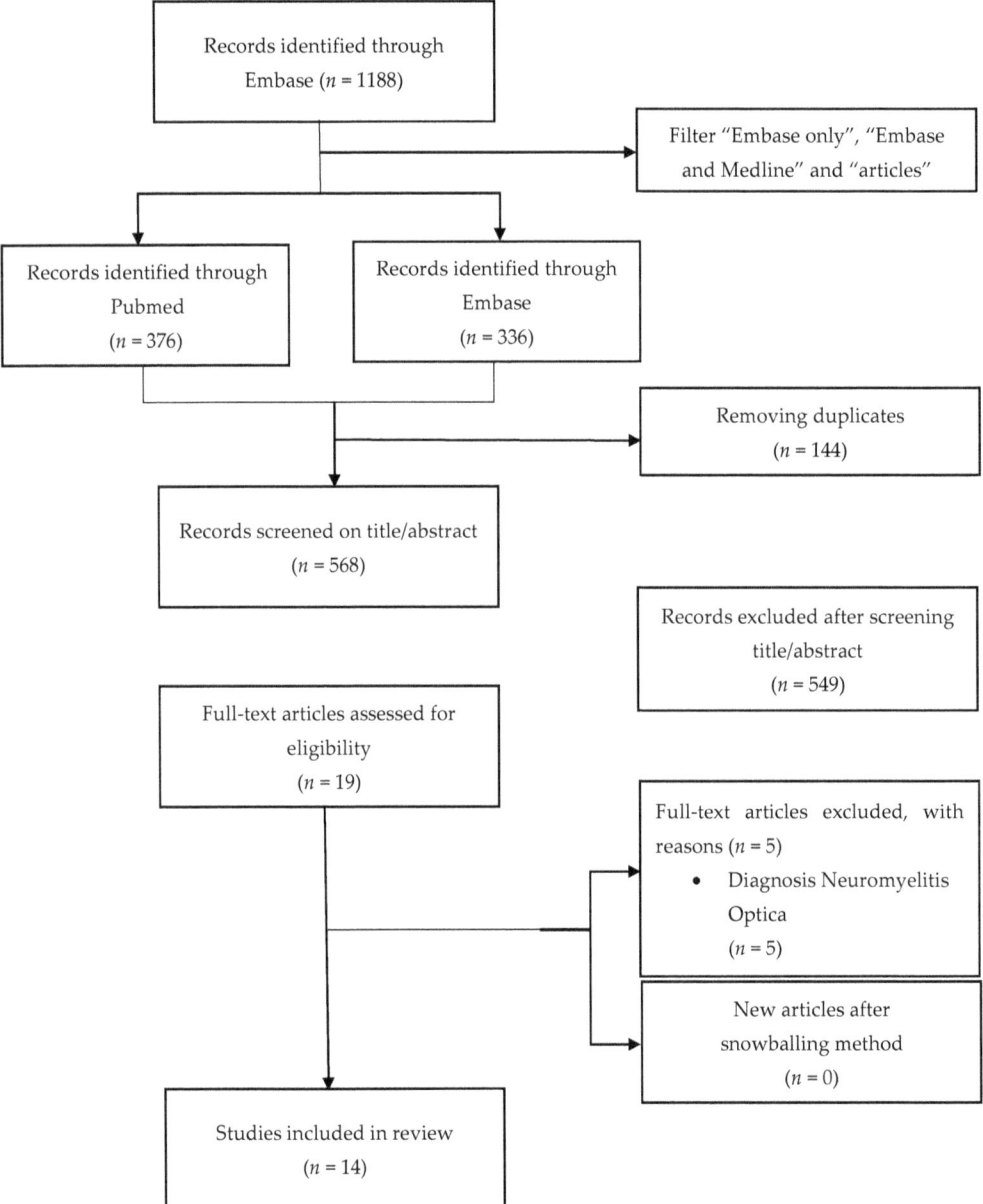

Figure 1. Flowchart of studies through the screening process.

2.4. Quality Assessment

The quality of the included studies was assessed with the Newcastle–Ottawa Quality Assessment Scale (NOS) [35]. The NOS contains eight categories in the selection of cases and controls, comparability of the groups, and establishment of outcome. A study can be awarded a maximum of one star for each numbered item within the Selection and Exposure categories, a maximum of two stars can be given for comparability. A score of 0–3 points is defined as a study of low quality, a score of 4–6 points represents a moderate quality study, and studies with 7–8 points are studies of high quality. The quality of the included studies was independently assessed by WF and JN. Both reviewers checked the article together in the event of discrepancies in scores in order to reach consensus on the score.

3. Results

3.1. Literature Search

The PubMed databank was searched with aforementioned terms. As a result, we came up with 376 articles. We also searched through Embase, which resulted in 1188 articles, and subsequently filtering on "Embase only" or "Embase and Medline" reduced this to 336 articles. After removing the duplicates from the total of 712 articles, we identified 568 articles that fulfilled the inclusion criteria.

Subsequent selection based on content described in the abstracts resulted in 19 articles that both reviewers agreed on their inclusion. We also checked the references lists but did not find any extra articles. Then, after reading the full articles, we excluded another five articles because of Neuromyelitis Optica diagnosis of the patients. In this category of MS patients, bowel problems are not very common. In total, we found four articles on SCI and ten articles on MS (Figure 1).

3.2. Description of Included Studies

Twelve papers were observational, cross-sectional studies; one study was an observational longitudinal study [36] and one study was an interventional, longitudinal study [37]. In Table 1, we included a description of the included studies looking at sample size, disease characteristics, HC characteristics, mean age and number of faecal samples. Most studies had small sample sizes, varying between 13 and 89 patients. The number of HC varied between 14 and 165. The age of most patients and HC was between 30 and 40 years. In the four SCI articles [38–41], all studies described how long the injury existed. In the MS articles, some described the time since diagnosis but did not correct this for the outcomes. All MS articles included if their patients suffered from Relapsing Remitting MS (RRMS) or Primary Progressive MS (PPMS). Only some described if their patients were in an active disease state or in remission.

Twelve studies looked at just one faecal sample. One study looked at two samples of all the participants within a two-month interval. Finally, one study looked at samples of the HC every two weeks.

The recruitment of HC was different in every study. In seven studies, there were no specific descriptions of HC recruitment [39–45]. In three studies, HC were recruited from databases (Metabolic Department University Hospital Brussels [46], Norwegian Bone Marrow Donor Registry [37], Brigham and Women's Hospital PhenoGenetic project [47]). In four studies, HC were recruited from hospital staff or students (Hospital Brussels (para)medical staff [46], University of Manitoba Health Sciences Centre [36], Turkish hospital employees [38], Azabu University [48]). In one study, family members were recruited [49] and in one study, the participants' proxies were included as HC [46].

Table 1. Description of the included articles arranged by date.

Authors	Objectives	Sample Size & Mean Age	Disease Characteristics	Healthy Controls	No. Faeces Samples per Subject	Outcome Measures	Microbiome Analyses
							Study Design
Li [39]	Compare the gut microbiome composition among individuals with A-SCI, Chron-SCI, vs. able-bodied controls	7 A-SCI (36 ± 12 years) 25 Chron-SCI (46 ± 13 years) 25 HC (42 ± 13 years)	- Time since injury - Level of lesion	- No specifics about recruitment - Age-matched - Generally healthy	1	- α diversity - β diversity - compositional differences	• Stool collection: Para-pak (non-nutritive solution) • Store temp: −80 °C • DNA extraction: Zymo research Fecal DNA isolation kit • Targeted 16S rRNA gene region: V4
Reynders [46]	Microbiota alterations in MS versus HC	89 MS (48 ± 13.8 years) 120 HC (49 ± 14.3 years)	- Benign MS - Untreated active RRMS - Untreated active RRMS with relapse - Interferon treated RRMS - PPMS	- Recruited among participants' proxies & database Metabolic Department University Hospital Brussels & paramedical staff - Same geographical regions - Matched for age, sex, BMI, BSS	1	- α diversity - β diversity - compositional differences	• Stool collection: Faecal collection kits (not specified) • Store temp: −80 °C • DNA extraction: Mo-bioPowerMicrobiome • Targeted 16S rRNA gene region: V4
Choileain [43]	Association between the gut microbiome and inflammatory T cells subsets in RRMS patients and HC	26 MS (42 ± 13 years) 39 HC (45 ± 12 years)	RRMS	- No specifics about recruitment	1	- α diversity - inflammatory T cell subsets - compositional differences	• Stool collection: Kit (not specified) • Store temp: −70 °C • DNA extraction: Mo-bioPowerMicrobiome • Targeted 16S rRNA gene region: V4
Zhang [40]	Neurogenic bowel management and changes in the gut microbiota and associations between serum biomarkers	20 SCI (39.9 ± 10.6 years) 23 HC (40 ± 9.0 years)	- Cervical traumatic, complete - Male - Time since injury >6 months	- No specifics about recruitment - 18-60 y; no antibiotic/probiotics 1-month prior study; no history of diabetes, gastrointestinal system diseases, MS, immune metabolic diseases	1	- α diversity - compositional differences	• Stool collection: no transport (at hospital, not specified) • Store temp: −80 °C • DNA extraction: EZNA Stool DNA kit • Targeted 16S rRNA gene region: V3–V4
Ventura [49]	Compare the microbiome between MS patients and HC	45 MS (37.1 ± 12.7 years) 44 HC (31.8 ± 9.0 years)	- RRMS - Ethnic groups: Caucasian, Hispanic, African American	- family members & responders to advertisement - ethnicity matched - 18-70y; no antibiotic therapy <3 months prior, no extreme diet, no inflammatory bowel disease, GI tract surgery	1	- α diversity - β diversity - compositional differences	• Stool collection: Stool collection containers (not specified) • Store temp: −80 °C • DNA extraction: PowerSoil bacterial DNA extraction kit • Targeted 16S rRNA gene region: V4

Table 1. *Cont.*

Authors	Objectives	Sample Size & Mean Age	Disease Characteristics	Healthy Controls	No. Faeces Samples per Subject	Study Design	
						Outcome Measures	Microbiome Analyses
Storm-Larsen [37]	Determine if dimethyl fumarate alters the abundance and diversity of microbiota, and if these changes are associated with gastrointestinal side-effects	36 MS (46 ± 7 years) 165 HC (47 ± 6 years)	RRMS	- previously collected samples from the Norwegian Bone Marrow Donor Registry, same geographic distribution	>1	- α diversity - β diversity - compositional differences	- Stool collection: PSP tubes - Store temp: −80 °C - DNA extraction: PSP Spin Stool DNA kit - Targeted 16S rRNA gene region: V3-V4
Oezguen [45]	Analyze and compare faecal microbiota signatures between HC, MS and NBD	13 MS (39.1 ± 11.6 years) 14 HC (37.8 ± 8.6 years)	RRMS in remission	- no specifics about recruitment - no history of autoimmune disease	1	- α diversity - compositional differences	- Stool collection: self-collected (not specified) - Store temp: −80 °C - DNA extraction: PowerSoil Isolation Kit - Targeted 16S rRNA gene region: V3-V5
Kozhieva [44]	Compare the composition and structure of faecal bacterial assemblage in patients with PPMS and HC	15 MS (45: 25-56 years) 15 HC (23: 20-73 years)	PPMS	- no specifics about recruitment	1	- α diversity	- Stool collection: Sterile faecal specimen containers - Store temp: −80 °C - DNA extraction: MetaHIT protocol - Targeted 16S rRNA gene region: V3-V4
Zhang [44]	Document neurogenic bowel management of male patients with chronic traumatic complete SCI and perform a comparative analysis of the gut microbiota between patients and healthy males	43 SCI (39.9 ± 10.6 years) 23 HC (40 ± 9.0 years)	Complete, traumatic Time since injury >6 months	- no specifics about recruitment - 18-60y; no history of antibiotics/probiotics 1 month prior to study; no history of diabetes, GI system diseases, MS, immune metabolic diseases	1	- neurogenic bowel management - α diversity	- Stool collection: no transport (at hospital, not specified) - Store temp: −80 °C - DNA extraction: EZNA Stool DNA kit - Targeted 16S rRNA gene region: V3-V4
Forbes [36]	Compare the gut microbiota in patients with Crohn's disease, ulcerative colitis, multiple sclerosis, rheumatoid arthritis and HC	19 MS (average 47.3 years) 23 HC (average 32.4 years)	MS Crohn's disease ulcerative colitis rheumatoid arthritis	- recruitment at University of Manitoba health Sciences centre - no antibiotics in the previous 8 weeks - no GI, neurological of joint disease	2	- α diversity - compositional differences	- Stool collection: self-collected (not specified) - Store temp: −80 °C - DNA extraction: ZR-96 Fecal DNA Kit - Targeted 16S rRNA gene region: V4

Table 1. *Cont.*

Authors	Objectives	Sample Size & Mean Age	Disease Characteristics	Healthy Controls	No. Faeces Samples per Subject	Outcome Measures	Microbiome Analyses
						Study Design	
Gungor [38]	Characterize the gut microbiota in adult SCI patients with different types of bowel dysfunction	30 SCI: 15 LMN (34 ± 8.9 years) 15 UMN (35 ± 9.5 years) 10 HC (34.4 ± 8.0 years)	- Complete or cauda equina - Time since injury >12 months - traumatic - UMN or LMN	- recruitment from hospital employees	1	- compositional differences	• Stool collection: no transport (at hospital, not specified) • Store temp: −80 °C • DNA extraction: PowerSoil bacterial DNA extraction kit • Targeted 16S rRNA gene region: V4
Chen [42]	Investigate whether gut microbiota are altered in MS by comparing the faecal microbiota in RRMS to that of HC	31 MS: 12 active MS (39.3 ± 10.6 years) 19 remission MS (45.2 ± 10.2 years) 36 HC (40.3 ± 7.3 years)	RRMS: - Active - Remission	- no specifics about recruitment - age, sex-matched cohort, no known disease symptoms - no prior bowel surgery, no antibiotics/probiotics use, no autoimmune disease, diabetes or IBD	1	- α diversity - compositional differences	• Stool collection: Commode Specimen collection kit • Store temp: −70 °C • DNA extraction: MoBio PowerSoil • Targeted 16S rRNA gene region: V3–V5
Jangi [47]	Investigate the gut microbiome in subjects with MS and HC	60 MS (49.7 ± 8.5 years) 43 HC (42.2 ± 9.6 years)	RRMS	- recruited from the Brigham and Women's Hospital PhenoGenetic project - age-matched - no corticosteroids, history of gastroenteritis, travel outside the country in prior month, no IBD, bowel surgery, inflammatory bowel disease of autoimmune disease	1	- α diversity - β diversity - compositional differences	• Stool collection: Collection containers (not specified) • Store temp: −80 °C • DNA extraction: PowerSoil Isolation Kit • Targeted 16S rRNA gene region: V3–V5
Miyake [48]	Investigate whether gut microbiota in patients with MS is altered compared to HC	20 MS (36 ± years) 50 HC (27.2 ± years)	RRMS	- recruitment at Azabu University - no antibiotics during collection of faecal samples	In some multiple	- α diversity - compositional differences	• Stool collection: Plastic bag (not specified) • Store temp: −80 °C • DNA extraction: Enzymatic lysis method • Targeted 16S rRNA gene region: V1–V2

A-SCI:Acute Spinal Cord Injury LMN: Lower Motor Neuron Bowel Syndrome; RRMS: Relapsing Remitting Multiple Sclerosis Chron-SCI: Chronic-Spinal Cord Injury; UMN: Upper Motor Neuron Bowel Syndrome; PPMS:Primary ProgressiveMultiple Sclerosis; BMI:Body Mass Index; BSS:Bristol Stool Scale; IBD:Inflammatory Bowel Disease.

In four studies, HC and patients are matched for age [39,42,46,47]. In four studies, they were matched for geographical region [37,46,47,49]. Seven articles [36,40–42,45,47,49] were matched for medical history, including former diseases and medical conditions. There was only one study that matched for Body Mass Index [46]. The exclusion criteria for patients and HC within a study were mostly the same.

All studies determined the gut microbiota composition by 16S rRNA gene sequencing. Not all studies collected the faeces samples in the same way. Most samples were collected by participants at home, whilst some were collected at the hospital [38,40,41]. There were different kits and different storage temperatures. All samples in the articles were stored at −80 °C, with the exception of two articles, which were stored at −70 °C [42,43]. For DNA extraction, different kits were used. There were also differences in the targeted variable (V) region of the 16 rRNA. Six studies targeted V4 ([36,38,39,43,46,49]), four studies V3–V4 ([37,40,41,44]), three studies V3-V5 ([42,45,47]) and one study targeted V1–V2 ([48]). All of these methodological differences are big confounders, hampering a detailed comparative gut microbiota analysis between the different studies.

3.3. Quality Assessment within Studies

We used the Newcastle–Ottawa Quality Assessment Scale to assess the methodological quality of the case-control studies in this systematic review (Table A2. According to this scale, we did not find an article of low quality (0–3 points). Twelve articles were of moderate quality (4–6 points), with most studies (seven in total) scoring five points. There were only two articles of high quality: one article [41] with seven points and one article [49] with eight points. When we compared these articles, we did not find the same outcomes. Both articles excluded antibiotic use before the start of the study. But in none of these articles were the participants put on the same diet. Because none of the articles scored as low quality, we did not exclude any articles after completing this scale. The conclusion could be that the NOS is not specific enough, because the great majority scored moderate. On the category "comparability", only two factors can be scored. In gut microbiota studies this might not be enough for comparability of cases and controls.

3.4. Alpha Diversity

When comparing the alpha diversity between groups of participants in the 14 publications, we found that six articles [36,40,41,43,46,48] showed a lower alpha diversity of bacteria in SCI and MS compared to HC, five articles [37,42,45,47,49] showed a comparable alpha diversity, while two articles [39,44] showed a higher alpha diversity. In one article there was no conclusion about alpha diversity [38] (Table 2).

When we looked at the SCI and MS group separately, we found in two articles [40,41] a lower alpha diversity in the SCI group compared to HC. In one article [39], there was a higher alpha diversity. In this last article patients had an acute spinal cord injury.

In the MS group, we found in five articles [37,42,45,47,49] a similar alpha diversity between MS and HC. Four articles [36,43,46,48] found a lower alpha diversity in MS compared to HC. In one study [44], a higher alpha diversity in MS compared to HC was found. This last study only had four stars on the NOS, which is the lowest score out of the fourteen articles (Table A2). In one article [46] a downward trend was found in alpha diversity from benign, active untreated MS to RRMS treated with interferon and untreated RRMS during relapse.

In conclusion, there is not an overall outcome that is unambiguous. However, there seems to be a lower or comparable alpha diversity in patients compared to HC.

Table 2. Alpha Diversity.

Article	Diagnosis	Diversity
Jia Li [39]	SCI	α diversity SCI > HC (A-SCI highest)
Reynders [46]	MS	α diversity MS < HC
Choileain [43]	MS	α diversity: RRMS < HC
Zhang [40]	SCI	α diversity SCI < HC
Ventura [49]	MS	No differences in α diversity
Storm-Larsen [37]	MS	α diversity MS = HC
Oezguen [45]	MS	Overall richness MS = HC
Kozhieva [44]	MS	α diversity MS > HC
Zhang [41]	SCI	α diversity SCI < HC
Forbes [36]	MS	α diversity MS < HC
Gungor [38]	SCI	-
Chen [42]	MS	α diversity RRMS = HC
Jangi [47]	MS	α diversity MS = HC
Miyake [48]	MS	α diversity MS < HC
		Alpha Diversity per Article
SCI vs. HC		[39] ↑ [40] ↓ [41] ↓ [38] unknown
MS vs. HC		[46] ↓ [43] ↓ [49] = [37] = [45] = [44] ↑ [36] ↓ [42] = [47] = [48] ↓

↑: patient-group is higher than HC ↓: HC is higher than patients =: no differences. SCI: Spinal Cord Injury, HC: Healthy Controls, MS: Multiple Sclerosis, RRMS: Relapsing Remitting Multiple Sclerosis.

3.5. Taxonomic Differences

Overall, all studies compared and contrasted gut microbiota composition at various levels and depth of analyses, but only some of them reported beta diversity observations. When looking at specific taxonomic differences in the respective articles, we did not find uniform observations between the studies. At the phylum level, however, we observed that Firmicutes and Bacteroidetes were the most dominant in all studies, the variation between studies is large and independent of the health status of the individual. Both lower and higher relative abundances of these phyla were observed in SCI and MS patients compared to HC. In five studies [36,39,40,45,49] we came across a higher relative abundance of Firmicutes and in four studies [41–43,46] a higher relative abundance of Bacteroidetes. Not surprisingly, higher taxonomic resolution up to genus level did not reveal consistent differences when comparing MS and SCI patients to HC. We speculate that these inconsistent observations are not only due to subject-specificity of the gut microbiota composition, but also to the result of many confounders between the studies (as will be discussed in the next section) that hamper a detailed comparison.

3.6. Variation in Design and Methodology between Studies

When comparing the different articles, we discovered differences between participant selection, the method of stool storage, DNA isolation and 16S rRNA gene sequencing (Table 1). There were different stool collection methods, storage temperatures and DNA extraction kits. Because of the variability across studies listed in Table 1, it is possible that the results may differ just because of the discrepancies in the above-mentioned topics. That is why in-depth comparison between the studies is hampered.

There were also different targeting regions of the bacterial 16S rRNA gene (Table 1). The chosen targeted 16S rRNA gene region and primers to use for amplification can also have a major impact on depth of taxonomic resolution for classification and overall gut microbiota profiles [50]. When we compared the six articles [36,38,39,43,46,49] with V4 being the targeted 16S rRNA gene region, in three of them [36,39,49] we found comparability with a higher relative abundance of the genus *Clostridium* (Phylum Firmicutes) in patients compared to HC. When we compared the four articles [36,43,46,49] with MS subjects and V4 being the targeted 16S rRNA gene region, we found in two articles [43,46] a similarity of a higher relative abundance of the genus *Bacteroides* (Phylum Bacteroidetes). When we compared the four articles [37,40,41,44], with V3–V4 being the targeted gene region, we found in two articles [37,40], a lower relative abundance of the genus *Faecalibacterium* (Phylum Firmicutes) in patients compared to HC. Furthermore, in two articles [40,44], we observed a higher relative abundance of Phylum Verrucomicrobia. When we compared the two articles [37,44] with MS patients and V3–V4 being the targeted gene region, we did not find uniform taxonomic differences between MS patients and HC. When we compared the three articles [42,45,47], with V3–V5 being the targeted gene region, we found in two articles [42,45] a higher relative abundance of Phylum Firmicutes and *Genus Dorea* (Phylum Firmicutes) in patients compared to HC. Overall, these observations indicate that the targeted 16S rRNA gene region impacts the findings of the different studies.

We also found variability between the cases and controls recruited in the different studies. In only four articles [39,42,46,47] participants were age-matched. In three articles [37,46,49] participants lived in the same geographical region. In seven articles [36,40–42,45,47,49], participants are matched for (part of their) medical history.

In light of our research question, we were especially interested in bowel function, diet and antibiotic use (Table 3).

Four articles [37,40,41,46] scored the bowel function of their participants. Only one article [41] collected NBD symptom dates in their patients and formed subgroups. They divided their patients into a "with constipation" group or "without constipation" group; they also formed a "bloating" and a "without bloating" group. The constipation group showed a higher relative abundance of the genus *Bifidobacterium* (Phylum Actinobacteria), the bloating group showed a higher number of the genus *Megamonas* (Phylum Firmicutes) and the without bloating group showed a higher number of the genus *Alistipes*.(Phylum Bacteroidetes). This specific article also gave their participants the same hospital food and excluded antibiotics.

Four articles [37,46,47,49] collected dietary intake data using a dietary survey, but provided only limited information about the exact method and findings, apart from one study [49], that concluded that yoghurt intake did not influence alpha diversity. Three studies [38,40,41] gave their participants the same hospital food (not further specified) for a certain period, prior to faeces collection. In two of these articles [40,41], a lower number of Phylum Firmicutes in patients compared to HC became apparent. In all three articles, we found a lower number of the genera *Megamonas* and *Dialister* (both Phylum Firmicutes) in patients compared to HC.

All studies but two [44,45] excluded antibiotic use before faeces collection. There were a lot of differences in the antibiotic exclusion period. We looked at the four articles [36,43,47,49] that excluded antibiotics for the longest period: more than eight weeks. In two of these studies [36,49], a higher number of the genus *Clostridium* (Phylum Firmicutes) was found in patients compared to HC. However, in a third study [43], a lower number of *Clostridium* in patients compared to HC was discovered. In this last study, the period without antibiotics was longer than the two studies with a higher number of *Clostridium*. The study [47] with the longest period without antibiotics (6 months) showed a higher number of phylum Verrucomicrobia and genus *Akkermansia* in patients compared to HC.

Table 3. Overview of how the individual studies addressed or assessed bowel function, diet and antibiotic use. An empty cell means the studies did not provide this information.

Article	Bowel Function	Diet	No Antibiotic Use for
Jia Li [39]	-	-	A-SCI: no antibiotic use but not clear for how long Chron-SCI & HC: not clear at all
Reynders [46]	Participants scored time since last defaecation & stool consistency (not being used in analysis)	Dietary habits assessed (no further details & not being used in analysis)	4 weeks
Choileain [43]	-	-	>than 3 months
Zhang [40]	Patients: NBD symptoms & management data HC: no information (not being used in analysis)	Participants: 2 weeks before stool collection standard hospital food (no specifications)	4 weeks
Ventura [49]	-	Participants: dietary survey: assessment of general diet type and duration, current weekly estimate of consumption of variety of foods (e.g., yogurt, red meat, bread, fatty foods, fruits and vegetables)	3 months
Storm-Larsen [37]	Participants: GI scoring records (Gastrointestinal Symptoms Rating Scale) (not used in baseline analyses)	Participants: Norwegian Food Frequency questionnaires (not used in baseline analyses)	30 days
Oezguen [45]	-	-	-
Kozhieva [44]	-	-	-
Zhang [41]	Patients: NBD symptom dates: 2 groups: constipation & without constipation 2 groups: Bloating & without bloating	Participants: 2 weeks before stool collection standard hospital food (not specified)	4 weeks
Forbes [36]	-	-	8 weeks
Gungor [38]	-	Participants: 1–3 weeks before stool collection standard hospital food (not specified)	3 weeks
Chen [42]	-	-	during study
Jangi [47]	-	Participants: Dietary survey before collection of samples (not used in analyses)	6 months
Miyake [48]	-	-	During trial

SCI: Spinal Cord Injury, HC: Healthy Controls, MS: Multiple Sclerosis A-SCI: Acute Spinal Cord Injury, Chron-SCI: Chronic Spinal Cord Injury; NBD: Neurogenic Bowel Dysfunction.

4. Discussion

Studies in the field of gut microbiota analysis are always difficult to perform because of general limitations. The composition is subject to a complex interplay and there are many factors that can influence the gut microbiota.

Our systematic literature review retrieved fourteen studies. Based on those studies, we cannot draw strong conclusions on differences between SCI or MS patients and HC about composition of the gut microbiota. Putatively, the chronic SCI group may have a lower alpha diversity compared to HC, while there are also some indications that the MS group shows mainly a compatible or a lower alpha diversity compared to HC. Taxonomic differences in both groups are too diverse to draw strong conclusions. The limited information about dietary intake, antibiotic use and NBD further limits our ability to draw conclusions about the possible role of those factors in any differences in gut microbiota.

This review retrieved fourteen articles that included relatively small datasets. Moreover, all studies but two were cross-sectional. Since microbial composition in individuals can shift over time [51], the collection of multiple samples over a prolonged time is essential to obtain a better understanding of how microbial composition changes over time, and how changes interact with changes in diet, antibiotic use and bowel problems.

The studies we retrieved varied largely in terms of methodological aspects, the extensiveness of the description of the recruitment of patients and controls, the extensiveness of the information collected about the patients and controls, and the factors that could affect microbiological composition. First of all, methodologically, the studies used different protocols with regards to the amount of faeces samples, stool collection, DNA extraction and amplification of the targeted 16S rRNA gene V region, all of which will impact variability of findings between studies.

Secondly, in regard to recruitment, the information provided on how patients and controls were recruited was not always clearly described. It is important to have a clear understanding of how those participants were recruited: how long had they been a patient, how many bowel complaints had they been experiencing, and (with respect to controls) were they family members, suffering from a specific illness, matched for age, weight, gender? Knowing about these factors is important in assessing the validity of the findings of a study. Thirdly, the information provided about patients and controls was very brief. It did not always include clinical metadata on whether the illness was sub-acute or chronic (for SCI), whether patients suffered from RRMS or PPMS (for MS patients), or whether the disease was active or in remission (MS patients). This clinical metadata is relevant as chronic patients with SCI or MS suffer more often from constipation and usually have a history of infections and multiple antibiotic use, which all could impact microbial composition. Thus, extensive collection and reporting of those metadata is important for the correct interpretation of findings of studies.

Fourthly, not all the studies reported extensively on diet, use of antibiotics and NBD. When they did, they showed a wide variation in their descriptions. In the fourteen articles, we found an inconsistent way in which diet was taken into account, varying from no attention to diet at all, to giving all participants the same hospital food without further nutritional details. Antibiotic use can cause modification of the gut microbiota for at least two months [52]. Most studies excluded antibiotic use, but they all differed in the exclusion period. Only a minority of articles discussed the participants' bowel function and only one article [41] included the collection of NBD symptom dates in patients. Literature shows that differences in intestinal transit time and constipation can affect the gut microbiota composition [53]. A very recent published article, about the effects of bowel management on the gut microbiota in patients with NBD, excluded the confounding effects of age, diet, obesity and intestinal mobility [54]. This study was a longitudinal, intervention study and concluded that bowel management by transanal irrigation can influence gut microbiota. The collection of and reporting on information on bowel function and management is therefore important.

All named factors have a significant impact on the ability to draw strong conclusions from this review.

Clinical consequences of these results are also difficult to draw at this point. The lower alpha diversity might lead to bowel problems and, in our population, to some of the symptoms of NBD. In these patients, supplementing with probiotics or diet adjustments might have a positive effect [3,28]. But more, longitudinal, research is needed to get a better understanding of possible clinical consequences or therapy options.

5. Conclusions

We conclude that only few studies assessed the composition of the gut microbiota of patients with SCI or MS; most studies were cross-sectional and were hampered in terms of the methodological aspects and information reported on participants that could influence the composition of the gut microbiota.

Future studies should collect multiple faecal samples over time. Moreover, the accurate collection and reporting of information about dietary intake, antibiotic use, NBD and changes in those factors should be required, as well as better reporting on patients' characteristics/clinical metadata to draw rational conclusions.

Author Contributions: Conceptualization, W.F., J.S.-S., J.N. and B.W.; methodology, W.F., F.v.G., J.S.-S. and J.N.; software, W.F. and F.v.G.; validation, W.F. and J.N.; formal analysis, W.F., F.v.G. and J.N.; investigation, W.F., F.v.G. and J.N.; resources, W.F., F.v.G. and J.N.; data curation, W.F., F.v.G. and J.N.; writing—original draft preparation W.F., F.v.G., J.N., J.S.-S., R.W., E.Z. and B.W.; writing—review and editing, W.F., F.v.G., J.N., J.S.-S., R.W., E.Z. and B.W.; visualization, W.F., F.v.G., J.N., J.S.-S., R.W., E.Z. and B.W.; supervision, E.Z., R.W. and B.W.; project administration, W.F.; funding acquisition, W.F. All authors have read and agreed to the published version of the manuscript.

Funding: This research received no external funding. The cost of publication was supported by an educational grant from Coloplast, Denmark.

Institutional Review Board Statement: Not applicable.

Informed Consent Statement: Not applicable.

Data Availability Statement: section "MDPI Research Data Policies" at https://www.mdpi.com/ethics (accessed on 11 February 2021).

Conflicts of Interest: The authors declare no conflict of interest. The funders had no role in the design of the study; in the collection, analyses, or interpretation of data; in the writing of the manuscript, or in the decision to publish the results.

Appendix A

Table A1. Full search syntax.

(((((((((((Multiple Sclerosis(MeSH Terms)) OR (Spinal Cord Injuries(MeSH Terms))) OR (Spinal Cord Diseases (MeSH Terms))) OR (Spinal Dysraphism (MeSH Terms))) OR (Multiple sclerosis(Title/Abstract))) OR (Spinal cord disease * (Title/Abstract))) OR (Spinal cord injury * (Title/Abstract))) OR (SCI(Title/Abstract))) OR (Spinal Dysraphism(Title/Abstract))) AND ((((((((Gastrointestinal Microbiome(MeSH Terms)) OR (dysbiosis (MeSH Terms))) OR (Microbiom* (Title/Abstract))) OR (dysbiosis (Title/Abstract))) OR (dysbacteriosis(Title/Abstract))) OR (intestine flora(Title/Abstract))) OR (stool sample (Title/Abstract))) On 08-07-2020 Embase databank was searched combining the following terms: 'multiple sclerosis'/exp OR 'spinal cord injury'/exp OR 'spinal cord disease'/exp OR 'neurogenic bowel'/exp OR 'spinal dysraphism'/exp OR 'multiple sclerosis': ab,ti OR 'spinal cord injury*':ab,ti OR 'spinal cord disease*':ab,ti OR 'sci':ab,ti OR 'spinal dysraphism':ab,ti
AND
'intestine flora'/exp OR 'dysbiosis'/exp OR microbiom*:ab,ti OR 'intestine flora':ab,ti OR dysbiosis:ab,ti OR dysbacteriosis:ab,ti OR 'stool sample':ab,ti
AND [embase]/lim AND 'article'/it

Table A2. Results of the Newcastle–Ottawa Quality Assessment Scale.

Article	Selection				Comparability Cases/Control	Exposure			Stars
	Case Definition	Repre Sentativeness Cases	Selection Controls	Definition Controls		Ascer Tainment. Exposure	Same Method Ascer Tainment Cases and Controls	Non-Response Rate	
[39]	*	-	*	*	*	*	*	-	6
[46]	*	-	*	*	*	*	*	-	6
[43]	*	-	-	*	*	*	*	-	5
[40]	*	-	-	*	**	*	*	-	6
[49]	*	-	*	*	**	*	*	*	8
[37]	*	-	-	*	*	*	*	-	5
[45]	*	-	*	*	-	*	*	-	5
[44]	*	-	-	*	-	*	*	-	4
[41]	*	*	-	*	**	*	*	-	7
[36]	*	-	-	*	*	*	*	-	5
[38]	*	-	-	*	**	*	*	-	6
[42]	*	-	-	*	*	*	*	-	5
[47]	*	-	-	*	*	*	*	-	5
[48]	*	-	-	*	*	*	*	-	5

*: one star: one point in the scoring system; **: two stars: two points in the scoring system.

Table A3. Diversity and Taxonomic outcomes per study.

Study	Major Differences in Composition
Jia Li [39]	α diversity SCI > HC (A-SCI highest)
	A-SCI more unique bacteria communities but not well-represented (low relative abundances)
	SCI higher relative abundance: **Family:** Erysipelotrichaceae, Acidaminococcaceae, Rikencellaceae, Lachnospiraceae, Rikenellaceae, Ruminococcaceae *Genera: Lachnoclostridium. Eisenbergiella* *Genera: Alistipes* *Genera: Oscillibacter, Anaerotruncus*
	Chron-SCI higher relative abundance: **Order:** Clostridiales **Family:** Lachnospiraceae, Eggerthellaceae, Chron-SCI lower relative abundance: **Order:** Bacillales *Genus: Campylobacter*
	A-SCI: higher **Family:** Desulfovibrionaceae, Burkholderiaceae, Marinifilacceae *Genus: Sutterella* *Genus: Odoribacter*
	Chron-SCI lower relative abundance: **Family:** Burkholderiaceae

Table A3. *Cont.*

Study	Major Differences in Composition
Reynders [46]	α diversity: downward trend: benign, active untreated MS, RRMS interferon, untreated RRMS during relapse MS interferon & untreated RRMS during relapse: microbial richness < benign & primary progressive MS HC & active untreated MS: intermediate microbial richness
	RRMS interferon more prevalent: *Genus: bacteroides*
	Relative abundance primary progressive MS < active untreated MS < HC *Genus: Butyricicoccus* (from the Clostridium cluster IV – produces short-chain fatty acids which can initiate anti-inflammatory effects) global microbial composition differed between MS & HC
	MS lower relative abundance: *Alistipes, Anaerotroncus Lactobacillus, Parabacteroides, Sporobacter and Clostridium cluster IV*
Choileain [43]	α diversity: RRMS < HC β diversity: significant different Altered gut microbiome in MS, suggestive of dysbiosis
	Decreased relative abundance: *Genus: Coprococcus, Clostridium and unidentified Ruminococcaceae*
	Increased in MS: **Phylum:** Bacteroidetes
	Reduced in MS: *Genus: multiple Firmicutes:* *Coprococcus, Clostridium and Ruminococcaceae* (short chain fatty acids producing bacteria) Also reductions: **Phylum:** Bacteriodetes *Genus: paraprevotella* **Phylum:** Euryarchaeota *Genus: methanobrevibacter* *Genus: Proteobacteria*
Chao Zhang [40]	α diversity SCI < HC Diversity lower in SCI
	SCI decreased: **Phylum:** Firmicutes (butyrate producing) *Genus: Faecalibacterium, Megamonas, Prevotella_9, Dialister, Subdoligranulum*
	SCI more abundant: **Phylum:** Proteobacteria, Verrucomicrobia *Genus: Bacteroides, Blautia (produces short chain fatty acids), Escherichia-Shigella, Lactobacillus and Akkermansia (Genus: Lactobacillus (probiotic) and dialister less abundant?)*
Ventura [49]	No differences in α diversity & β diversity
	MS Increased relative abundance *Genus: Clostridium*
	MS Caucasian: Increase **Phylum** Verrucomicrobiales Increase *Genus Akkermansia*

Table A3. *Cont.*

Study	Major Differences in Composition
Storm-Larsen [37]	β diversity MS > HC α diversity MS = HC
	MS lower relative abundance *Genus: Faecalibacterium*
Oezguen [45]	Overall richness MS = HC **Genus** level no significant differences MS and HC
	MS decrease *Genus: mainly Prevotella,* *Succinivibrio, (Burytricimonas, Erysipelotrichaceae not significant)*
	MS Increase *Genus: Clostridium XVIII, Ruminococcus2, Coriobacteriaceae, Coprococcus,* *Butyricicoccus, Dorea and Escherichia/Shigella. Parabacteroides and Gemmiger*
	MS increase **Phylum:** Actinobacteria, Firmicutes
	Larger microbiota community shifts in MS
Kozhieva [44]	MS α diversity > HC
	Relative lower abundance MS **Class:** Clostridia
	Relative abundance increase MS **Phylum:** Verrucomicrobiae (Akkermansia muciniphila)
	More abundant MS: **Order:** Desulfovibrionales **Family:** Desulfovibrionaceae *Genus: Bilophila, Desulfovibtio* **Order** level:minimal differences **Family** level: some differences
Zhang [41]	Diversity gut microbiota SCI reduces Structural composition different
	SCI relative abundance lower: *Genus: Megamonas, Prevotella_9, (Eubacterium)_rectale_group, Dialister,* *Subdoligranulum*
	SCI relative abundance higher: *Genus: Bacteroides, Blautea, Lachnoclostridium, Escherichia-Shigella,* *Bifidobacterium*
	SCI:enriched *Genus: Veillonellaceae and Prevotellaceae,* HC enriched: *Genus: Bacteroidaceae and Bacteroides*
	Constipation group: *Genus: Bifidobacterium* Bloating group: *Genus: Megamonas significantly higher* Without bloating: *Genus: Alistipes significantly higher*
	Paraplegia: Decrease in intestinal flora diversity *Genus: Firmicutes higher compared to quadriplegia*

Table A3. *Cont.*

Study	Major Differences in Composition
Forbes [36]	Richness en diversity lower in MS compared to HC
	MS higher relative abundance *Genus: Actinomyces, Eggerthella, Clostridium III, Faealicoccus and Streptococcus*
	MS lower relative abundance of *Genus: Gemmiger, Lachnospira and Sporobacter*
	MS higher relative abundance *Genus: Anaerofustis*
	MS higher relative abundance: *Genus: Erysipelotrichaceae, unclassified Clostridiales incertae sedis XIII*
	MS lower relative abundance *Genus: Dialister*
Gungor [38]	**Phylum**: Butyrate producing members SCI < HC
	UMN bowel dysfunction lower: *Genus: Pseudobutyrivibrio (=butyrate, lactic acid and formic acid producer),* *Dialister,& Megamonas (=Bacteroides members – interactions with intestine)* *Genus: Marvinbryantia (fam Lachnospiraceae – produce butyrate) UMN < LMN*
	LMN bowel dysfunction lower: *Genus: Roseburia (fam Lachnospiraceae – produce butyrate), Pseudobutyrivibrio,* *Megamonas*
Jun Chen [42]	α diversity RRMS = HC
	RRMS active disease decreased species richness compared to RRMS remission
	MS increased relative abundance: **Pylum:** Proteobactreia *Genus: Pseudomonas, Mycoplana, Haemophilus, Blautia and Dorea*
	MS lower relative abundance: **Phylum:** Actinobacteria *Genus: Adlercreutzia, Collinsella*
	MS higher relative abundance: **Phylum:** Bacteroidetes *Genus: Pedobacter, Flavobacterium* Lower relative abundance: *Genus: Parabacteroides*
	MS enriched: **Phylum:** Firmicutes *Genus: Blautia, Dorea*
	MS lower relative abundance **Phylum:** Firmicutes **Fam:** Erysipelotrichaceae, Lachnospiraceae, Veillonellaceae *Genus: Lactobacillus, Coprobacillus*
	MS more abundant: **Phylum:** Proteobacteria *Genus: Pseudomonas, Mycoplana*
	HC increased relative abundance/MS decreased **Phylum:** Bacteroidetes *Genus: Parabacteroides, Prevotella* **Phylum:** Actinobacteria *Genus: Adlercreutzia, Collinsella* **Phylum:** Firmicutes *Genus: Erysipelotrichaceae*
	MS: gut microbial dysbiosis

Table A3. *Cont.*

Study	Major Differences in Composition
Jangi [47]	α diversity MS = HC
	MS + disease modifying treatment: increase relative abundance: *Genus: Prevotella and Sutterella* Decrease of: *Genus: Sarcina* (in treated MS pt; Untreated MS = HC Treatment associated effect)
	MS: increased relative abundance: **Phylum** Euryarchaeota *Genus: Methanobrevibacter* **Phylum** Verrucomicrobia *Genus: Akkermansia*
	MS: reduces relative abundance **Phylum** Bacteroidetes (Butyrate, short chain fatty acid, producing) *Genus: Butyricimonas*
	Untreated MS: decreased **Phylum** Actinobacteria *Genus: Collinsella and Slackia* **Phylum** Bacteroidetes *Genus: Prevotella*
Miyake [48]	MS lower number of species Difference in number of species and richness not significant Shannon index not significant different Overall gut microbiota structure difference MS > inter-individual variability gut microbiota Moderate dysbiosis in structure of gut microbiota MS
	MS higher relative abundance: *Species: unknown bacteria*
	MS relative depletion: *Species: Clostridia XIV en IV*
	MS more prevalent: **Phylum:** Actinobacteria
	MS less abundant: **Phylum:** Bacteroidetes, Firmicutes *Genus: Bacteroides, Faecalibacterium, Prevotella, Anaerostipes. Suterella*
	MS more abundant: *Genus: Bifidobacterium, Streptococcus*
	MS significant increase: *Genus: Coprococcus* *Species: Streptococcus thermophilus, Eggerthella lenta*

SCI: Spinal Cord Injury; MS: Multiple Sclerosis, HC: Healthy Controls, A-SCI: Acute Spinal Cord Injury, LMN: Lower Motor Neuron, RRMS: Relapsing Remitting Multiple Sclerosis, Chron-SCI: Chronic Spinal Cord Injury; UMN: Upper Motor Neuron Bowel Syndrome; PPMS: Primary Progressive Multiple Sclerosis.

Table A4. Taxonomic outcomes per diagnosis.

SCI lower	SCI Higher	MS Lower	MS Higher
Phylum Firmicutes Class Negativicutes, *Genus Dialister, Megamonas,* Class Clostridia *Genus Subdoligranulum,* *Pseudobutyrivibrio,* *Marvinbryantia, Roseburia,* *Faecalibacterium*	Phylum Verrucomicrobia Class Verrucomicrobiae *Genus Akkermansia*	Phylum Bacteroidetes Class Bacteroidia *Genus Parabacteroides,* *Prevotella, Bacteriodes,* *Paraprevotella, Butyricimonas*	Phylum Actinobacteria Class Actinobacteria *Genus Bifidobacterium,* *Coriobacterium, Actinomyces* *Eggerthella,*

Table A4. *Cont.*

SCI lower	SCI Higher	MS Lower	MS Higher
Phylum Bacteriodetes Class Bacteroidia *Genus Prevotella*	Phylum Proteobacteria Class Gammaproteobacteria *Genus Escherichia-Shigella* Class Epsilonproteobacteria *Genus Campylobacter* Class Betaproteobacteria *Genus Suterella,*	Phylum Firmicutes Class Bacilli *Genus Lactobacillus* Class Erysipelotrichaceae, *Genus Coprobacillus,* Class Clostridia *Genus Coprococcus, Clostridium,* *Ruminococcaceae* *Clostridia XIV en IV* *Genus Faecalibacterium,* *Anaerostipes, Roseburia,* *Gemmiger, Lachnospira,* *Sporobacter,* Class Negativicutes *Genus Dialister*	Phylum Verrucomicrobiales Class Verrucomicrobiae *Genus Akkermansia*
Phylum Proteobacteria Class Epsilonproteobacteria *Genus Campylobacter*	Phylum Bacteriodetes Class Bacteroidales *Genus Bacterioidetes* Class Bacteroidia *Genus Alistipes, Odoribacter*	Phylum Actinobacteria Class Actinobacteria *Genus Adlercreutzia, Collinsella,* *Slackia*	Phylum Proteobacteria Class Gammaproteobacteria *Genus Pseudomonas,* *Haemophilus,* *Escherichia/Shigella* Class Deltaproteobacteria *Genus Desulfovibrio, Bilophila*
	Phylum Firmicutes Class Clostridia *Genus Blautia,* *Lachnoclostridium,* *Eisenbergiella, Oscillobacter* *Anaerotruncus* Class Bacilli *Genus Lactobacillus*	Phylum Euryarchaeota Class Methanobacteria *Genus Methanobrevibacter*	Phylum Tenericutes Class Mollicutes *Genus Mycoplasma*
	Phylum Actinobacteria *Class Actinobacteria* *Genus Bifidobacterium*	Phylum Proteobacteria Class Betaproteobacteria *Genus Suterella,* Class Gammaproteobacteria *Genus Succinivibrio*	Phylum Bacteroidetes Class Sphingobacteriia *Genus Pedobacter* Class Flavobacteriia *Genus Flavobacterium* Class Bacteroidia *Genus Parabacteroides,* *Bacteroides*
			Phylum Firmicutes Class Clostridia *Genus Blautia, Dorea,* *Coprococcus, Clostridium,* *Clostridium XVIII* *Eubacterium halii, Eubacterium* *cylindroides, Anaerofustis,* *Butyricicoccus* *Gemmiger* Class Bacilli *Genus Streptococcus,* *Lactobacillus, Enterococcus,* *Ruminococcus, Faelicoccus* Class Erysipelotrichia *Genus Erysipelotrichaceae,*
			Phylum Euryarchaeota Class Methanobacteria *Genus Methanobrevibacter*

SCI: Spinal Cord Injury, MS: Multiple Sclerosis.

References

1. Browne, P.; Chandraratna, D.; Angood, C.; Tremlett, H.; Baker, C.; Taylor, B.V.; Thompson, A.J. Atlas of Multiple Sclerosis 2013: A growing global problem with widespread inequity. *Neurology* **2014**, *83*, 1022–1024. [CrossRef]
2. Wyndaele, M.; Wyndaele, J. Incidence, prevalence and epidemiology of spinal cord injury: What learns a worldwide literature survey? *Spinal Cord* **2006**, *44*, 523–529. [CrossRef]
3. Faber, W.X.M.; Nachtegaal, J.; Stolwijk-Swuste, J.M.; Achterberg-Warmer, W.J.; Koning, C.J.M.; Der Vaart, I.B.-V.; Van Bennekom, C.A.M. Study protocol of a double-blind randomised placebo-controlled trial on the effect of a multispecies probiotic on the incidence of antibiotic-associated diarrhoea in persons with spinal cord injury. *Spinal Cord* **2020**, *58*, 149–156. [CrossRef]
4. Krassioukov, A.; Eng, J.J.; Claxton, G.; Sakakibara, B.M.; Shum, S.; the SCIRE Research Team. Neurogenic bowel management after spinal cord injury: A systematic review of the evidence. *Spinal Cord* **2010**, *48*, 718–733. [CrossRef]
5. Adriaansen, J.J.E.; Ruijs, L.E.M.; Van Koppenhagen, C.F.; Van Asbeck, F.W.A.; Snoek, G.J.; Van Kuppevelt, D.; Visser-Meily, J.M.A.; Post, M.W.M. Secondary health conditions and quality of life in persons living with spinal cord injury for at least ten years. *J. Rehabil. Med.* **2016**, *48*, 853–860. [CrossRef]
6. Adriaansen, J.J.; Van Asbeck, F.W.; Van Kuppevelt, D.; Snoek, G.J.; Post, M.W. Outcomes of Neurogenic Bowel Management in Individuals Living with a Spinal Cord Injury for at Least 10 Years. *Arch. Phys. Med. Rehabil.* **2015**, *96*, 905–912. [CrossRef] [PubMed]
7. Emmanuel, A. Neurogenic bowel dysfunction. *F1000Research* **2019**, *8*, 1800. [CrossRef] [PubMed]
8. Coggrave, M.; Norton, C.; Wilson-Barnett, J. Management of neurogenic bowel dysfunction in the community after spinal cord injury: A postal survey in the United Kingdom. *Spinal Cord* **2009**, *47*, 323–333. [CrossRef]
9. Johns, J.; Krogh, K.; Ethans, K.; Chi, J.; Querée, M.; Eng, J.; Spinal Cord Injury Research Evidence Team. Pharmacological Management of Neurogenic Bowel Dysfunction after Spinal Cord Injury and Multiple Sclerosis: A Systematic Review and Clinical Implications. *J. Clin. Med.* **2021**, *10*, 882. [CrossRef] [PubMed]
10. Mekhael, M.; Kristensen, H.; Larsen, H.; Juul, T.; Emmanuel, A.; Krogh, K.; Christensen, P. Transanal Irrigation for Neurogenic Bowel Disease, Low Anterior Resection Syndrome, Faecal Incontinence and Chronic Constipation: A Systematic Review. *J. Clin. Med.* **2021**, *10*, 753. [CrossRef]
11. Preziosi, G.; Gordon-Dixon, A.; Emmanuel, A. Neurogenic bowel dysfunction in patients with multiple sclerosis: Prevalence, impact, and management strategies. *Degener. Neurol. Neuromuscul. Dis.* **2018**, *8*, 79–90. [CrossRef]
12. Bakke, A.; Myhr, K.M.; Grønning, M.; Nyland, H. Bladder, bowel and sexual dysfunction in patients with multiple sclerosis–a cohort study. *Scand. J. Urol. Nephrol. Suppl.* **1996**, *179*, 61–66. [PubMed]
13. Hinds, J.P.; Eidelman, B.H.; Wald, A. Prevalence of bowel dysfunction in multiple sclerosis: A population survey. *Gastroenterology* **1990**, *98*, 1538–1542. [CrossRef]
14. Hinds, J.P.; Wald, A. Colonic and anorectal dysfunction associated with multiple sclerosis. *Am. J. Gastroenterol.* **1989**, *84*, 587–595.
15. Munteis, E.; Andreu, M.; Téllez, M.J.; Mon, D.; Ois, A.; Roquer, J. Anorectal dysfunction in multiple sclerosis. *Mult. Scler. J.* **2006**, *12*, 215–218. [CrossRef] [PubMed]
16. Sun, W.M.; Katsinelos, P.; Horowitz, M.; Read, N.W. Disturbances in anorectal function in patients with diabetes mellitus and faecal incontinence. *Eur. J. Gastroenterol. Hepatol.* **1996**, *8*, 1007–1012. [CrossRef] [PubMed]
17. Lawthom, C.; Durdey, P.; Hughes, T. Constipation as a presenting symptom. *Lancet* **2003**, *362*, 958. [CrossRef]
18. Lynch, A.C.; Antony, A.; Dobbs, B.R.; Frizelle, F.A. Bowel dysfunction following spinal cord injury. *Spinal Cord* **2001**, *39*, 193–203. [CrossRef]
19. Mazzawi, T.; Lied, G.A.; Sangnes, D.A.; El-Salhy, M.; Hov, J.R.; Gilja, O.H.; Hatlebakk, J.G.; Hausken, T. The kinetics of gut microbial community composition in patients with irritable bowel syndrome following fecal microbiota transplantation. *PLoS ONE* **2018**, *13*, e0194904. [CrossRef]
20. O'Hara, A.M.; Shanahan, F. The gut flora as a forgotten organ. *EMBO Rep.* **2006**, *7*, 688–693. [CrossRef]
21. Flores, R.; Shi, J.; Gail, M.H.; Gajer, P.; Ravel, J.; Goedert, J.J. Assessment of the human faecal microbiota: II. Reproducibility and associations of 16S rRNA pyrosequences. *Eur. J. Clin. Investig.* **2012**, *42*, 855–863. [CrossRef]
22. Nicholson, J.K.; Holmes, E.; Kinross, J.; Burcelin, R.; Gibson, G.; Jia, W.; Pettersson, S. Host-Gut Microbiota Metabolic Interactions. *Science* **2012**, *336*, 1262–1267. [CrossRef]
23. Spor, A.; Koren, O.; Ley, R.E. Unravelling the effects of the environment and host genotype on the gut microbiome. *Nat. Rev. Microbiol.* **2011**, *9*, 279–290. [CrossRef] [PubMed]
24. Wu, W.-K.; Chen, C.-C.; Panyod, S.; Chen, R.-A.; Wu, M.-S.; Sheen, L.-Y.; Chang, S.-C. Optimization of fecal sample processing for microbiome study—The journey from bathroom to bench. *J. Formos. Med. Assoc.* **2019**, *118*, 545–555. [CrossRef] [PubMed]
25. Falony, G.; Joossens, M.; Vieira-Silva, S.; Wang, J.; Darzi, Y.; Faust, K.; Kurilshikov, A.; Bonder, M.J.; Valles-Colomer, M.; Vandeputte, D.; et al. Population-level analysis of gut microbiome variation. *Science* **2016**, *352*, 560–564. [CrossRef] [PubMed]
26. Tottey, W.; Feria-Gervasio, D.; Gaci, N.; Laillet, B.; Pujos, E.; Martin, J.-F.; Sebedio, J.-L.; Sion, B.; Jarrige, J.-F.; Alric, M.; et al. Colonic Transit Time Is a Driven Force of the Gut Microbiota Composition and Metabolism: In Vitro Evidence. *J. Neurogastroenterol. Motil.* **2017**, *23*, 124–134. [CrossRef] [PubMed]
27. Beuret-Blanquart, F.; Weber, J.; Gouverneur, J.; Demangeon, S.; Denis, P. Colonic transit time and anorectal manometric anomalies in 19 patients with complete transection of the spinal cord. *J. Auton. Nerv. Syst.* **1990**, *30*, 199–207. [CrossRef]

28. David, L.A.; Maurice, C.F.; Carmody, R.N.; Gootenberg, D.B.; Button, J.E.; Wolfe, B.E.; Ling, A.V.; Devlin, A.S.; Varma, Y.; Fischbach, M.A.; et al. Diet rapidly and reproducibly alters the human gut microbiome. *Nature* **2014**, *505*, 559–563. [CrossRef] [PubMed]

29. Pérez-Cobas, A.E.; Gosalbes, M.J.; Friedrichs, A.; Knecht, H.; Artacho, A.; Eismann, K.; Otto, W.; Rojo, D.; Bargiela, R.; Von Bergen, M.; et al. Gut microbiota disturbance during antibiotic therapy: A multi-omic approach. *Gut* **2013**, *62*, 1591–1601. [CrossRef]

30. Rabadi, M.H.; Mayanna, S.K.; Vincent, A.S. Predictors of mortality in veterans with traumatic spinal cord injury. *Spinal Cord* **2013**, *51*, 784–788. [CrossRef]

31. Bonfill, X.; Rigau, D.; Jáuregui-Abrisqueta, M.L.; Chacón, J.M.B.; De La Barrera, S.S.; Alemán-Sánchez, C.M.; Bea-Muñoz, M.; Pérez, S.M.; Duran, A.B.; Quirós, J.R.E.; et al. A randomized controlled trial to assess the efficacy and cost-effectiveness of urinary catheters with silver alloy coating in spinal cord injured patients: Trial protocol. *BMC Urol.* **2013**, *13*, 38. [CrossRef]

32. Marin, J.; Nixon, J.; Gorecki, C. A systematic review of risk factors for the development and recurrence of pressure ulcers in people with spinal cord injuries. *Spinal Cord* **2013**, *51*, 522–527. [CrossRef] [PubMed]

33. Moher, D.; Liberati, A.; Tetzlaff, J.; Altman, U.G. Preferred reporting items for systematic reviews and meta-analyses: The PRISMA Statement. *Open Med.* **2009**, *3*, e123–e130. [PubMed]

34. Ouzzani, M.; Hammady, H.; Fedorowicz, Z.; Elmagarmid, A. Rayyan—A web and mobile app for systematic reviews. *Syst. Rev.* **2016**, *5*, 1–10. [CrossRef]

35. Stang, A. Critical evaluation of the Newcastle–Ottawa scale for the assessment of the quality of nonrandomized studies in meta-analyses. *Eur. J. Epidemiol.* **2010**, *25*, 603–605. [CrossRef]

36. Forbes, J.D.; Chen, C.-Y.; Knox, N.C.; Marrie, R.-A.; El-Gabalawy, H.; De Kievit, T.; Alfa, M.; Bernstein, C.N.; Van Domselaar, G. A comparative study of the gut microbiota in immune-mediated inflammatory diseases—Does a common dysbiosis exist? *Microbiome* **2018**, *6*, 1–15. [CrossRef] [PubMed]

37. Storm-Larsen, C.; Myhr, K.-M.; Farbu, E.; Midgard, R.; Nyquist, K.; Broch, L.; Berg-Hansen, P.; Buness, A.; Holm, K.; Ueland, T.; et al. Gut microbiota composition during a 12-week intervention with delayed-release dimethyl fumarate in multiple sclerosis—A pilot trial. *Mult. Scler. J. Exp. Transl. Clin.* **2019**, *5*. [CrossRef]

38. Gungor, B.; Adigüzel, E.; Gürsel, I.; Yilmaz, B.; Gursel, M. Intestinal Microbiota in Patients with Spinal Cord Injury. *PLoS ONE* **2016**, *11*, e0145878. [CrossRef] [PubMed]

39. Li, J.; Van Der Pol, W.; Eraslan, M.; McLain, A.; Cetin, H.; Cetin, B.; Morrow, C.; Carson, T.; Yarar-Fisher, C. Comparison of the gut microbiome composition among individuals with acute or long-standing spinal cord injury vs. able-bodied controls. *J. Spinal Cord Med.* **2020**, 1–9. [CrossRef]

40. Zhang, C.; Jing, Y.; Zhang, W.; Zhang, J.; Yang, M.; Du, L.; Jia, Y.; Chen, L.; Gong, H.; Li, J.; et al. Dysbiosis of gut microbiota is associated with serum lipid profiles in male patients with chronic traumatic cervical spinal cord injury. *Am. J. Transl. Res.* **2019**, *11*, 4817–4834.

41. Zhang, C.; Zhang, W.; Zhang, J.; Jing, Y.; Yang, M.; Du, L.; Gao, F.; Gong, H.; Chen, L.; Li, J.; et al. Gut microbiota dysbiosis in male patients with chronic traumatic complete spinal cord injury. *J. Transl. Med.* **2018**, *16*, 1–16. [CrossRef] [PubMed]

42. Chen, J.; Chia, N.; Kalari, K.R.; Yao, J.Z.; Novotna, M.; Soldan, M.M.P.; Luckey, D.H.; Marietta, E.V.; Jeraldo, P.R.; Chen, X.; et al. Multiple sclerosis patients have a distinct gut microbiota compared to healthy controls. *Sci. Rep.* **2016**, *6*, 28484. [CrossRef]

43. Choileáin, S.N.; Kleinewietfeld, M.; Raddassi, K.; Hafler, D.A.; Ruff, W.E.; Longbrake, E.E. CXCR3+ T cells in multiple sclerosis correlate with reduced diversity of the gut microbiome. *J. Transl. Autoimmun.* **2020**, *3*, 100032. [CrossRef] [PubMed]

44. Kozhieva, M.; Naumova, N.; Alikina, T.; Boyko, A.; Vlassov, V.; Kabilov, M.R. Primary progressive multiple sclerosis in a Russian cohort: Relationship with gut bacterial diversity. *BMC Microbiol.* **2019**, *19*, 309. [CrossRef] [PubMed]

45. Oezguen, N.; Yalçınkaya, N.; Kücükali, C.I.; Dahdouli, M.; Hollister, E.B.; Luna, R.A.; Türkoglu, R.; Kürtüncü, M.; Eraksoy, M.; Savidge, T.C.; et al. Microbiota stratification identifies disease-specific alterations in neuro-Behcet's disease and multiple sclerosis. *Clin. Exp. Rheumatol.* **2019**, *37* (Suppl. 121), 58–66.

46. Reynders, T.; Devolder, L.; Valles-Colomer, M.; Van Remoortel, A.; Joossens, M.; De Keyser, J.; Nagels, G.; D'Hooghe, M.; Raes, J. Gut microbiome variation is associated to Multiple Sclerosis phenotypic subtypes. *Ann. Clin. Transl. Neurol.* **2020**, *7*, 406–419. [CrossRef]

47. Jangi, S.; Gandhi, R.; Cox, L.M.; Li, N.; Von Glehn, F.; Yan, R.; Patel, B.; Mazzola, M.A.; Liu, S.; Glanz, B.L.; et al. Alterations of the human gut microbiome in multiple sclerosis. *Nat. Commun.* **2016**, *7*, 12015. [CrossRef]

48. Miyake, S.; Kim, S.; Suda, W.; Oshima, K.; Nakamura, M.; Matsuoka, T.; Chihara, N.; Tomita, A.; Sato, W.; Kim, S.-W.; et al. Dysbiosis in the Gut Microbiota of Patients with Multiple Sclerosis, with a Striking Depletion of Species Belonging to Clostridia XIVa and IV Clusters. *PLoS ONE* **2015**, *10*, e0137429. [CrossRef]

49. Ventura, R.E.; Iizumi, T.; Battaglia, T.; Liu, M.; Perez-Perez, G.I.; Herbert, J.; Blaser, M.J. Gut microbiome of treatment-naïve MS patients of different ethnicities early in disease course. *Sci. Rep.* **2019**, *9*, 1–10. [CrossRef]

50. Rintala, A.; Pietilä, S.; Munukka, E.; Eerola, E.; Pursiheimo, J.-P.; Laiho, A.; Pekkala, S.; Huovinen, P. Gut Microbiota Analysis Results Are Highly Dependent on the 16S rRNA Gene Target Region, Whereas the Impact of DNA Extraction Is Minor. *J. Biomol. Tech. JBT* **2017**, *28*, 19–30. [CrossRef]

51. Johnson, A.J.; Vangay, P.; Al-Ghalith, G.A.; Hillmann, B.M.; Ward, T.L.; Shields-Cutler, R.R.; Kim, A.D.; Shmagel, A.K.; Syed, A.N.; Walter, J.; et al. Daily Sampling Reveals Personalized Diet-Microbiome Associations in Humans. *Cell Host Microbe* **2019**, *25*, 789–802.e5. [CrossRef] [PubMed]
52. De La Cochetiere, M.F.; Durand, T.; Lepage, P.; Bourreille, A.; Galmiche, J.P.; Dore, J. Resilience of the Dominant Human Fecal Microbiota upon Short-Course Antibiotic Challenge. *J. Clin. Microbiol.* **2005**, *43*, 5588–5592. [CrossRef] [PubMed]
53. Vandeputte, D.; Falony, G.; Vieira-Silva, S.; Tito, R.Y.; Joossens, M.; Raes, J. Stool consistency is strongly associated with gut microbiota richness and composition, enterotypes and bacterial growth rates. *Gut* **2016**, *65*, 57–62. [CrossRef]
54. Furuta, A.; Suzuki, Y.; Takahashi, R.; Jakobsen, B.P.; Kimura, T.; Egawa, S.; Yoshimura, N. Effects of Transanal Irrigation on Gut Microbiota in Pediatric Patients with Spina Bifida. *J. Clin. Med.* **2021**, *10*, 224. [CrossRef] [PubMed]

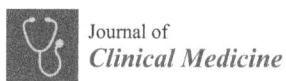

Journal of
Clinical Medicine

Article

Effects of Transanal Irrigation on Gut Microbiota in Pediatric Patients with Spina Bifida

Akira Furuta [1,*], Yasuyuki Suzuki [2], Ryosuke Takahashi [3], Birte Petersen Jakobsen [4], Takahiro Kimura [1], Shin Egawa [1] and Naoki Yoshimura [5]

[1] Department of Urology, Jikei University School of Medicine, Tokyo 105-8471, Japan; tkimura@jikei.ac.jp (T.K.); s-egpro@jikei.ac.jp (S.E.)
[2] Department of Urology, Tokyo Metropolitan Rehabilitation Hospital, Tokyo 131-0034, Japan; ysuro@jikei.ac.jp
[3] Department of Urology, Spinal Injuries Center, Fukuoka 820-0053, Japan; r-taka@uro.med.kyushu-u.ac.jp
[4] Consultant MD, MedDevHealth, Geelsvej, 15 2840 Holte, Denmark; birte@meddevhealth.com
[5] Department of Urology, University of Pittsburgh School of Medicine, Pittsburgh, PA 15261, USA; nyos@pitt.edu
* Correspondence: a-furuta@jikei.ac.jp; Tel.: +81-3-3433-1111

Abstract: Recent studies using 16S rRNA-based microbiota profiling have demonstrated dysbiosis of gut microbiota in constipated patients. The aim of this study was to investigate the changes in gut microbiota after transanal irrigation (TAI) in patients with spina bifida (SB). A questionnaire on neurogenic bowel disfunction (NBD), Bristol scale, and gut microbiota using 16S rRNA sequencing were completed in 16 SB patients and 10 healthy controls aged 6–17 years. Then, 11 of 16 SB patients with moderate to severe NBD scores received TAI for 3 months. Changes in urine cultures were also examined before and after the TAI treatments. In addition, correlation of gut microbiota and Bristol scale was analyzed. Significantly decreased abundance in *Faecalibacterium*, *Blautia* and *Roseburia*, and significantly increased abundance in *Bacteroides* and *Roseburia* were observed in the SB patients compared with controls and after TAI, respectively. The abundance of *Roseburia* was significantly correlated positively with Bristol scale. Urinary tract infection tended to decrease from 82% to 55% after TAI ($p = 0.082$) despite persistent fecal incontinence. Butyrate-producing bacteria such as *Roseburia* play a regulatory role in the intestinal motility and host immune system, suggesting the effects of TAI on gut microbiota.

Keywords: constipation; gut microbiota; spina bifida; transanal irrigation; urinary tract infection

Citation: Furuta, A.; Suzuki, Y.; Takahashi, R.; Jakobsen, B.P.; Kimura, T.; Egawa, S.; Yoshimura, N. Effects of Transanal Irrigation on Gut Microbiota in Pediatric Patients with Spina Bifida. *J. Clin. Med.* **2021**, *10*, 224. http://doi.org/10.3390/jcm10020224

Received: 13 December 2020
Accepted: 5 January 2021
Published: 10 January 2021

Publisher's Note: MDPI stays neutral with regard to jurisdictional claims in published maps and institutional affiliations.

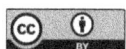

Copyright: © 2021 by the authors. Licensee MDPI, Basel, Switzerland. This article is an open access article distributed under the terms and conditions of the Creative Commons Attribution (CC BY) license (https://creativecommons.org/licenses/by/4.0/).

1. Introduction

Patients with neurogenic diseases affecting the spinal cord such as spina bifida (SB) and spinal cord injury (SCI) often present disturbance of bladder and bowel function. To date, treatments of neurogenic bowel dysfunction (NBD) have been largely empirical, and individual solutions have been sought, whereas clean intermittent catheterization (CIC) has commonly been used to treat neurogenic bladder due to spinal cord lesions. Patients with SB or SCI often suffer from both urinary and bowel symptoms, and expect to undergo the treatments of NBD at the same time. The Peristeen® transanal irrigation system (Coloplast A/S, Humlebaek, Denmark) was for the first time permitted for use in the treatments of intractable neurogenic constipation from March 2018 in Japan. A randomized controlled trial found that SCI patients treated with the Peristeen® transanal irrigation system showed improvements in constipation, fecal incontinence, and symptom-related quality of life compared with patients treated with conservative bowel management as the best supportive bowel care without irrigation [1]. It has also been reported that about 60% (36/60) of SB patients aged 8–17 years showed relief from neurogenic constipation three months after transanal irrigation (TAI) [2].

The human intestinal tract is colonized by hundreds of trillions of bacteria whose number exceeds that of the host cells by ten-fold or more [3]. Gut microbiota act as a barrier against pathogens, stimulate the host immune system, and produce a great variety of compounds from the metabolism of diet that could affect the host [4,5]. Immune function in patients with spinal cord lesions is crucial because of the increased incidence of urinary tract infection (UTI), probably due to the increased residual urine volume [6]. Therefore, the CIC maneuver has been introduced to reduce the incidence of UTI [7]. On the other hand, the growth and composition of gut microbiota are affected by a plethora of factors, including age [8], diet [9], obesity [10], and intestinal motility [11]. Recent studies using 16S rRNA-based microbiota profiling have demonstrated dysbiosis of gut microbiota in constipated patients [11]. However, to the best of our knowledge, there have been no reports concerning the effects of TAI on gut microbiota in constipated patients. Therefore, the aim of this study was to investigate the changes in gut microbiota after TAI in SB patients using 16S rRNA sequencing, which detects microbes that have not yet been cultured but can be assigned as relatives of cultured representatives with known function.

2. Experimental Section

2.1. Study Design

Sixteen pediatric SB patients aged 6–17 years treated with self or helped CIC due to neurogenic bladder were recruited from the Jikei University Hospital, and 10 age- and sex-matched healthy controls without any disease were included from the same hospital employees' children between July 2018 and June 2019. SB patients with myelomeningocele at lumbosacral or sacral lesion levels were included. Obese children whose body mass index (BMI) was over 25 kg/m^2 were excluded. All participants completed the Bristol scale (range 1–7; 1 = separate hard lumps, 4 = like a smooth, soft sausage or snake, 7 = liquid consistency with no solid pieces) and NBD score (range 0–47; 0–6 = very minor, 7–9 = minor, 10–13 = moderate, 14–47 = severe), which consists of 10 questions including frequency of bowel movements (range 0–6; 0 = daily, 6 = less than once a weak), time used for defecation (range 0–7; 0 = 0–30 min, 7 = more than 1 h), headache or perspiration during defecation (range 0–2; 0 = no, 2 = yes), use of tablets against constipation (range 0–2; 0 = no, 2 = yes), use of drops against constipation (range 0–2; 0 = no, 2 = yes), digital stimulation or evacuation (range 0–6; 0 = daily, 6 = less than once a week), frequency of fecal incontinence (range 0–13; 0 = less than once a week, 13 = daily), use of tablets against fecal incontinence (range 0–4; 0 = no, 4 = yes), flatus incontinence (range 0–2; 0 = no, 2 = yes), and perianal skin problems (range 0–3; 0 = no, 3 = yes) in cooperation with their parents.

Eleven of the sixteen intractable constipated SB patients with moderate to severe NBD score then received TAI using the Peristeen® anal irrigation system every two days for 3 months. Changes in urine cultures (10^4 colony forming units/mL or larger was regarded as bacteriuria) in addition to the Bristol scale and NBD score were also examined before and after the TAI treatments. The use of new gastrointestinal interventions including prebiotics, probiotics, antibiotics, modifications to their diet, or medication for the treatment of constipation were prohibited during the study.

All participants gave their written informed consent to the protocol and were permitted to withdraw from the study at any time. The study was approved by the Ethics Committee of the Jikei University School of Medicine (9156).

2.2. Fecal Sample Collection and 16S rRNA Gene Sequencing

Fecal samples were collected from 10 healthy controls without TAI, 16 SB patients before TAI, and 11 SB patients after TAI using dedicated containers (Techno Suruga Laboratory, Shizuoka, Japan) for the analysis of 16S rRNA sequencing and stored at 4 °C in refrigerators until further processing. DNA was isolated with Isospin fecal DNA (Nippon Gene Co., LTD, Tokyo, Japan) according to manufacturer's instructions.

The exacted DNA was analyzed in Repertoire Genesis Inc. (Osaka, Japan). The V1V2 region of 16S rRNA genes was amplified using FOH-27Fmod (5′-AGRGTTTGATYMTGGCT CAG-3′) and ROH-338R (5′-TGCTGCCTCCCGTAGGAGT-3′) under the following polymerase chain reaction (PCR) conditions: one cycle of denaturation at 95 °C for 3 min,

25 cycles at 95 °C for 30 s, 55 °C for 30 s, 72 °C for 30 s, and final extension at 72 °C for 5 min. The PCR products were sequenced by MiSeq Deep sequencer using MiSeq Reagent Kit v3 (Illumina, San Diego, CA, USA) following the manufacturer's instructions. The sequence data were preprocessed and analyzed using the "Flora Genesis software" (Repertoire Genesis Inc.). In brief, the R1 and R2 read pairs were joined and chimera sequences were removed. The operational taxonomic unit (OTU) picking was performed by the open-reference method using the 97% identity prefiltered Greengenes database and the UCLUST. The representative sequences of each OTU were chosen and taxonomy assignment was performed by Ribosomal Database Project (RDP) classifier using a threshold score of 0.5 or more. The OTUs were grouped if their annotation was the same regardless of their RDP score.

2.3. Statistical Analysis

All data were represented as mean values ± standard deviation of the mean. Statistical analysis software (Prism, GraphPad Software, San Diego, CA, USA) was used to perform the data analysis.

Significant differences in the age, BMI, Bristol scale, and NBD score in the controls and SB patients were analyzed using Mann–Whitney U-test, whereas the sex differences were detected by Chi-square test. Meanwhile, changes in the Bristol scale, NBD score, and UTI after TAI in the SB patients were examined using Wilcoxon signed rank test.

All microbes at the phylum level were compared, whereas the microbes at the genus level with low relative abundances (<0.1%) were filtered and the remaining top 50 different types were analyzed. Significant differences in the relative abundance of microbes in the controls and SB patients were detected using Mann–Whitney U-test. Changes in the relative abundance of microbes after TAI in the SB patients were examined by Wilcoxon signed rank test. In addition, the correlation of the microbes and Bristol scale was analyzed by Spearman rank correlation.

3. Results

3.1. Characteristics in the SB Patients Compared with Healthy Controls

There were not significant differences in the sex, age, and BMI between the controls and SB patients, as shown in Table 1. On the other hand, the Bristol scale was significantly decreased and the NBD score was significantly increased in the SB patients compared with the controls. All of the SB patients had mild (3), moderate (4), or severe (9) neurogenic constipation.

Table 1. Characteristics of the study groups. BMI: body mass index; CIC: clean intermittent catheterization; NBD: neurogenic bowel dysfunction.

	Healthy Control	Spina Bifida	*p* Value
Participants (Number)	10	16	
Male/Female (Number)	5/5	5/11	0.339
Age (Mean ± SD)	12.6 ± 2.5	10.8 ± 3.3	0.223
BMI (Mean ± SD)	17.5 ± 1.6	18.9 ± 3.8	0.429
CIC (Number)	0	16	
Bristol scale (Mean ± SD)	3.8 ± 0.4	1.8 ± 1.0	0.001
NBD score (Mean ± SD)	0.5 ± 1.0	14.1 ± 4.7	0.001
Very mild (Number)	10	0	
Mild (Number)	0	3	
Moderate (Number)	0	4	
Severe (Number)	0	9	

3.2. Comparison of Gut Microbiota in the SB Patients and Healthy Controls

At the phylum level, there were no significant differences in the relative abundance of microbes in the controls and SB patients, although a total of 15 microbes were detected

(Figure 1A, Table 2). On the other hand, at the genus level, the relative abundance of *Faecalibacterium*, *Blautia*, *Roseburia*, *Lachnospira*, and *Dialister* was significantly decreased and that of *Oscillospira* was significantly increased in the SB patients before TAI compared with the controls (Figure 1B, Table 2).

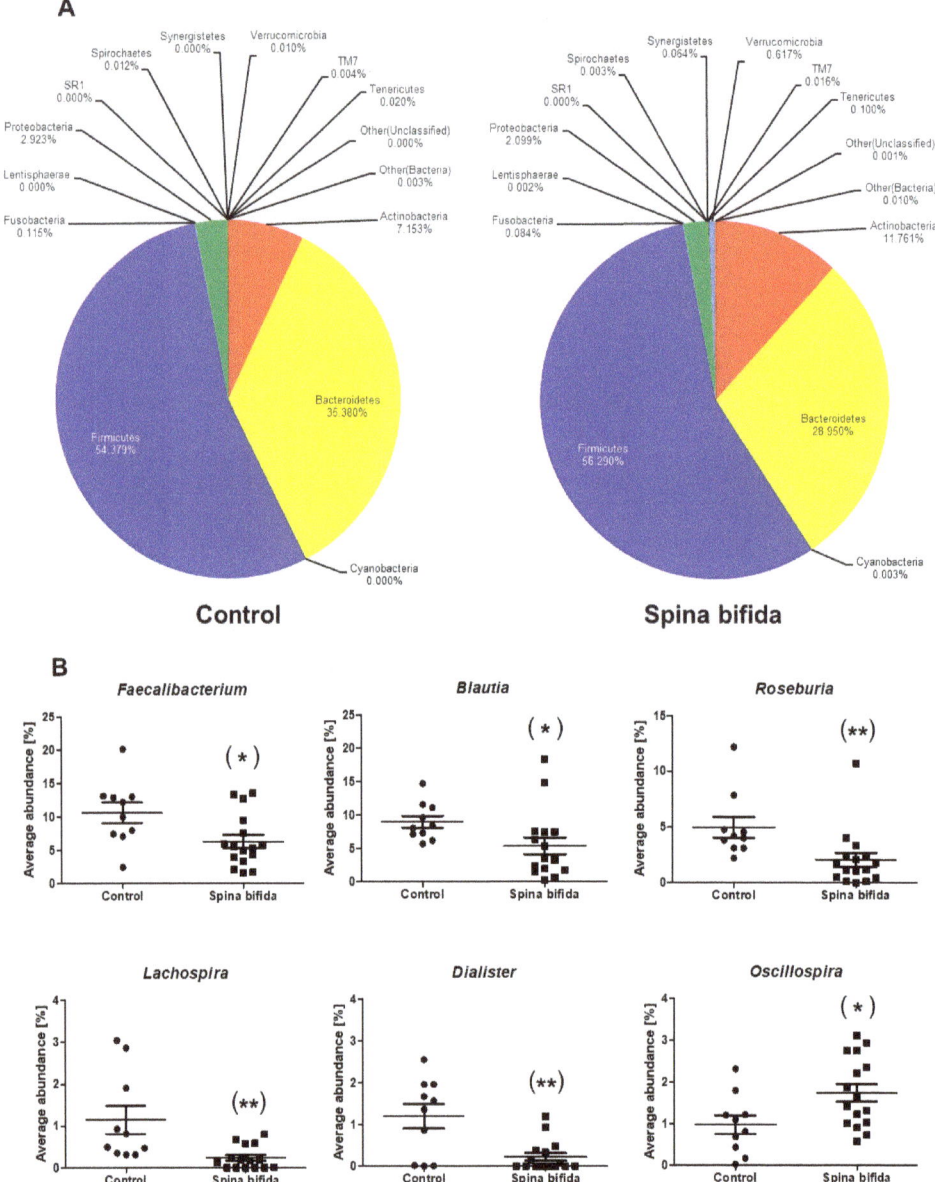

Figure 1. Comparison of gut microbiota in the spina bifida (SB) patients and healthy controls at the phylum level (**A**) and the genus level (**B**). *; $p < 0.05$, **; $p < 0.01$ vs. Control.

Table 2. Differences between gut microbiota in the SB patients and healthy controls.

Phylum Level	Control (Mean)	Spina Bifida (Mean)	*p* Value
Family Level / Genus Level			
Firmicutes/Bacteroidetes ratio	1.58	2.38	0.246
Firmicutes	54.38	56.29	0.654
Ruminococcaceae			
Ruminococcus	2.79	6.30	0.108
Faecalibacterium	10.64	6.33	0.033
Oscillospira	0.98	1.74	0.029
Lachospiraceae			
Blautia	9.00	5.38	0.017
Ruminococcus	8.44	8.53	0.693
Roseburia	4.99	2.06	0.001
Dorea	1.71	1.73	0.937
Lachnospira	1.15	0.24	0.002
Coprococcus	1.07	0.55	0.654
Lactobacillus	0.03	1.18	0.346
Streptococcaceae			
Streptococcus	1.98	1.82	0.304
Clostridiaceae			
SMB53	1.15	2.50	0.120
Veillonellaceae			
Veillonella	1.22	0.97	0.051
Dialister	1.20	0.22	0.003
Bacillaceae			
Bacillus	0.04	1.89	0.593
Erysipelotrichaceae			
Eubacterium	0.20	0.61	0.055
Turicibacteraceae			
Turicibacter	0.24	0.80	0.144
Bacteroidetes	35.38	28.95	0.147
Bacteroidaceae			
Bacteroides	27.66	20.11	0.087
Porphyromonadaceae			
Parabacteroides	2.34	3.69	0.257
Prevotellaceae			
Prevotella	3.05	0.06	0.477
Actinobacteria	7.15	11.76	0.133
Bifidobacteriaceae			
Bifidobacterium	5.89	8.67	0.280
Coriobacteriaceae			
Collinsella	0.96	2.01	0.684
Proteobacteria	2.92	2.09	0.414
Alcaligenaceae			
Sutterella	1.81	1.07	0.087
Enterobacteriaceae			
Trabulsiella	0.36	0.41	0.385

3.3. Outcome Measures before and after TAI in the SB Patients

Significant changes in the Bristol scale and total NBD score were observed after the TAI treatments in the constipated SB patients. The results analyzing the sub-NBD score showed that use of tablets against constipation was significantly decreased without significant changes in the frequency of fecal incontinence. Asymptomatic bacteriuria caused by *Escherichia coli* tended to decrease from 82% to 55% after TAI, although the difference was not statistically significant (*p* = 0.082) (Table 3).

Table 3. Influence of transanal irrigation (TAI) on outcome measures.

	Before TAI	After TAI	*p* Value
Bristol scale (Mean ± SD)	1.9 ± 1.2	3.6 ± 1.2	0.001
Total NBD score (Mean ± SD)	15.6 ± 4.1	11.1 ± 4.6	0.009
Frequency of bowel movements (Mean ± SD)	1.7 ± 2.4	1.0 ± 0.0	0.279
Time used for defecation (Mean ± SD)	0.9 ± 2.1	1.1 ± 1.5	0.828
Headache or perspiration during defecation (Mean ± SD)	0.6 ± 0.9	0.1 ± 0.5	0.082
Use of tablets against constipation (Mean ± SD)	1.1 ± 1.0	0.4 ± 0.9	0.019
Use of drops against constipation (Mean ± SD)	0.4 ± 0.9	0.0 ± 0.0	0.082
Digital stimulation or evacuation (Mean ± SD)	4.3 ± 2.8	3.4 ± 3.1	0.336
Frequency of fecal incontinence (Mean ± SD)	5.0 ± 3.7	3.7 ± 3.4	0.108
Use of tablets against fecal incontinence (Mean ± SD)	0.3 ± 1.1	0.0 ± 0.0	0.336
Flatus incontinence (Mean ± SD)	2.0 ± 0.0	2.0 ± 0.0	1.000
Perianal skin problems (Mean ± SD)	0.9 ± 1.4	0.2 ± 0.8	0.083
Urinary tract infection (Number, %)	9 (82%)	6 (55%)	0.082
Causative bacteria (Number) *Escherichia coli*	9	6	

3.4. Changes in Gut Microbiota after TAI in the SB Patients

At the phylum level, there were no significant changes in the relative abundance of 15 microbes after the TAI treatments (Figure 2A, Table 4). At the genus level, the relative abundance of *Bacteroides* and *Roseburia* was significantly increased and that of *Turicibacter* was significantly decreased after TAI in SB patients (Figure 2B, Table 4).

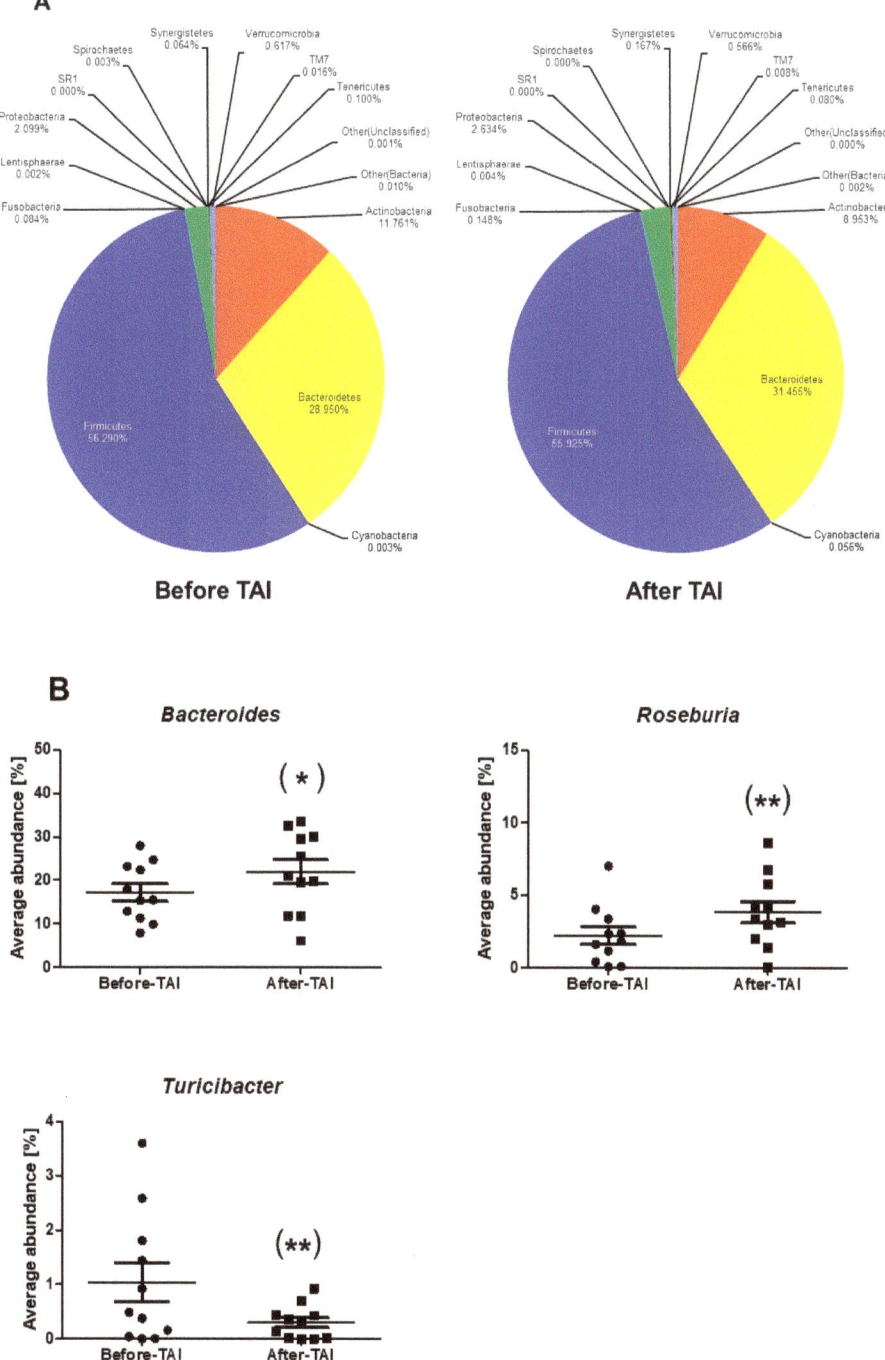

Figure 2. Changes in gut microbiota after TAI in the SB patients at the phylum level (**A**) and the genus level (**B**). *; $p < 0.05$, **; $p < 0.01$ vs. before TAI.

Table 4. Changes in gut microbiota after TAI in the SB patients.

Phylum Level			
Family Level Genus Level	Before TAI (Mean)	After TAI (Mean)	*p* Value
Firmicutes/Bacteroidetes ratio	2.53	2.36	0.638
Firmicutes	58.57	57.28	0.638
Ruminococcaceae			
Ruminococcus	7.48	7.48	1.000
Faecalibacterium	7.30	9.27	0.320
Oscillospira	1.72	1.83	0.700
Lachospiraceae			
Blautia	6.11	7.45	0.240
Ruminococcus	8.70	8.05	0.966
Roseburia	2.22	3.86	0.007
Dorea	2.28	2.12	0.638
Coprococcus	0.75	0.54	1.000
Streptococcaceae			
Streptococcus	1.49	2.00	0.700
Clostridiaceae			
SMB53	2.98	1.00	0.067
02d06	0.90	0.53	0.695
Veillonellaceae			
Phascolarctobacterium	0.50	0.47	0.938
Erysipelotrichaceae			
Eubacterium	0.74	0.83	0.898
Turicibacteraceae			
Turicibacter	1.04	0.30	0.003
Bacteroidetes	28.92	31.65	0.638
Bacteroidaceae			
Bacteroides	17.35	21.92	0.048
Porphyromonadaceae			
Parabacteroides	3.03	3.34	0.831
Prevotellaceae			
Prevotella	1.96	2.33	0.557
Odoribacteraceae			
Odoribacter	0.51	0.49	0.922
Actinobacteria	9.74	7.67	0.320
Bifidobacteriaceae			
Bifidobacterium	6.79	5.93	0.413
Coriobacteriaceae			
Collinsella	1.65	1.43	0.250
Proteobacteria	1.84	2.52	0.175
Alcaligenaceae			
Sutterella	0.71	1.35	0.059

3.5. Correlation of Gut Microbiota and Bristol Scale

The relative abundance of *Roseburia* was significantly correlated positively with the Bristol scale, although a significant correlation was not detected in *Bacteroides*, *Faecalibacterium*, or *Blautia* (Table 5).

Table 5. Correlation of gut microbiota and Bristol scale.

Bacteria	Bristol Scale	*p* Value
(Genus level)	(Correlation coefficient)	
Bacteroides	0.262	0.147
Faecalibacterium	0.239	0.187
Blautia	0.264	0.144
Roseburia	0.486	0.005

4. Discussion

The results of this study indicate that Bristol scale and total NBD score were significantly deteriorated in the SB patients compared with healthy controls and then significantly improved after TAI in the SB patients, which is consistent with previous reports [1,2] It was also observed that 82% of the SB patients had asymptomatic UTI predominantly caused by *E. coli* before TAI, which then tended to decrease after TAI ($p = 0.082$). Therefore, it is assumed that TAI, by improving bowel habit and washing of the colorectal tract, can reduce the risk of bladder contamination by *E. coli* [2], although persistent fecal incontinence after TAI due to atonic sphincters remained after TAI in this study.

An innovative point of the present study was to investigate the changes in gut microbiota before and after TAI in the constipated SB patients, with the exclusion of probable confounding effects of age, diet, and intestinal motility on gut microbiota. In addition, we decided to enroll non-obese patients with a body mass index of 25 kg/m^2 or less because obesity has a large impact on gut microbial composition (based on a previous report demonstrating that an increased *Firmicutes/Bacteroidetes* ratio is associated with obesity) [10].

Firmicutes and *Bacteroidetes* were the most predominant bacteria at the phylum level in the gut, in accordance with a previous report [12]. They ferment indigestible carbohydrates and generate short-chain fatty acids (SCFAs) including acetate, propionate, and butyrate. It has been reported that *Bacteroidetes* produce high levels of acetate and propionate, whereas *Firmicutes* produce high amounts of butyrate [13]. The most numerous butyrate-producing bacteria are highly oxygen-sensitive anaerobes belonging to the *Clostridial* clusters IV, including *Faecalibacterium*, and XIVa, including *Roseburia* and *Lachnospira* [14,15]. The abundance of *Faecalibacterium* has significantly been decreased in patients with functional constipation [16]. Significantly decreased abundance in *Roseburia* was also observed in patients with functional constipation [16,17] or in constipated patients with irritable bowel syndrome (IBS) as well as in SCI patients compared with healthy controls [18–20]. In addition, *Blautia* or *Dialister* has been reported to produce acetate or propionate, respectively [21,22]. In the present study, the abundance of *Blautia* and *Dialister* as well as *Faecalibacterium*, *Roseburia*, and *Lachnospira* was significantly decreased in the SB patients.

Gut microbiota obtained from constipated patients with IBS were observed to produce more sulfides and hydrogen and less butylate from starch fermentation than healthy controls [18]. This study showed that the abundance of *Roseburia* was significantly correlated positively with Bristol scale, which is possibly because butyrate plays a regulatory role in the transepithelial fluid transport and intestinal motility via release of 5-hydroxytryptamine [23]. On the other hand, the anti-inflammatory effects of SCFAs are mediated through binding of the G-protein-coupled receptor 41 and 43, which are both expressed on immune cells, suggesting that SCFAs are involved in the activation of leucocytes [23]. Significantly decreased levels of butylate and acetate has been previously reported in patients with irritable bowel diseases compared with health controls [24]. In the present study, significantly increased abundance in *Roseburia and Bacteroides* was observed after TAI, which may contribute to the tendency for UTIs to be reduced in the constipated SB patients treated with CIC despite the persistent fecal incontinence remaining. Furthermore, as mentioned above, significantly increased abundance in *Bacteroides* was observed after TAI in this study, whereas significantly decreased abundance in *Bacteroides* and *Prevotella* has been reported in constipated patients with IBS [25]. Three enterotypes, including *Bacteroides*, *Prevotella*, and *Ruminococcus* at the genus level, have recently been defined in a global collection of gut microbiota [26]. The results of this study therefore suggested the contribution of TAI to the changes in *Bacteroides*, one of the enterotypes.

It has been reported that *Oscillospira* is closely related to human health because its abundance is negatively correlated with systolic and diastolic blood pressure, fasting blood glucose, triglyceride, uric acid, and Bristol scale, suggesting that *Oscillospira* is a predictor of low BMI and constipation [27]. In addition, an association between *Turicibacter* and exercise has been reported in mice. A previous study showed that the percentage of *Turicibacter* in controls was 0.22%, whereas that of *Turicibacter* in voluntary wheel running groups was 0% [28]. In the present study, significantly decreased abundance in *Turicibacter* was observed after TAI, suggesting the recovery of intestinal motility possibly due to butyrate in the SB patients.

Psyllium is widely used for the treatment of constipation. It is capable of retaining water in the small intestine, and thereby increasing water flow into the ascending colon. The increases in the fluidity of colonic content may explain the success of psyllium in treating constipation [29]. Interestingly, psyllium supplementation increased fecal water, resulting in the significant increases in *Faecalibacterium, Roseburia*, and *Lachnospira* in the patients with functional constipation [30]. Similarly, the present study for the first time suggested the effects of TAI on gut microbiota, especially butyrate-producing bacteria such as *Roseburia*.

A major limitation of this study was the small number of patients, but confounding effects of age, diet, obesity, and intestinal motility on gut microbiota were excluded by comparing gut microbial composition before and after the TAI treatment. In addition, we only characterized gut microbiota without investigating their metabolites, such as SCFAs. Further studies are needed to clarify this point.

5. Conclusions

TAI significantly improved constipation in addition to significantly increasing the abundance in *Roseburia*, which may contribute to improvements in the host immune system, resulting in the tendency for UTIs to be reduced, despite persistent fecal incontinence. Therefore, TAI combined with CIC could be beneficial for improving bowel dysfunction in constipated patients with spinal cord lesions such as SB.

Author Contributions: Conceptualization: A.F. and B.P.J.; methodology: A.F. and R.T.; formal analysis: T.K.; writing—original draft preparation: A.F. and Y.S.; writing—review and editing: S.E. and N.Y. All authors have read and agreed to the published version of the manuscript.

Funding: Analysis cost of gut microbiota using 16S rRNA sequencing was supported by Coloplast Japan. Coloplast Japan had no influence on the study design, data analysis, or data interpretation.

Institutional Review Board Statement: The study was conducted according to the guidelines of the Declaration of Helsinki, and approved by the Institutional Ethics Committee of Jikei University School of Medicine (protocol code: 9156 and date of approval: 12 September 2018).

Informed Consent Statement: Informed consent was obtained from all subjects involved in the study.

Data Availability Statement: The data that support the findings are available from the corresponding author (A.F.) upon reasonable request.

Acknowledgments: The authors thank Yukio Nakamura (Repertoire Genesis Inc.) for 16S rRNA sequencing of the fecal samples.

Conflicts of Interest: The authors declare no conflict of interest.

J. Clin. Med. **2021**, *10*, 224

Abbreviations

BMI	body mass index
CIC	clean intermittent catheterization
IBS	irritable bowel syndrome
NBD	neurogenic bowel dysfunction
OUT	operational taxonomic unit
PCR	polymerase chain reaction
RDP	Ribosomal Database Project
SCFAs	short-chain fatty acids
SCI	spinal cord injury
TAI	transanal irrigation
UTI	urinary tract infection.

References

1. Christensen, P.; Bazzocchi, G.; Coggrave, M.; Abel, R.; Hultling, C.; Krogh, K.; Media, S.; Laurberg, S. A randomized, controlled trial of transanal irrigation versus conservative bowel management in spinal cord-injured patients. *Gastroenterology* **2006**, *131*, 738–747. [CrossRef] [PubMed]
2. Ausili, E.; Focarelli, B.; Tabacco, F.; Murolo, D.; Sigismondi, M.; Gasbarrini, A.; Rendeli, C. Transanal irrigation in myelomeningocele children: An alternative, safe and valid approach for neurogenic constipation. *Spinal Cord.* **2010**, *48*, 560–565. [CrossRef] [PubMed]
3. Dethlefsen, L.; McFall-Ngai, M.; Relman, D.A. An ecological and evolutionary perspective on human-microbe mutualism and disease. *Nature* **2007**, *449*, 811–818. [CrossRef] [PubMed]
4. Round, J.L.; Mazmanian, S.K. The gut microbiota shapes intestinal immune responses during health and disease. *Nat. Rev. Immunol* **2009**, *9*, 313–323. [CrossRef] [PubMed]
5. Arpaia, N.; Campbell, C.; Fan, X.; Dikiy, S.; van der Veeken, J.; deRoos, P.; Liu, H.; Cross, J.R.; Pfeffer, K.; Coffer, P.J.; et al. Metabolites produced by commensal bacteria promote peripheral regulatory T-cell generation. *Nature* **2013**, *504*, 451–455. [CrossRef] [PubMed]
6. Merritt, J.L. Residual urine volume: Correlate of urinary tract infection in patients with spinal cord injury. *Arch. Phys. Med. Rehabil.* **1981**, *62*, 558–561.
7. Weld, K.J.; Dmochowski, R.R. Effect of bladder management on urological complications in spinal cord injured patients. *J. Urol.* **2000**, *163*, 768–772. [CrossRef]
8. Yatsunenko, T.; Rey, F.E.; Manary, M.J.; Trehan, I.; Dominguez-Bello, M.G.; Contreras, M.; Magris, M.; Hidalgo, G.; Baldassano, R.N.; Anokhin, A.P.; et al. Human gut microbiome viewed across age and geography. *Nature* **2012**, *486*, 222–227. [CrossRef]
9. Nishijima, S.; Suda, W.; Oshima, K.; Kim, S.W.; Hirose, Y.; Morita, H.; Hattori, M. The gut microbiome of healthy Japanese and its microbial and functional uniqueness. *DNA Res.* **2016**, *23*, 125–133. [CrossRef]
10. Ley, R.E.; Turnbaugh, P.J.; Klein, S.; Gordon, J.I. Microbial ecology: Human gut microbes associated with obesity. *Nature* **2006**, *444*, 1022–1023. [CrossRef]
11. Ohkusa, T.; Koido, S.; Nishikawa, Y.; Sato, N. Gut Microbiota and Chronic Constipation: A Review and Update. *Front. Med.* **2019**, *6*, 19. [CrossRef] [PubMed]
12. Cho, I.; Blaser, M.J. The human microbiome: At the interface of health and disease. *Nat. Rev. Genet.* **2012**, *13*, 260–270. [CrossRef]
13. Macfarlane, S.; Macfarlane, G.T. Regulation of short-chain fatty acid production. *Proc. Nutr. Soc.* **2003**, *62*, 67–72. [CrossRef] [PubMed]
14. Pryde, S.E.; Duncan, S.H.; Hold, G.L.; Stewart, C.S.; Flint, H.J. The microbiology of butyrate formation in the human colon. *FEMS Microbiol. Lett.* **2002**, *217*, 133–139. [CrossRef] [PubMed]
15. Meehan, C.J.; Beiko, R.G. A phylogenomic view of ecological specialization in the Lachnospiraceae, a family of digestive tract-associated bacteria. *Genome Biol. Evol.* **2014**, *6*, 703–713. [CrossRef]
16. Zhuang, M.; Shang, W.; Ma, Q.; Strappe, P.; Zhou, Z. Abundance of Probiotics and Butyrate-Production Microbiome Manages Constipation via Short-Chain Fatty Acids Production and Hormones Secretion. *Mol. Nutr. Food Res.* **2019**, *63*, e1801187. [CrossRef]
17. Mancabelli, L.; Milani, C.; Lugli, G.A.; Turroni, F.; Mangifesta, M.; Viappiani, A.; Ticinesi, A.; Nouvenne, A.; Meschi, T.; van Sinderen, D.; et al. Unveiling the gut microbiota composition and functionality associated with constipation through metagenomic analyses. *Sci. Rep.* **2017**, *7*, 9879. [CrossRef]
18. Chassard, C.; Dapoigny, M.; Scott, K.P.; Crouzet, L.; Del'homme, C.; Marquet, P.; Martin, J.C.; Pickering, G.; Ardid, D.; Eschalier, A.; et al. Functional dysbiosis within the gut microbiota of patients with constipated-irritable bowel syndrome. *Aliment. Pharmacol. Ther.* **2012**, *35*, 828–838. [CrossRef]
19. Gobert, A.P.; Sagrestani, G.; Delmas, E.; Wilson, K.T.; Verriere, T.G.; Dapoigny, M.; Del'homme, C.; Bernalier-Donadille, A. The human intestinal microbiota of constipated-predominant irritable bowel syndrome patients exhibits anti-inflammatory properties. *Sci. Rep.* **2016**, *6*, 39399. [CrossRef]

20. Gungor, B.; Adiguzel, E.; Gursel, I.; Yilmaz, B.; Gursel, M. Intestinal Microbiota in Patients with Spinal Cord Injury. *PLoS ONE* **2016**, *11*, e0145878. [CrossRef]
21. Liu, C.; Li, J.; Zhang, Y.; Philip, A.; Shi, E.; Chi, X.; Meng, J. Influence of glucose fermentation on CO_2 assimilation to acetate in homoacetogen Blautia coccoides GA-1. *J. Ind. Microbiol. Biotechnol.* **2015**, *42*, 1217–1224. [CrossRef] [PubMed]
22. Morotomi, M.; Nagai, F.; Sakon, H.; Tanaka, R. Dialister succinatiphilus sp. nov. and Barnesiella intestinihominis sp. nov., isolated from human faeces. *Int. J. Syst. Evol. Microbiol.* **2008**, *58*, 2716–2720. [CrossRef] [PubMed]
23. Canani, R.B.; Costanzo, M.D.; Leone, L.; Pedata, M.; Meli, R.; Calignano, A. Potential beneficial effects of butyrate in intestinal and extraintestinal diseases. *World J. Gastroenterol.* **2011**, *17*, 1519–1528. [CrossRef] [PubMed]
24. Huda-Faujan, N.; Abdulamir, A.S.; Fatimah, A.B.; Anas, O.M.; Shuhaimi, M.; Yazid, A.M.; Loong, Y.Y. The impact of the level of the intestinal short chain Fatty acids in inflammatory bowel disease patients versus healthy subjects. *Open Biochem. J.* **2010**, *4*, 53–58. [CrossRef]
25. Rajilić-Stojanović, M.; Biagi, E.; Heilig, H.G.; Kajander, K.; Kekkonen, R.A.; Tims, S.; de Vos, W.M. Global and deep molecular analysis of microbiota signatures in fecal samples from patients with irritable bowel syndrome. *Gastroenterology* **2011**, *141*, 1792–1801. [CrossRef]
26. Arumugam, M.; Raes, J.; Pelletier, E.; Le Paslier, D.; Yamada, T.; Mende, D.R.; Fernandes, G.R.; Tap, J.; Bruls, T.; Batto, J.M.; et al. Enterotypes of the human gut microbiome. *Nature* **2011**, *473*, 174–180. [CrossRef]
27. Chen, Y.R.; Zheng, H.M.; Zhang, G.X.; Chen, F.L.; Chen, L.D.; Yang, Z.C. High Oscillospira abundance indicates constipation and low BMI in the Guangdong Gut Microbiome Project. *Sci. Rep.* **2020**, *10*, 9364. [CrossRef]
28. Allen, J.M.; Berg Miller, M.E.; Pence, B.D.; Whitlock, K.; Nehra, V.; Gaskins, H.R.; White, B.A.; Fryer, J.D.; Woods, J.A. Voluntary and forced exercise differentially alters the gut microbiome in C57BL/6J mice. *J. Appl. Physiol.* **2015**, *118*, 1059–1066. [CrossRef]
29. Erdogan, A.; Rao, S.S.; Thiruvaiyaru, D.; Lee, Y.Y.; Coss Adame, E.; Valestin, J.; O'Banion, M. Randomised clinical trial: Mixed soluble/insoluble fibre vs. psyllium for chronic constipation. *Aliment. Pharmacol. Ther.* **2016**, *44*, 35–44. [CrossRef]
30. Jalanka, J.; Major, G.; Murray, K.; Singh, G.; Nowak, A.; Kurtz, C.; Silos-Santiago, I.; Johnston, J.M.; de Vos, W.M.; Spiller, R. The Effect of Psyllium Husk on Intestinal Microbiota in Constipated Patients and Healthy Controls. *Int. J. Mol. Sci.* **2019**, *20*, 433. [CrossRef]

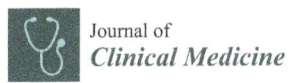

Journal of
Clinical Medicine

MDPI

Review

Laxative Use in the Community: A Literature Review

Barry L. Werth * and Sybèle-Anne Christopher

Susan Wakil School of Nursing and Midwifery, Faculty of Medicine and Health, The University of Sydney,
Camperdown, NSW 2006, Australia; sybele.christopher@sydney.edu.au
* Correspondence: bwer8557@uni.sydney.edu.au; Tel.: +61-428-115-866

Abstract: Laxatives are widely available without prescription and, as a consequence, they are commonly used for self-management of constipation by community-dwelling adults. However, it is not clear to what extent laxatives are used. Nor is it clear how laxatives are chosen, how they are used and whether consumers are satisfied with their performance. This review of published literature in the last 30 years shows the prevalence of laxative use in community-dwelling adults varied widely from 1% to 18%. The prevalence of laxative use in adults with any constipation (including both chronic and sporadic constipation) also varied widely from 3% to 59%. Apart from any geographical differences and differences in research methodologies, this wide range of estimated prevalence may be largely attributed to different definitions used for laxatives. This review also shows that laxative choice varies, and healthcare professionals are infrequently involved in selection. Consequently, satisfaction levels with laxatives are reported to be low and this may be because the laxatives chosen may not always be appropriate for the intended use. To improve constipation management in community and primary healthcare settings, further research is required to determine the true prevalence of laxative use and to fully understand laxative utilisation.

Keywords: laxatives; constipation; adults; prevalence; utilisation

1. Introduction

Laxatives accelerate or induce defecation [1] and are often used in the management of constipation in the community [2]. Constipation, a common community problem globally [3,4], is frequently self-diagnosed and self-managed by community-dwelling adults [5]. Constipation represents a substantial cost in the community [6], particularly chronic constipation which is usually defined by a set of clinical symptoms known as the Rome criteria [7]; these criteria have been revised several times since their introduction in 1994 as Rome I criteria. Constipation also includes both chronic and sporadic constipation [8]. Most adults attempt to self-manage their constipation before consulting a healthcare professional [9]. Self-management often includes the use of laxative products, most of which may be purchased in pharmacies and elsewhere without prescription. However, failures in the self-management of constipation are frequent and lead to additional costs which add considerably to the financial burden of constipation in the community [10].

Laxative pharmaceutical products available without prescription are generally referred to as over-the-counter (OTC) laxatives. Classification of laxatives is based on the mode of action and the four main classes of OTC laxatives are bulk-forming laxatives, softeners/lubricants, contact/stimulant laxatives and osmotic laxatives [1]. This classification is commonly used worldwide and is incorporated in the World Health Organization's list of drugs for constipation as defined by the Anatomical Therapeutic Classification (ATC) [11]. For optimal management of constipation, healthcare professionals working in primary healthcare settings need to understand the extent of OTC laxative use in the community and how laxatives are used by community-dwelling adults. Because OTC laxatives are widely available without prescription, it is not clear which laxative agents are being used, why and how they are selected, and for what purpose they are used. OTC laxatives are intended for

Citation: Werth, B.L.; Christopher, S.-A. Laxative Use in the Community: A Literature Review. *J. Clin. Med.* **2021**, *10*, 143. https://doi.org/10.3390/jcm10010143

Received: 7 December 2020
Accepted: 30 December 2020
Published: 4 January 2021

Publisher's Note: MDPI stays neutral with regard to jurisdictional claims in published maps and institutional affiliations.

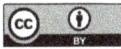

Copyright: © 2021 by the authors. Licensee MDPI, Basel, Switzerland. This article is an open access article distributed under the terms and conditions of the Creative Commons Attribution (CC BY) license (https://creativecommons.org/licenses/by/4.0/).

use in the management of constipation although they are sometimes used by consumers for other purposes such as weight loss [12]. In managing constipation, OTC laxatives may be used in two ways—either for treatment or for prevention of constipation [13]. Treatment of constipation refers to the use of a laxative to relieve constipation symptoms. Prevention of constipation refers to use of a laxative to prevent the symptoms of constipation from occurring. In the context of constipation management, it is also important to understand consumer satisfaction regarding OTC laxative effectiveness [14]. Although laxatives feature prominently in constipation management, rigorous scientific evidence for their efficacy is scarce because most OTC laxatives have been in use for several decades [15]. Nevertheless, therapeutic outcomes of OTC laxative usage in the community are not necessarily reflected in clinical trials [16].

The aims of this review are to report the prevalence of laxative use, and to report on the choice and utilisation of laxatives as well as satisfaction with laxatives, in community-dwelling adult populations.

2. Methods

Relevant literature published in the period 1989 to 2019 was located using Medline and Embase databases. Search terms in various combinations using the AND Boolean operator were applied using keywords and combined terms to refine the search process: "constipation", "laxative", "prevalence", "survey", "adults", "population". In addition to electronic database searches, the search strategy employed for this review also included the "ancestry approach" [17] where the references of yielded articles were examined for relevant studies reporting laxative use in the community.

The search was limited to population-based studies which reported or described the prevalence of laxative use or laxative utilisation in community-dwelling adults. The search was also limited to English language articles. Studies were excluded if the sample size was fewer than 100 participants or if subpopulations such as older adults or only one gender were used.

Articles were identified and screened for their eligibility according to the inclusion and exclusion criteria (Table 1). An examination of journal titles and abstracts captured salient studies which were short listed as suitable for inclusion in the literature review. If the prevalence of laxative use was not specifically stated, it was calculated from the published data by dividing the number of participants using laxatives by the total number of participants in the sample and expressing the result as a percentage. This applied to both general community and constipated population samples. Articles reporting laxative use in constipated populations were segmented into chronic constipation and any constipation (self-defined constipation including both chronic and sporadic constipation).

Table 1. Literature inclusion and exclusion criteria.

Category	Inclusion	Exclusion
Population Sample	Community-dwelling adults (aged 15 and above)	Not residing in the community
	General population and/or constipated population	Sample size fewer than 100 participants
	Sample size greater than 100 participants	Samples of subpopulations e.g., only one gender or samples of older populations
Variables	Prevalence of laxative use	No data regarding laxative use
	Laxative utilisation	
	Self-defined constipation	
	Chronic constipation	
Period	1989–2019	Prior to 1989
Linguistic Range	English language	Non-English language
Type of Study	Population-based surveys	Qualitative studies
	Cross-sectional surveys	

3. Results

A total of 31 articles spanning 18 countries met the inclusion criteria. The prevalence of laxative use was reported in 22 studies. In addition, data were provided in 22 studies which enabled the prevalence in either general community or constipation population samples to be calculated (Table 2). Of notable interest, two studies [18,19] reported data for more than one country and one European study reported combined data for 10 countries [14]. In addition, one article [20] described laxative choice and utilisation but did not report any data relating to prevalence of use. The remaining 27 studies reported data for individual countries or regions. Interestingly, only four studies specifically surveyed the usage of laxatives with most studies focusing on constipation rather than laxative use.

Table 2. Range of prevalence of laxative use in community-dwelling adult populations.

Community-Dwelling Adults (General Population)			Community-Dwelling Adults Reporting Chronic Constipation			Community-Dwelling Adults Reporting Any Constipation		
No. of Studies Reporting Prevalence	No. of Studies Where Prevalence Calculated from Data	Prevalence Range	No. of Studies Reporting Prevalence	No. of Studies where Prevalence Calculated from Data	Prevalence Range	No. of Studies Reporting Prevalence	No. of Studies where Prevalence Calculated from Data	Prevalence Range
7	9	1 to 18%	9	2	3 to 72%	6	11	8 to 87%

3.1. Prevalence of Laxative Use

A total of 16 studies surveyed general community populations where the prevalence of laxative use was either reported or calculated. The overall prevalence of laxative use by adults in the community ranged from 1% to 18% in studies conducted in USA [21–25], Europe [5,26–30], Asia [31–33] and Brazil [34] (Tables 2 and 3). However, a definition of laxative was not provided in any of these studies. In addition to these studies, one US study provided a list of laxative products and 75% of participants aged from 40 to 80 years reported that they had used laxatives at some time in their life [35].

The prevalence of laxative use was either reported or calculated in 17 studies of constipated populations. The prevalence of laxative use in samples of constipated adults in the community varied widely from 3% to 87%. An extremely wide range was found for both chronic [9,14,22,23,29,36,38,41,42,45] and any constipation [5,18,19,21,36,37,40,43,46] (Tables 2 and 3). Only one study clearly defined laxative use and provided a list of products to survey participants [14]; in this European study, the prevalence of laxative use in chronic constipation was 68%. This contrasts with an Australian study where a prevalence of only 3% was reported for undefined laxatives in chronic constipation [45].

In most countries, laxative usage in females was higher than males [5,18,19,39] although male usage was higher than females in the USA, UK and Italy [18]. Laxative use generally increased with age [18,19,39] except in Spain, Korea, China, Indonesia and Brazil [5,19]. Laxative use was associated with lower education and lower income levels in the USA; however, no such associations were found in any other countries [18,19].

Table 3. Prevalence of laxative use in studies of community-dwelling adult populations.

Author (Reference)	Location	Sample Size	Age Range (Years)	Method	Laxative Definition	Time Period (months)	% Prevalence of Use— General	% Prevalence of Use— Constipated	Constipation Definition
Everhart 1989 [21]	USA (NHANES I)	5951	35–84	FTF interview	ND but included stool softener	Monthly or more	17.9 *	58.8 *	Self-report (NTP)
Talley 1991 [22]	USA (Olmsted)	835	30–64	Mail survey	ND but included bran & bulking agents	12	15.6 *	42.9	CC (BDQ)
Talley 1993 [23]	USA (Olmsted)	690	30–64	Mail survey	ND but included enemas	12	6.8 *	20	CC (Rome I)
Harari 1996 [24]	USA (NHIS)	42,375	18+	FTF interview	ND but included stool softener	Monthly or more	11.5	NR	N/A
Wald 2008 [18]	USA	2000	15+	FTF interview	ND	12	NR	40.2 *	Self-report (12 months)
Pare 2001 [36]	Canada	1149	18+	Phone survey	ND	3	NR	34.3 / 26.3	Self-report (3 months) / CC (Rome II)
Ferrazzi 2002 [37]	Canada	200	18+	Phone survey	ND but included herbal, homeopathic, fibre & foods	12	NR	86.5	Self-report (12 months)
Choung 2012 [25]	USA (Olmsted)	2853	20+	Mail survey	Laxative (ND) or fibre	12	13.7 *	52 / 28	Persistent CC / Non-persistent CC
Johanson 2007 [38]	USA	553	18+	Internet survey	Laxative (ND) or fibre	Current	NR	72	CC (Rome II mod)
Roberts 2003 [35]	USA (North Carolina)	1651	40–80	FTF interview	All laxatives including fibre	Lifetime	70.9 (cancer) / 74.6 (controls)	NR	N/A

J. Clin. Med. 2021, 10, 143

Table 3. Cont.

Author (Reference)	Location	Sample Size	Age Range (Years)	Method	Laxative Definition	Time Period (months)	% Prevalence of Use—General	% Prevalence of Use—Constipated	Constipation Definition
Harris 2017 [9]	USA	1223	18+	Internet survey	All laxatives including fibre	Current	NR	40 (OTC) 16 (Rx)	CC (Rome IV or doctor diagnosed)
Heaton 1993 [39]	UK (East Bristol)	1892	25–69 (females) 40–69 (males)	FTF interview	ND excluding bulking agents and bran	NTP	NR	46.2	Self-report (Often/always)
Siproudhis 2006 [40]	France	7196	15+	Mail survey	ND	12	NR	35.3 43.4	FDD OC
Enck 2016 [30]	Germany	15,002	18+	Phone interview	ND	NTP	4.4	NR	N/A
Wald 2008 [18]	UK	2000	15+	FTF interview	ND	12	NR	35.8 *	Self-report (12 months)
Wald 2008 [18]	France	2000	15+	FTF interview	ND	12	NR	32.9 *	Self-report (12 months)
Wald 2008 [18]	Germany	2000	15+	FTF interview	ND	12	NR	30.8 *	Self-report (12 months)
Wald 2008 [18]	Italy	2000	15+	FTF interview	ND	12	NR	34.6 *	Self-report (12 months)
Bassotti 2004 [26]	Italy	298	Adults (ages not reported)	Written questionnaire	ND	1	5	NR	N/A
Galvez 2006 [5]	Spain	349	18–65	Mail survey	ND (but including suppositories & enemas)	NTP	14	40	Self-report (12 months)
Rey 2014 [29]	Spain	1500	18+	Phone interview	ND	12	11.3	38.9 *	CC (Rome III)
Carrasco-Garrido 2008 [27]	Spain	19,514	16+	FTF interview	ND	2 weeks	1.16 *	NR	N/A
Carrasco-Garrido 2010 [28]	Spain	30,428	16+	FTF interview	ND	2 weeks	3.0 *	NR	N/A

Table 3. *Cont.*

Author (Reference)	Location	Sample Size	Age Range (Years)	Method	Laxative Definition	Time Period (months)	% Prevalence of Use—General	% Prevalence of Use—Constipated	Constipation Definition
Muller-Lissner 2013 [14]	Europe (10 countries)	1255	18+	Internet survey	All classes including fibre and rectal products	Current	NR	68	CC (Self-report)
Jeong 2008 [32]	Korea	1417	18–69	FTF interview	ND	Current	4.7 *	NR	N/A
Wald 2008 [18]	Korea	2000	15+	Phone survey	ND	12	NR	16 *	Self-report (12 months)
Wald 2010 [19]	China	2000	15–60	Phone survey	ND	12	NR	39 *	Self-report (12 months)
Wald 2010 [19]	Indonesia	2000	15+	FTF interview	ND	12	NR	40 *	Self-report (12 months)
Adibi 2007 [31]	Iran	995	14–41	Written questionnaire	ND including bulking agents	NTP	7.7 *	NR	N/A
Herz 1996 [41]	Israel	531	21+	Written questionnaire	ND including suppositories	NTP	NR	41	Self-report (NTP)
Rooprai 2017 [42]	India	925	18+	FTF interview	ND	NTP	NR	40.1 *	CC (Rome III)
Kubota 2016 [33]	Japan	72,014	40–79	Written questionnaire	ND	12	10.5 *	NR	N/A
Tamura 2016 [43]	Japan	5155	20–79	Internet survey	ND (OTC)	NTP	NR	7.9	Self-report (NTP)
Song 2019 [41]	China	6318	18+	Internet survey	ND	NTP	NR	25.2	CC (Self-report)
Wald 2008 [18]	Brazil	2000	15+	FTF interview	ND	12	NR	21.9 *	Self-report (12 months)
Wald 2010 [19]	Argentina	2000	15+	FTF interview	ND	12	NR	31.9 *	Self-report (12 months)

Table 3. *Cont.*

Author (Reference)	Location	Sample Size	Age Range (Years)	Method	Laxative Definition	Time Period (months)	% Prevalence of Use—General	% Prevalence of Use—Constipated	Constipation Definition
Wald 2010 [19]	Colombia	2000	15+	FTF interview	ND	12	NR	28.4 *	Self-report (12 months)
Chinzon 2015 [34]	Brazil (Sao Paulo)	3028	18+	Phone interview	ND	NTP	13.4	NR	N/A
Lynch 2001 [44]	New Zealand (Canterbury)	717	18–70	Mail survey	ND	NTP	4.7	NR	N/A
Ng 2014 [45]	Australia (Western Sydney)	396	18+	Written questionnaire	ND	NTP (regular use)	NR	3.1	CC (Rome III modified)

Notes: * Calculated from data published; NR = not reported; ND = not defined; CC = chronic constipation; FTF = face to face; BDQ = bowel disease questionnaire; OTC = over the counter; Rx = prescription; NTP = no time period reported; N/A = not applicable; + = greater than or equal to.

3.2. Laxative Choice, Utilisation and Satisfaction

The popularity of laxatives chosen by adults to manage chronic or any constipation varied by country and/or region. In North America [9,37,38], fibre/bulk-forming laxatives such as ispaghula were the most popular; stool softeners such as docusate were also popular, and prescription products featured prominently in US studies [9,38]. In Europe and certainly in Italy [14,20], contact laxatives such as senna and bisacodyl, and osmotic laxatives such as lactulose, were more popular than bulk-forming laxatives. Products administered by the rectal route also appeared to be popular in Italy [20].

The involvement of healthcare professionals in laxative product selection appears to be limited. A Spanish study found that only 39.4% of those with self-reported constipation or using laxatives in the last year had sought consultation [29]. An Italian study found that only 58.2% of laxative purchases were made on healthcare professional recommendation [20]; the choice of product was influenced by several sources: doctor (37.7%), pharmacist (20.5%), relatives (14%), acquaintances (12.1%) and advertising (11.7%). A Canadian study reported that 59.5% of adults had attempted self-management of constipation for more than a year before consulting a doctor [37] while in the USA an average of three laxative products are used prior to consulting a healthcare professional [9].

The purpose for using laxatives has not been studied, although it is apparent in some studies that the purpose may not always be for treatment of constipation. For example, in a survey of 1417 adults in Korea [32], the total prevalence of laxative use was 4.7% but only 2.6% of the sample were identified as having chronic constipation according to Rome II criteria. This indicates that 2.1% of adults were using laxatives to either prevent chronic constipation, or treat other forms of constipation, or for some other purpose, such as weight loss [12]. Using laxatives for purposes other than treatment is also evident in UK and Spanish studies where up to 4% of laxative users appear to have no constipation whatsoever [5,39] which suggests that laxatives are either being used successfully for prevention of constipation or being used for some other purpose. Italian researchers were concerned about inappropriate use when they found that that 40% of adults were using laxatives when having three or more bowel motions per week [20]. Usage of laxatives on a daily basis was reported in two studies [5,20].

A high proportion of adults with chronic constipation have reported dissatisfaction with laxatives. A US study reported 47% of 533 adults with chronic constipation were not completely satisfied with laxatives or fibre, 82% of which was related to dissatisfaction with efficacy [38]. Another US study found that, of 1223 adults with chronic constipation, only 40% were satisfied with OTC laxatives [9]. A European study of 793 adults with chronic constipation found that only 28% were satisfied with laxatives used, with 44% being neutral and 28% dissatisfied [14]; satisfaction ratings were similar for all laxative classes.

Adults with any constipation are also dissatisfied with laxatives. In a Canadian study of 200 adults using laxatives for self-reported constipation, 50% were satisfied, 18% were neutral and 32% were dissatisfied [37]. In an Italian study of 7324 laxative purchasers in pharmacies, only 30% purchased the same product that they had purchased in the past, whilst all others chose another product because of "reduced effect" [20]. This indicates that 70% were dissatisfied with the efficacy of laxatives purchased previously.

4. Discussion

4.1. Prevalence of Laxative Use

There are a number of possible explanations for the wide range of results in studies estimating the prevalence of laxative use. Firstly, any differences in prevalence between countries might be explained by the same factors as differences in prevalence of constipation, i.e., differences in culture, diet, environment and genetics may be partly responsible [8]. For laxatives in particular, socioeconomic differences and differences in healthcare systems may be important considerations as they may impact the availability and affordability of laxative products in different countries. Particular aspects of healthcare systems which may differ between countries include differences in product availability with and without prescription, and differences in product reimbursement.

It is difficult to compare prevalence when different studies have used different study designs. One research group has conducted multinational studies in 11 countries using the same methodology and questionnaire [18,19]. In each country, the sample size was 2000 subjects, aged 15 years or older and representative of the country's population (except China where the sample size was 2100 and subjects aged over 60 years were excluded). Using the same sample size and data collection method in each country should ensure consistent data and enable comparisons between countries. However, because the term "laxative" was not defined and no list of laxative products was provided, the legitimacy of such comparisons is weakened. Nevertheless, calculation of the prevalence of laxative use in the community shows that prevalence ranged from 16% in Korea to 40% in USA and Indonesia.

Within one country, it might be expected that the prevalence of laxative use would fall within a narrow range, but this has not been the case in the studies reviewed. For example, two Canadian studies have reported different prevalence rates. In a phone survey of 1149 adults with self-reported constipation over three months [36], 34.3% had used laxatives (laxatives were not defined other than the use of prescribed or OTC medication for constipation during the past three months). However, in another Canadian survey 86.5% of 200 participants self-reporting constipation over the last 12 months had used some form of laxative products which included herbal or homeopathic products, fibre and foods [37]. This disparity illustrates that vastly different results may be obtained from the same country when different survey methods, different sample sizes, different constipation definitions, different time periods and no standard laxative definitions are used.

Differences in study design will influence prevalence results. For example, various data collection methods have been used in studies, the most common being face-to-face (FTF) interviews. Similar to constipation prevalence studies [8], the research method used may influence survey results. Because of participant embarrassment, FTF interviews may result in lower prevalence rates compared to mail or internet surveys. For example, in North America [18,36,38] and Europe [14,18,29] internet surveys have reported prevalence rates that were up to twice those of surveys conducted by FTF or phone interviews. Another aspect of study design relates to the sample. As with constipation prevalence [8], the sample size may affect the prevalence of laxative use. Study samples have ranged in size from 200 [37] to 72,000 [33] participants. Because sample size calculations have usually not been provided, it is not clear if the chosen sample sizes are appropriate. It is also not clear in most surveys if the sample used was nationally representative; in over half of the studies, regional populations were surveyed. Nationally representative samples are preferred for estimation of prevalence, along with some evidence of representativeness. Similar to constipation prevalence [8], the age range of the sample is another important consideration. In most studies of the general adult population, participants sampled were at least 15 or 18 years old with no upper limit but in some studies [5,21–23,31–33,39,44], the age of participants was restricted, therefore not all adults in the community were included.

Unfortunately, the majority of studies have not provided definitions of the term "laxative" which means it was self-defined by survey participants. One study of adults with chronic constipation [14] defined the term precisely and included a product list to aid recall; the prevalence was 30% or more higher than most other comparable studies where the meaning was self-defined [22,23,29,36,42,45].

Provision of a product list not only aids definition but also improves recall by providing a useful memory aid [47]. If not defined, it is possible that participants may not regard products such as bulk-forming laxatives and herbal products as laxatives. Also, in some studies where laxatives have not been precisely defined, certain products such as bulk-forming (fibre) products have been either specifically included [22,31,38] or excluded [39]. The ATC laxative definition (A06A: Drugs for constipation) is an international drug classification system, that could be used as a standard definition [11]. The ATC definition includes all OTC laxative agents including bulk-forming laxatives and herbal laxatives, oral and rectal forms, as well as prescription laxatives. In studies reporting the prevalence of laxative use in constipated populations, the definition of constipation is an important consideration as this will also influence the result [8]. Differentiation is usually made between chronic and any constipation. For chronic constipation, most studies used one of the Rome criteria definitions. The majority of studies have reported laxative use with only one definition of constipation.

The recall period used in surveys is an important consideration when estimating prevalence of laxative use [47]. Most studies did not specify any time period. Yet, some studies enquired about current laxative use [9,14,38], and others defined a time period for laxative use such as the past two weeks [27,28], one month [21,26], 3 months [36] or 12 months [18,19,22,23,29,33,37,40]. Clearly the recall period should be defined, and different recall periods will influence the estimated prevalence of laxative usage [47]. Whenever information is elicited from participants, a potential for recall bias exists.

4.2. Laxative Choice, Utilisation and Satisfaction

Laxative choice varied by country. In North America, stool softeners such as docusate were popular despite a lack of evidence regarding efficacy [48–50], and prescription products feature prominently in US studies [9,38], possibly because more new products have been approved there than elsewhere. An important consideration with laxative choice is the year in which the study was conducted. Many studies were over ten years old and older studies may be less relevant because of changes in product preference and availability. For example, the increasing world-wide use of macrogol as an OTC osmotic laxative and the recent availability of new prescription laxatives in some countries need to be considered [51].

Most adults attempt self-management in the first instance [9,37]. In most cases, healthcare professionals are not consulted [29,36,52] and importantly, healthcare professionals are usually not involved with OTC laxative product selection [20,53]. It has been postulated that this might be the result of advertising and other media as well as the possibility of patient embarrassment in discussing constipation [54]. Consequently, OTC laxative choice and use may not always be appropriate [20]. Without advice from healthcare professionals, appropriate product selection and directions for use are challenging for the consumer [53] who may be influenced by other less reliable sources of information [20] such as advertising, acquaintances, or relatives.

High levels of dissatisfaction with laxatives have been reported mainly because of poor efficacy with no differences noted in laxative classes. This may be related to how laxatives are being used. Daily use of laxatives indicates use for prevention rather than treatment. Another indication of preventive use is that some adults report laxative use but not constipation. It seems clear that there is a dual purpose for laxative use—prevention and treatment of constipation, apart from any use not related to constipation. However, no studies have investigated this aspect. In particular, no studies have assessed the perceived effectiveness of laxative agents used for treatment compared to those used for prevention of constipation. Appropriate OTC laxative choice for the intended purpose should be based on the onset of action [55]. The high levels of dissatisfied laxative users in several studies suggest that laxatives are not being used appropriately [9,14,37,38]. Knowledge of the effectiveness of laxatives in practice is essential for improving the management of constipation in the community.

4.3. Limitations

A limitation of the literature review is the risk of bias, whereby the studies included were conducted in an English-speaking context and written in English and were further refined according to the inclusion/exclusion criteria. The risk of bias is acknowledged since some relevant studies may have been excluded from the literature reviewed. The authors also acknowledge potential recall bias because survey results were based on recall

J. Clin. Med. **2021**, *10*, 143

of participants, the period of which varied in different studies. Furthermore, differences in healthcare systems in different countries will also influence the results obtained in different studies.

5. Conclusions

It is difficult to determine the true prevalence of laxative use in the community. Estimates of laxative prevalence in community-dwelling adults vary greatly, whether in general community populations or in constipated populations. Apart from any country differences, a number of other factors may explain the wide variation. One important factor is the lack of a precise laxative definition in most studies which makes it difficult to determine what agents have been included or excluded. Other factors to consider are different recall periods, study designs and sampling differences. For studies in constipated populations, different constipation definitions also affect laxative prevalence estimates.

To estimate the prevalence of laxative use more accurately, an internationally accepted laxative definition such as the ATC definition, a specified recall time period, a nationally representative sample of appropriate size and a questionnaire which includes a list of laxative product names to facilitate recall are recommended. In constipated populations, it is recommended that universally accepted constipation definitions are used such as the Rome criteria for chronic constipation, or self-reported constipation in a specified time period for any constipation.

Few published studies have investigated the choice and utilisation of laxatives, and whether users are satisfied with their use. It appears that laxatives are not always being used for treatment of constipation and that they are also used for prevention of constipation. This distinction in the purpose of laxative use requires investigation along with the sources of influence for choice of laxative. It seems that healthcare professionals are not always involved in laxative choice, but this also needs to be further researched particularly with regard to the dual purpose of laxative use. Studies regarding laxative choice are now outdated and new studies investigating currently available laxatives are required, particularly to assess their effectiveness in preventing and treating constipation in the community.

To improve constipation management in community and primary healthcare settings, knowledge of the true prevalence and utilisation of laxative use is required, and this review indicates the need for further research in these areas.

Author Contributions: Conceptualization, B.L.W. and S.-A.C.; methodology, B.L.W. and S.-A.C.; writing—original draft preparation, B.L.W.; writing—review and editing, B.L.W. and S.-A.C. All authors have read and agreed to the published version of the manuscript.

Funding: This research did not receive any funding.

Acknowledgments: The authors acknowledge guidance received from Murray Fisher, University of Sydney, and Lisa Pont and Kylie Williams, University of Technology Sydney.

Conflicts of Interest: The authors declare no conflict of interest regarding publication of this review.

References

1. Klaschik, E.; Nauck, F.; Ostgathe, C. Constipation—Modern laxative therapy. *Supportive Care Cancer* **2003**, *11*, 679–685. [CrossRef] [PubMed]
2. Jones, M.P.; Talley, N.J.; Nuyts, G.; Dubois, D. Lack of objective evidence of efficacy of laxatives in chronic constipation. *Dig. Dis. Sci.* **2002**, *47*, 2222–2230. [CrossRef] [PubMed]
3. Sbahi, H.; Cash, B.D. Chronic constipation: A review of current literature. *Curr. Gastroenterol. Rep.* **2015**, *17*, 47. [CrossRef] [PubMed]
4. Rao, S.S.; Rattanakovit, K.; Patcharatrakul, T. Diagnosis and management of chronic constipation in adults. *Nat. Rev. Gastroenterol. Hepatol.* **2016**, *13*, 295–305. [CrossRef] [PubMed]
5. Galvez, C.; Garrigues, V.; Ortiz, V.; Ponce, M.; Nos, P.; Ponce, J. Healthcare seeking for constipation: A population-based survey in the Mediterranean area of Spain. *Aliment. Pharmacol. Ther.* **2006**, *24*, 421–428. [CrossRef]
6. Dennison, C.; Prasad, M.; Lloyd, A.; Bhattacharyya, S.K.; Dhawan, R.; Coyne, K. The health-related quality of life and economic burden of constipation. *Pharmacoeconomics* **2005**, *23*, 461–476. [CrossRef]

7. Drossman, D.A. Functional gastrointestinal disorders: History, pathophysiology, clinical features, and Rome IV. *Gastroenterology* **2016**, *150*, 1262–1279. [CrossRef]
8. Werth, B.L. Epidemiology of constipation in adults: Why estimates of prevalence differ. *J. Epidemiol. Res.* **2019**, *5*, 37–49. [CrossRef]
9. Harris, L.A.; Horn, J.; Kissous-Hunt, M.; Magnus, L.; Quigley, E.M.M. The better understanding and recognition of the disconnects, experiences, and needs of patients with chronic idiopathic constipation (BURDEN-CIC) study: Results of an online questionnaire. *Adv. Ther.* **2017**, *34*, 2661–2673. [CrossRef]
10. Guerin, A.; Carson, R.T.; Lewis, B.; Yin, D.; Kaminsky, M.; Wu, E. The economic burden of treatment failure amongst patients with irritable bowel syndrome with constipation or chronic constipation: A retrospective analysis of a Medicaid population. *J. Med. Econ.* **2014**, *17*, 577–586. [CrossRef]
11. WHO. ATC/DDD Index. Collaborating Centre for Drug Statistics Methodology. 2017. Available online: https://www.whoccno/atc_ddd_index/ (accessed on 4 September 2017).
12. Roerig, J.; Steffen, K.J.; Mitchell, J.E.; Zunker, C. Laxative abuse: Epidemiology, diagnosis and management. *Drugs* **2010**, *70*, 1487–1503. [CrossRef] [PubMed]
13. Werth, B.L.; Williams, K.A.; Pont, L.G. A longitudinal study of constipation and laxative use in a community-dwelling elderly population. *Arch. Gerontol. Geriatr.* **2015**, *60*, 418–424. [CrossRef] [PubMed]
14. Muller-Lissner, S.; Tack, J.; Feng, Y.; Schenck, F.; Specht Gryp, R. Levels of satisfaction with current chronic constipation treatment options in Europe—An internet survey. *Aliment. Pharmacol. Ther.* **2013**, *37*, 137–145. [CrossRef] [PubMed]
15. Collins, B.R.; O'Brien, L. Prevention and management of constipation in adults. *Nurs. Stand.* **2015**, *29*, 49–58. [CrossRef] [PubMed]
16. WHO. *Introduction to Drug Utilization Research*; World Health Organisation: Oslo, Norway, 2003.
17. Morrison, S.M.; Symes, L. An integrative review of expert nursing practice. *J. Nurs. Scholarsh.* **2011**, *32*, 163–170. [CrossRef] [PubMed]
18. Wald, A.; Scarpignato, C.; Mueller-Lissner, S.; Kamm, M.A.; Hinkel, U.; Helfrich, I.; Schuijt, C.; Mandel, K.G. A multinational survey of prevalence and patterns of laxative use among adults with self-defined constipation. *Aliment. Pharmacol. Ther.* **2008**, *28*, 917–930. [CrossRef] [PubMed]
19. Wald, A.; Mueller-Lissner, S.; Kamm, M.A.; Hinkel, U.; Richter, E.; Schuijt, C.; Mandel, K.G. Survey of laxative use by adults with self-defined constipation in South America and Asia: A comparison of six countries. *Aliment. Pharmacol. Ther.* **2010**, *31*, 274–284. [CrossRef]
20. Motola, G.; Mazzeo, F.; Rinaldi, B.; Capuano, A.; Rossi, S.; Russo, F.; Vitelli, M.R.; Rossi, F.; Filippelli, A. Self-prescribed laxative use: A drug-utilization review. *Adv. Ther.* **2002**, *19*, 203–208. [CrossRef]
21. Everhart, J.E.; Go, V.L.; Johannes, R.S.; Fitzsimmons, S.C.; Roth, H.P.; White, L.R. A longitudinal survey of self-reported bowel habits in the United States. *Dig. Dis. Sci.* **1989**, *34*, 1153–1162. [CrossRef]
22. Talley, N.J.; Zinsmeister, A.R.; van Dyke, C.; Melton, L.J., III. Epidemiology of colonic symptoms and the irritable bowel syndrome. *Gastroenterology* **1991**, *101*, 927–934. [CrossRef]
23. Talley, N.J.; Weaver, A.L.; Zinsmeister, A.R.; Melton, L.J., III. Functional constipation and outlet delay: A population-based study. *Gastroenterology* **1993**, *105*, 781–790. [CrossRef]
24. Harari, D.; Gurwitz, J.H.; Avorn, J.; Bohn, R.; Minaker, K.L. Bowel habit in relation to age and gender. Findings from the National Health Interview survey and clinical implications. *Arch. Intern. Med.* **1996**, *156*, 315–320. [CrossRef] [PubMed]
25. Choung, R.S.; Locke, G.R., III; Rey, E.; Schleck, C.D.; Baum, C.; Zinsmeister, A.R.; Talley, N.J. Factors associated with persistent and nonpersistent chronic constipation, over 20 years. *Clin. Gastroenterol. Hepatol.* **2012**, *10*, 494–500. [CrossRef] [PubMed]
26. Bassotti, G.; Bellini, M.; Pucciani, F.; Bocchini, R.; Bove, A.; Alduini, P.; Battaglia, E.; Bruzzi, P. Italian Constipation Study, G. An extended assessment of bowel habits in a general population. *World J. Gastroenterol.* **2004**, *10*, 713–716. [CrossRef] [PubMed]
27. Carrasco-Garrido, P.; Jimenez-Garcia, R.; Barrera, V.H.; de Miguel, A.G. Predictive factors of self-medicated drug use among the Spanish adult population. *Pharmacoepidemiol. Drug Saf.* **2008**, *17*, 193–199. [CrossRef] [PubMed]
28. Carrasco-Garrido, P.; Hernandez-Barrera, V.; Lopez de Andres, A.; Jimenez-Trujillo, I.; Jimenez-Garcia, R. Sex—Differences on self-medication in Spain. *Pharmacoepidemiol. Drug Saf.* **2010**, *19*, 1293–1299. [CrossRef] [PubMed]
29. Rey, E.; Balboa, A.; Mearin, F. Chronic constipation, irritable bowel syndrome with constipation and constipation with pain/discomfort: Similarities and differences. *Am. J. Gastroenterol.* **2014**, *109*, 876–884. [CrossRef]
30. Enck, P.; Leinert, J.; Smid, M.; Kohler, T.; Schwille-Kiuntke, J. Prevalence of constipation in the German population—A representative survey (GECCO). *United Eur. Gastroenterol. J.* **2016**, *4*, 429–437. [CrossRef]
31. Adibi, P.; Behzad, E.; Pirzadeh, S.; Mohseni, M. Bowel habit reference values and abnormalities in young Iranian healthy adults. *Dig. Dis. Sci.* **2007**, *52*, 1810–1813. [CrossRef]
32. Jeong, J.J.; Choi, M.G.; Cho, Y.S.; Lee, S.G.; Oh, J.H.; Park, J.M.; Cho, Y.K.; Lee, I.S.; Kim, S.W.; Han, S.W.; et al. Chronic gastrointestinal symptoms and quality of life in the Korean population. *World J. Gastroenterol.* **2008**, *14*, 6388–6394. [CrossRef]
33. Kubota, Y.; Iso, H.; Tamakoshi, A. Bowel movement frequency, laxative use, and mortality from coronary heart disease and stroke among Japanese men and women: The Japan collaborative cohort (JACC) study. *J. Epidemiol.* **2016**, *26*, 242–248. [CrossRef] [PubMed]
34. Chinzon, D.; Dias-Bastos, T.R.P.; Medeiros da Silva, A.; Eisig, J.N.; de Oliveira Latorre, M.D.R.D. Epidemiology of constipation in Sao Paulo, Brazil: A population-based study. *Curr. Med. Res. Opin.* **2015**, *31*, 57–64. [CrossRef] [PubMed]

35. Roberts, M.C.; Millikan, R.C.; Galanko, J.A.; Martin, C.; Sandler, R.S. Constipation, laxative use, and colon cancer in a North Carolina population. *Am. J. Gastroenterol.* **2003**, *98*, 857–864. [CrossRef] [PubMed]
36. Pare, P.; Ferrazzi, S.; Thompson, W.G.; Irvine, E.J.; Rance, L. An epidemiological survey of constipation in Canada: Definitions, rates, demographics, and predictors of health care seeking. *Am. J. Gastroenterol.* **2001**, *96*, 3130–3137. [CrossRef] [PubMed]
37. Ferrazzi, S.; Thompson, G.W.; Irvine, E.J.; Pare, P.; Rance, L. Diagnosis of constipation in family practice. *Can. J. Gastroenterol.* **2002**, *16*, 159–164. [CrossRef]
38. Johanson, J.F.; Kralstein, J. Chronic constipation: A survey of the patient perspective. *Aliment. Pharmacol. Ther.* **2007**, *25*, 599–608. [CrossRef]
39. Heaton, K.W.; Cripps, H.A. Straining at stool and laxative taking in an English population. *Dig. Dis. Sci.* **1993**, *38*, 1004–1008. [CrossRef]
40. Siproudhis, L.; Pigot, F.; Godeberge, P.; Damon, H.; Soudan, D.; Bigard, M.A. Defecation disorders: A French population survey. *Dis. Colon Rectum* **2006**, *49*, 219–227. [CrossRef]
41. Song, J.; Bai, T.; Zhang, L.; Hou, X.H. Clinical features and treatment options among Chinese adults with self-reported constipation: An internet-based survey. *Dig. Dis.* **2019**, *20*, 409–414. [CrossRef]
42. Rooprai, R.; Bhat, N.; Sainani, R.; Mayabhate, M.M. Prevalence of functional constipation and constipation-predominant irritable bowel syndrome in Indian patients with constipation. *Int. J. Basic Clin. Pharmacol.* **2017**, *6*, 275–285. [CrossRef]
43. Tamura, A.; Tomita, T.; Oshima, T.; Toyoshima, F.; Yamasaki, T.; Okugawa, T.; Kondo, T.; Kono, T.; Tozawa, K.; Ikehara, H.; et al. Prevalence and self-recognition of chronic constipation: Results of an internet survey. *J. Neurogastroenterol. Motil.* **2016**, *22*, 677–685. [CrossRef] [PubMed]
44. Lynch, A.C.; Dobbs, B.R.; Keating, J.; Frizelle, F.A. The prevalence of faecal incontinence and constipation in a general New Zealand population; A postal survey. *N. Z. Med. J.* **2001**, *114*, 474–477. [PubMed]
45. Ng, K.S.; Nassar, N.; Hamd, K.; Nagarajah, A.; Gladman, M.A. Prevalence of functional bowel disorders and faecal incontinence: An Australian primary care survey. *Colorectal Dis.* **2015**, *17*, 150–159. [CrossRef] [PubMed]
46. Herz, M.J.; Kahan, E.; Zalevski, S.; Aframian, R.; Kuznitz, D.; Reichman, S. Constipation: A different entity for patients and doctors. *Fam. Pract.* **1996**, *13*, 156–159. [CrossRef] [PubMed]
47. Gama, H.; Correia, S.; Lunet, N. Questionnaire design and the recall of pharmacological treatments: A systematic review. *Pharmacoepidemiol. Drug Saf.* **2009**, *18*, 175–187. [CrossRef] [PubMed]
48. Ramkumar, D.; Rao, S.S.C. Efficacy and safety of traditional medical therapies for chronic constipation: Systematic review. *Am. J. Gastroenterol.* **2005**, *100*, 936–971. [CrossRef]
49. Tarumi, Y.; Wilson, M.P.; Szafran, O.; Spooner, G.R. Randomized, double-blind, placebo-controlled trial of oral docusate in the management of constipation in hospice patients. *J. Pain Symptom Manag.* **2013**, *45*, 2–13. [CrossRef]
50. Pare, P.; Fedorak, R.N. Systematic review of stimulant and nonstimulant laxatives for the treatment of functional constipation. *Can. J. Gastroenterol. Hepatol.* **2014**, *28*, 549–557. [CrossRef]
51. Luthra, P.; Camilleri, M.; Burr, N.E.; Quigley, E.M.M.; Black, C.J.; Ford, A.C. Efficacy of drugs in chronic idiopathic constipation: A systematic review and network meta-analysis. *Lancet Gastroenterol. Hepatol.* **2019**, *4*, 831–844. [CrossRef]
52. Heidelbaugh, J.J.; Stelwagon, M.; Miller, S.A.; Shea, E.P.; Chey, W.D. The spectrum of constipation-predominant irritable bowel syndrome and chronic idiopathic constipation: US survey assessing symptoms, care seeking, and disease burden. *Am. J. Gastroenterol.* **2015**, *110*, 580–587. [CrossRef]
53. Shibata, K.; Matsumoto, A.; Nakagawa, A.; Akagawa, K.; Nakamura, A.; Yamamoto, T.; Kurata, N. Use of pharmacist consultations for nonprescription laxatives in Japan: An online survey. *Biol. Pharm. Bull.* **2016**, *39*, 1767–1773. [CrossRef] [PubMed]
54. Bellini, M.; Gambaccini, D.; Usai-Satta, P.; De Bortoli, N.; Bertani, L.; Marchi, S.; Stasi, C. Irritable bowel syndrome and chronic constipation: Fact and fiction. *World J. Gastroenterol.* **2015**, *21*, 11362–11370. [CrossRef] [PubMed]
55. Selby, W.; Corte, C. Managing constipation in adults. *Aust. Prescr.* **2010**, *33*, 116–119. [CrossRef]

MDPI

St. Alban-Anlage 66

4052 Basel

Switzerland

Tel. +41 61 683 77 34

Fax +41 61 302 89 18

www.mdpi.com

Journal of Clinical Medicine Editorial Office

E-mail: jcm@mdpi.com

www.mdpi.com/journal/jcm

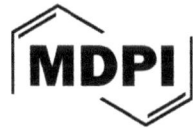

www.ingramcontent.com/pod-product-compliance
Lightning Source LLC
Chambersburg PA
CBHW042021080526
44654CB00092B/219

* 9 7 8 3 0 3 6 5 4 7 9 7 8 *